MW01283702

Minimally Invasive Foot and Ankle Surgery

Minimally Invasive Foot and Ankle Surgery

Series Editor

Paul Tornetta III, MD
Professor and Vice Chairman
Department of Orthopaedic Surgery
Boston University Medical Center
Director of Orthopaedic Trauma
Boston University Medical Center
Boston, Massachusetts

Editors

Eric M. Bluman, MD, PhD
Medical Director
Division of Foot and Ankle
Brigham and Women's Hospital
Harvard Medical School
Boston, Massachusetts

Christopher P. Chiodo, MD
Chief
Foot and Ankle Surgery Service
Brigham and Women's Hospital
Harvard Medical School
Boston, Massachusetts

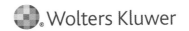

Philadelphia • Baltimore • New York • London
Buenos Aires • Hong Kong • Sydney • Tokyo

Acquisitions Editor: Brian Brown
Product Development Editor: Dave Murphy
Marketing Manager: Dan Dressler
Production Project Manager: Marian Bellus
Design Coordinator: Joan Wendt
Manufacturing Coordinator: Beth Welsh
Prepress Vendor: Aptara, Inc.

Copyright © 2016 Wolters Kluwer.

All rights reserved. This book is protected by copyright. No part of this book may be reproduced or transmitted in any form or by any means, including as photocopies or scanned-in or other electronic copies, or utilized by any information storage and retrieval system without written permission from the copyright owner, except for brief quotations embodied in critical articles and reviews. Materials appearing in this book prepared by individuals as part of their official duties as U.S. government employees are not covered by the above-mentioned copyright. To request permission, please contact Wolters Kluwer at Two Commerce Square, 2001 Market Street, Philadelphia, PA 19103, via email at permissions@lww.com, or via our website at lww.com (products and services).

9 8 7 6 5 4 3 2 1

Printed in China

978-1-45113-161-1

Library of Congress Cataloging-in-Publication Data
available upon request

This work is provided "as is," and the publisher disclaims any and all warranties, express or implied, including any warranties as to accuracy, comprehensiveness, or currency of the content of this work.

This work is no substitute for individual patient assessment based upon healthcare professionals' examination of each patient and consideration of, among other things, age, weight, gender, current or prior medical conditions, medication history, laboratory data and other factors unique to the patient. The publisher does not provide medical advice or guidance and this work is merely a reference tool. Healthcare professionals, and not the publisher, are solely responsible for the use of this work including all medical judgments and for any resulting diagnosis and treatments.

Given continuous, rapid advances in medical science and health information, independent professional verification of medical diagnoses, indications, appropriate pharmaceutical selections and dosages, and treatment options should be made and healthcare professionals should consult a variety of sources. When prescribing medication, healthcare professionals are advised to consult the product information sheet (the manufacturer's package insert) accompanying each drug to verify, among other things, conditions of use, warnings and side effects and identify any changes in dosage schedule or contraindications, particularly if the medication to be administered is new, infrequently used or has a narrow therapeutic range. To the maximum extent permitted under applicable law, no responsibility is assumed by the publisher for any injury and/or damage to persons or property, as a matter of products liability, negligence law or otherwise, or from any reference to or use by any person of this work.

LWW.com

RRS1509

To my mother, Phyllis, who found the best in people, had compassion for all, and whose insight, guidance, and love have always made me believe that anything is possible.

Paul Tornetta, III, MD

To my parents, whom I cannot thank enough for giving me all of the opportunities
I had growing up and are greatly responsible for where I am today.

Also to my wife Trimble Augur, MD and our children Adair, Tenney, and Everett who allow
me to take time away from them more often than they would like
to complete projects such as these.

Eric M. Bluman, MD, PhD

To my family, colleagues, and patients. Thank you for your love, wisdom, and inspiration.

Chistopher P. Chiodo, MD

Contributing Authors

Jorge I. Acevedo, MD
Department of Surgery
Wellington Regional Medical Center
Wellington, Florida
Associate Clinical Faculty
Department of Orthopaedics and Rehabilitation
University of Miami
Miami, Florida

Samuel B. Adams, MD
Assistant Professor of Orthopaedic Surgery
Director of Foot and Ankle Research
Duke University Medical Center
Durham, North Carolina

Robert B. Anderson, MD
OrthoCarolina
Charlotte, North Carolina

Paul Appleton, MD
Clinical Instructor in Orthopaedics
Harvard Medical School
Beth Israel Deaconess Medical Center
Boston, Massachusetts

Frank R. Avilucea, MD
Resident
Department of Orthopaedics
University of Utah
Salt Lake City, Utah

Lijkele Beimers, MD
Staff
Department of Orthopaedic Surgery
Academic Medical Center
University of Amsterdam
Amsterdam, The Netherlands

Brad D. Blankenhorn, MD
Assistant Professor
Department of Orthopaedics
Warren Alpert Medical School of Brown University
Providence, Rhode Island

Eric M. Bluman, MD, PhD
Medical Director
Division of Foot and Ankle
Brigham and Women's Hospital
Harvard Medical School
Boston, Massachusetts

Christopher P. Chiodo, MD
Chief
Foot and Ankle Surgery Service
Brigham and Women's Hospital
Harvard Medical School
Boston, Massachusetts

Woo Jin Choi, MD
Department of Orthopaedic Surgery
Yonsei University College of Medicine
Seoul, South Korea

Marcus P. Coe, MD, MS
Dartmouth Hitchcock Medical Center
The University of British Columbia
Vancouver, BC Canada

Bruce Cohen, MD
OrthoCarolina
Charlotte, North Carolina

Timothy C. Fitzgibbons, MD, FACS
GIKK Orthopaedic Specialist
Clinical Associate Professor
Department of Orthopaedics
University of Nebraska Medical Center
Omaha, Nebraska

David Flood, MD
Assistant Professor of Clinical Orthopaedic Surgery
Department of Orthopaedic Surgery
University of Missouri
Columbia, Missouri

John P. Furia, MD
Orthopaedist
Sun Orthopaedics Group
Lewisburg, Pennsylvania

Sandro Giannini, MD
Full Professor
Clinical Orthopaedic and Traumatology
Unit II, Rizzoli Orthopaedic Institute
Bologna University
Bologna, Italy

Eric Giza, MD
Chief
Foot & Ankle Surgery
Assistant Professor of Orthopaedic Surgery
Department of Orthopaedics
University of California, Davis
Sacramento, California

David J. Inda, MD
GIKK Orthopaedic Specialist
Omaha, Nebraska

John P. Ketz, MD
Assistant Professor
Department of Orthopaedics
University of Rochester Medical Center
Assistant Professor
Department of Orthopaedics
Strong Memorial Hospital
Rochester, New York

Markus Knupp, MD
Senior Consultant
Department of Orthopaedic Surgery
University of Basel
Senior Consultant
Basel, Switzerland
Department of Orthopaedic Surgery
Kantonsspital Liestal
Liestal, Switzerland

Jin Woo Lee, Prof. MD, PhD
Department of Orthopaedic Surgery
Yonsei University College of Medicine
Seoul, South Korea

Tun Hing Lui, MBBS (HK), FRCS (Edin),
FHKAM, FHKCOS
Consultant
Department of Orthopaedics and Traumatology
North District Hospital
Hong Kong SAR, China

Peter Mangone, MD
Co-Director
Foot and Ankle Center
Blue Ridge Bone and Joint Clinic
Asheville, North Carolina

Jeremy J. Miles, MD
Department of Orthopaedics and Sports Medicine
University of South Florida
Tampa, Florida

Stuart H. Myers, MD
Foot and Ankle Fellow
Department of Orthopaedic Surgery
MedStar Union Memorial Hospital
Baltimore, Maryland

Florian Nickisch, MD
Associate Professor
Department of Orthopaedics
University of Utah
Salt Lake City, Utah

Vinod K. Panchbhavi, MD
Professor of Orthopaedic Surgery
University of Texas Medical Branch
Galveston, Texas

Phinit Phisitkul, MD
Clinical Assistant Professor
Department of Orthopaedics and Rehabilitation
University of Iowa
Iowa City, Iowa

V. James Sammarco, MD
Cincinnati Sports Medicine and Orthopedic Center
Cincinnati, Ohio

Roy W. Sanders, MD
Director
Orthopaedic Trauma Service
Florida Orthopaedic Institute
Chief
Department of Orthopaedics
Tampa General Hospital
Tampa, Florida

Lew C. Schon, MD
Chief of Foot and Ankle Services
Director of Foot and Ankle Fellowship Program
Union Memorial Hospital
Assistant Professor of Orthopedic Surgery
Johns Hopkins University
Clinical Associate Professor of Orthopedic Surgery
Georgetown University School of Medicine
Baltimore, Maryland

Michael J. Shereff, MD
Department of Orthopaedics and Sports Medicine
University of South Florida
Tampa, Florida

Edward Shin, MD
Orthopaedic Surgery Resident
Department of Orthopaedics
University of California, Davis
Sacramento, California

Jeremy T. Smith
Fellow in Foot and Ankle Surgery
Department of Orthopaedics
Division of Foot and Ankle
Brigham and Women's Hospital
Boston, Massachusetts

C. Christopher Stroud, MD
Attending Physician
William Beaumont Hospital
Troy, Michigan

Saul G. Trevino, MD
Mansfield Orthopaedics
Morrisville, Vermont

Lung Fung Tse, MBChB, FRCS(Orth), FHKAM, FHKCOS
Associate Consultant
Department of Orthopaedics and Traumatology
Prince of Wales Hospital
Hong Kong SAR, China

Santaram Vallurupalli, MD
Assistant Professor
Department of Orthopaedic Surgery
University of Oklahoma
Oklahoma City, Oklahoma

C. Niek van Dijk, MD, PhD
Professor
Department of Orthopaedic Surgery
Academic Medical Center
University of Amsterdam
Amsterdam, The Netherlands

Francesca Vannini, MD, PhD
Clinical Orthopaedic and Traumatology
Unit II, Rizzoli Orthopaedic Institute
Bologna UniversityBologna, Italy

Emilio Wagner, MD
Traumatologist
Foot and Ankle Clinic
Clinica Alemana
Santiago, Chile

Markus Walther, MD
Professor for Orthopedic Surgery
University of Wuerzburg
Center for Foot and Ankle Surgery
Schoen Klinik Muenchen Harlaching
Munich, Bavaria, Germany

Kathryn L. Williams, MD
Assistant Professor
Department of Orthopedics and Rehabilitation
University of Wisconsin
Madison, Wisconsin

Kevin Wing, BSc, MD, FRCS(C)
Dartmouth Hitchcock Medical Center
The University of British Columbia
Vancouver, BC Canada

Stephanie E. Wong, BS
Medical Student
UC Davis School of Medicine
University of California, Davis
Sacramento, California

Alan Yan, MD
Resident House Staff
Department of Orthopedic Surgery
Johns Hopkins Hospital
Baltimore, Maryland

Alastair S.E. Younger, MB, ChB, MSc, ChM, FRCS(C)
Dartmouth Hitchcock Medical Center
The University of British Columbia
Vancouver, BC Canada

Series Preface

It is my pleasure to introduce the second volume of the series, *Minimally Invasive Orthopaedic Surgery*. This book builds on the tradition of advances that orthopaedic surgery has made and captures the exciting methods being introduced by current innovators. Obtaining faster recovery while minimizing risk is the goal of minimally invasive procedures.

This volume, edited by Chris Chiodo, will focus on minimally invasive foot and ankle surgery. Over the past 15 years, the advent of better instrumentation and innovations in technique has allowed previously done open procedures to be performed with soft tissue–sparing methods. The editor has gathered experts in minimally invasive procedures and has presented them in a uniform way including the indications, setup, technical aspects of surgery, and the problem areas.

I am proud to see this series advance with this volume on foot and ankle surgery.

Paul Tornetta, III, MD

Preface

Minimally invasive surgery has not had a static definition. Procedures evolve such that clinical efficacy increases while tissue insult decreases. This process is ongoing; as technology advances, surgeries that are minimally invasive in the current era will be modified so that they become even less invasive. These different stages of evolution are illustrated within this text. Indeed, the chapters we have included range from treatments that do not breach the skin to those using incisions previously described in non-MIS texts.

Currently, there are procedures which may be considered less invasive than some featured here. As editors we included procedures that would be of maximal benefit to patients while maintaining an adequate safety profile. In this vein, an important safety concern is the significant training challenges in performing some of these techniques. We leave it to the reader to determine whether each described technique is appropriate for their individual practice.

This text is targeted to the practicing orthopedic foot and ankle surgeon. However, it will be of value to all health care providers who participate in the care of orthopedic foot and ankle patients. Specifically, we expect surgical residents, fellows, and allied health providers to benefit from this book.

In preparing this book, we assembled an internationally diverse cadre of experts considered as authoritative surgeons on the cutting edge of minimally invasive orthopedic foot and ankle surgery. Many of them have been on the forefront of developing and teaching the methods described herein. We are indebted to them for the time and effort they put in preparing their chapters. We hope that the techniques detailed herein aid the clinician, the health care system and most importantly patients.

Eric M. Bluman, MD, PhD
Christopher P. Chiodo, MD

Acknowledgments

This project really has been a family affair on many levels. As such, we would like to thank several groups of individuals:

This book would not have been possible without the significant and sustained contributions of the authors. All of them are accomplished orthopedic surgeons and part of the Orthopedic Foot & Ankle family. Their patients are fortunate to have them as physicians.

Our academic family consisting of mentors, colleagues, fellows, and residents, all of whom ask challenging and critical questions. They continue to inspire us and remain our greatest source of education.

The Wolters-Kluwer family and Brian Brown who agreed with us that this was a needed resource for orthopedic surgeons. We especially want to thank David Murphy who has been with us through multiple staff changes and editorial teams from inception to composition and finally publication.

Eric M. Bluman, MD, PhD
Christopher P. Chiodo, MD

Contents

SECTION 1
Tendons and Ligaments

CHAPTER 1

Brisement and Related Procedures

Stuart H. Myers   Lew C. Schon

BACKGROUND

Brisement (French: "breaking") is the lysis of adhesions around a tendon by high-pressure fluid injection. It is distinct from brisement forcé (French: "forced breaking"), which is the lysis of intra-articular adhesions by joint manipulation.

Achilles tendon brisement, the most studied form of brisement in the foot and ankle, is performed by a wide variety of healthcare providers. Orthopedic surgeons, podiatrists, and interventional radiologists have described and validated a variety of techniques. The greatest variation among the different techniques is the composition of the injection. A second distinction is the presence or absence of ultrasound guidance. Despite these differences, all Achilles brisement is directed toward distention of the paratenon–tendon interface.[1]

The mechanism by which brisement is thought to work is the arresting or reversing of the process of tendon neovascularization. Zanetti et al.[2] showed that neovascularization is associated with painful Achilles tendinopathy. Humphrey et al.[3] further showed that brisement reverses this process while reducing tendon thickness, with decreased pain scores.

In dry needling, tissue is stimulated and blood flow is promoted through repeated needle puncture. The reparative process may be further stimulated with injection of platelet-rich plasma (PRP) during needling.

The addition of a steroid to the brisement cocktail is controversial. In a review article, Schepsis et al.[1] recommended against the use of an injectable steroid solution except in the case of retrocalcaneal bursitis. Although Read showed that peritendinous steroid injections in patients with achillodynia did not increase the risk of rupture,[4] most protocols do not include a steroid in their injection.[5,6] However, steroids are used by some investigators for peritendinous injections.[3,7]

INDICATIONS

The syndrome of Achilles tendon pain, inflammation, and degeneration is not completely understood. A distinction is often made between peritendinitis (paratenon disease) and tendinosis (tendon disease). Peritendinitis—possibly caused by repetitive injury to the paratenon—has an acute inflammatory phase and a chronic fibrotic stage. Tendinosis has an acute inflammatory stage and a chronic degenerative stage. These processes can coexist. Jones suggests that refractory peritendinitis can be successfully treated with brisement, whereas symptomatic tendinosis requires debridement.[6]

In our experience, peritendinitis tends to occur in younger patients and is often accompanied by squeaking and palpable nodules. Tendinosis tends to occur in older patients and is often associated with a more focal distribution of pain.

Investigations of brisement tend to group these entities together because of the difficulty in distinguishing them or the high rate of concurrence. Indications in the literature for brisement include insertional Achilles tendinitis,[1] chronic Achilles tendinopathy,[7] chronic resistant Achilles tendinopathy,[3] refractory mid-Achilles tendinosis,[5] achillodynia,[4] Achilles peritendinitis,[6] and Achilles tenosynovitis.[8] It is difficult to review the literature on this subject because the diagnostic language for Achilles tendon disease is heterogenous and the understanding of its pathophysiology is incomplete.

We perform brisement for chronic Achilles peritendinitis and for Achilles tendinosis if there is substantial concomitant peritendinitis and only after nonoperative measures have failed. Our initial treatment program consists of relative rest, stretching, and anti-inflammatory medication. If this is unsuccessful, we immobilize the patient with a boot brace. Brisement is considered if there is failure to achieve symptom control along this pathway.

Brisement can also be used to treat peritendinous adhesions of the Achilles tendon, posterior tibialis tendon, peroneal tendons, long toe extensors, tibialis anterior, and flexor hallucis longus. This procedure can be especially useful in the treatment of postsurgical peritendinitis of the peroneal and extensor tendons. We consider one-time addition of a steroid to the brisement solution in the brisement treatment of flexor hallucis longus tendinitis.

Dry needling is performed in the case of intrasubstance tendinopathy (insertional or noninsertional). Tendons most commonly affected include the Achilles, peroneal, and posterior tibialis. Plantar fasciitis is also amenable to this treatment. Mechanical integrity of the tendon is a prerequisite for needling. Tendons that are attenuated or stretched based upon clinical examination are not good candidates for needling. Failure of nonoperative measures similar to those used in tendinitis is required before we recommend dry needling.

PATIENT POSITIONING

Supine or lateral positioning is used, depending upon the tendon(s) being treated.

SURGICAL APPROACHES

For noninsertional Achilles tendon brisement, the injection is performed medially to avoid the sural nerve. The injection point is 1 cm anterior to medial border of the Achilles tendon and 2 to 6 cm proximal to its insertion (Figs. 1–1 and 1–2). We modify this injection point occasionally depending on the location of tendon nodularity. Our protocol does not include ultrasound guidance, although techniques for use of ultrasound have been described.[3,5,7]

A 10-cc solution consisting of 2.5 cc 1% lidocaine, 2.5 cc 0.25% marcaine, and 5.0 cc normal saline is drawn into a 10-cc syringe. The injection is then done with positive pressure through a 1.5-in 25-gauge needle. The pressure is titrated such that the injection rate is approximately 1 cc per second. Correct injection into the peritendinous space can be confirmed visually based upon circumferential swelling.

Weekly brisement injections (no more than three) can be performed until the patient's symptoms resolve. The utility of repeated injections has not been rigorously studied but has been described in the literature.[5]

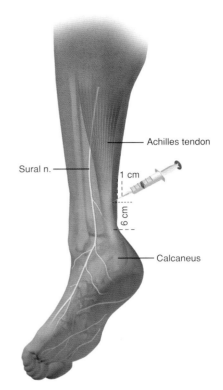

Figure 1–1. Illustration shows placement of needle 1 cm medial to the border of the Achilles tendon and 6 cm from the Achilles insertion.

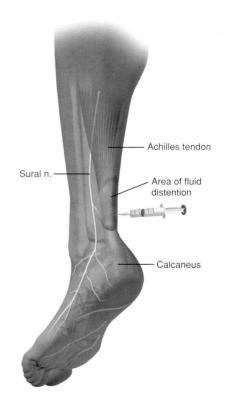

Figure 1–2. Illustration shows distention of paratenon after injection.

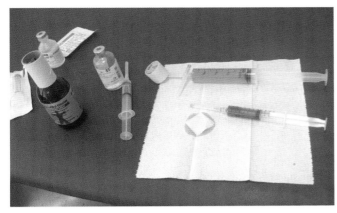

Figure 1–3. Creation and injection of platelet-rich plasma in the plantar fascia. Peripheral blood (60 cc) is drawn from a venipuncture in the antecubital fossa using a syringe with anticoagulant. The blood is placed sterilely in a specialized chamber, which is inserted into a centrifuge. The chamber allows for separation of the red blood cells from the PRP (red fluid) and platelet-poor plasma (yellow fluid). Long- and short-acting local anesthetics (6 cc) are also prepared.

Dry needling with PRP augmentation is preferred to brisement in the case of tendinosis and also plantar fasciopathy. We first harvest PRP from the peripheral blood (if the procedure is being done in the clinic) or from the bone marrow (if the procedure is being done in the OR) (Figs. 1–3–1–6). The plasma is then injected via a 25-gauge needle into the degenerated tendon or fascia in 15 to 20 fractionated doses. Skin punctures can be minimized by fanning the needle through the skin to allow several tendon punctures per skin puncture. The goal is to inject the plasma into and around the tendon (Figs. 1–7 and 1–8).

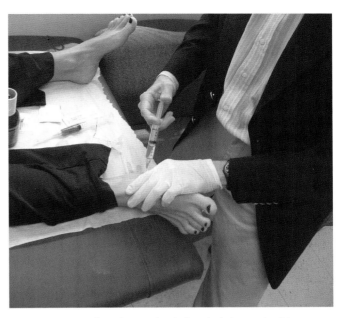

Figure 1–5. Local anesthetic is administered with a 25-gauge needle into the tender plantar fascia covering a broad circular area with a diameter of 3 to 4 cm.

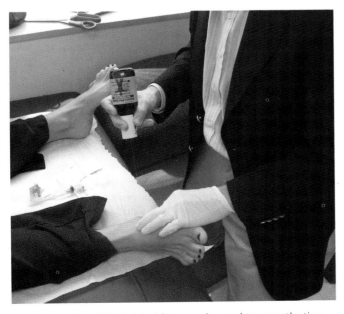

Figure 1–4. Ethyl chloride spray is used to anesthetize the skin.

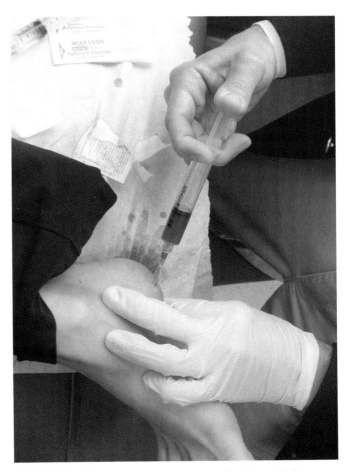

Figure 1–6. The PRP is then injected with multiple penetrating deep plantar fascia punctures using a 25-gauge needle.

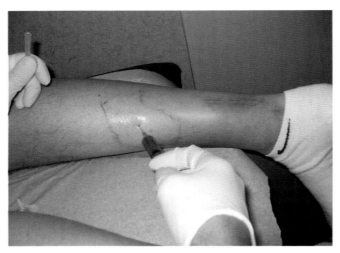

Figure 1–7. Injection of PRP into area of residual tendon tear following noninsertional Achilles tendon rupture that extended from midcalf to distal calf. Adjustment of trajectory will increase the zone of treatment.

COMPLICATIONS

Occasionally patients may experience some mild local irritation from the needle. Some bruising may occur. After the injection, patients may experience a flare of pain, local swelling, and warmth. This is particularly true if needling of the tendon is done. In these cases the flare of symptoms may last for up to 6 weeks. Complications such as infection are very rare. If the tendon is rupturing and this is not recognized, the injection may rarely be blamed for causing the final tearing.

REHABILITATION PROTOCOL

We keep patients immobilized in a boot brace for 1 week following the procedure. They are instructed to remove

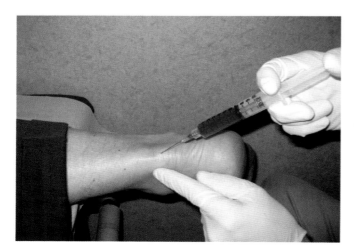

Figure 1–8. Injection of PRP in and around midsubstance (noninsertional) Achilles tendinopathy.

the brace for range-of-motion exercises. We ask that patients perform inversion, eversion, and dorsiflexion to avoid stiffness. We will occasionally prescribe theraband exercises. Patients are allowed to walk on the affected leg immediately. Unless the extensor tendons (anterior tibial, extensor hallucis longus, extensor digitorum longus tendons) are injected, we allow the patient to remove the brace at night. For the extensor tendons, it is often useful to use a night splint to minimize stretching of these tendons. We counsel patients that they will have reached 75% healing in 3 months and that we have a 50% to 75% success rate in relieving symptoms.

OUTCOME

Chan et al.[7] found short-term (4 weeks) and long-term (average of 30 weeks) statistically significant improvement in pain and function scores in reviewing 30 patients with chronic Achilles tendinopathy who had received high-volume steroid/bupivacaine/saline brisement. Using a similar brisement solution, Humphrey et al.[3] showed decreased neovascularization, reduced tendon thickness, and improved function scores in 11 athletes who underwent brisement for Achilles tendinopathy. In a retrospective review of chronic Achilles "tenosynovitis" patients, Johnston et al.[8] found that three of nine who received low-volume (5 cc) bupivacaine brisement had complete resolution of their symptoms.

Our experience is consistent with these findings, suggesting that properly selected patients will derive benefit from brisement and its related procedures.

REFERENCES

1. Schepsis AA, Jones H, Haas AL. Achilles tendon disorders in athletes. *Am J Sports Med*. 2002;30:287–305.
2. Zanetti M, Metzdorf A, Kundert HP, et al. Achilles tendons: Clinical relevance of neovascularization diagnosed with power Doppler US. *Radiology*. 2003;227:556–560.
3. Humphrey J, Chan O, Crisp T, et al. The short-term effects of high volume image guided injections in resistant noninsertional Achilles tendinopathy. *J Sci Med Sport*. 2010;13:295–298.
4. Read MT. Safe relief of rest pain that eases with activity in achillodynia by intrabursal or peritendinous steroid injection: The rupture rate was not increased by these steroid injections. *Br J Sports Med*. 1999;33:134–135.
5. Davidson J, Jayaraman S. Guided interventions in musculoskeletal ultrasound: What's the evidence? *Clin Radiol*. 2011;66:140–152.
6. Jones DC. Achilles tendon problems in runners. *Instr Course Lect*. 1998;47:419–427.
7. Chan O, O'Dowd D, Padhiar N, et al. High volume image guided injections in chronic Achilles tendinopathy. *Disabil Rehabil*. 2008;30:1697–1708.
8. Johnston E, Scranton P, Pfeffer GB. Chronic disorders of the Achilles tendon: Results of conservative and surgical treatments. *Foot Ankle Int*. 1997;18:570–574.

CHAPTER 2

Endoscopic Gastrocnemius Recession

Saul G. Trevino   Santaram Vallurupalli   David Flood

INTRODUCTION

Progressive deformities of the foot and ankle have been associated with contracture of the triceps surae. Historically, these contractures were addressed by distal release of the Achilles tendon.[1-3] Complications of this approach include calcaneal gait, plantar flexion weakness, and wound-healing problems. Isolated contracture of the gastrocnemius was first identified in the early 20th century. The first open procedure to release primarily the gastrocnemius contracture was described in 1913 by Vulpius[4] and modified in 1950 by Strayer.[5] Unfortunately, open procedures can be complicated by overlengthening, poor cosmesis, sural nerve damage, skin contractures, and wound-healing problems. Endoscopic gastrocnemius recession (EGR) has been developed to address these concerns.

The EGR has several advantages over open procedures. It can be done under local anesthetic without use of a tourniquet. The short surgical time (usually 10 to 15 minutes) allows ample time to perform associated reconstructions under the same anesthetic. The procedure has a small learning curve and can be mastered by the general orthopedic surgeon.[6,7] It can also be performed in pediatric patients. The short incisions are excellent from a cosmetic perspective.

INDICATIONS

EGR is indicated in cases of demonstrable gastrocnemius contracture. Isolated gastrocnemius contracture must be distinguished from contracture associated with tightness of the gastrocsoleus unit, as well as contracture associated with anatomic bone or joint pathology such as posttraumatic arthrosis.[7-11] Anatomical equinus may be defined as an ankle with less than 0 degrees of dorsiflexion. Functional ankle equinus has been defined as a limitation of ankle dorsiflexion of less than 10 degrees. Most authors agree that normal gait after toe off requires at least 10 degrees of dorsiflexion. Barrett described passive dorsiflexion less than 10 degrees with the leg extended as pathologic.[10] DiGiovanni et al.[12] proposed that passive dorsiflexion less than 5 degrees to be considered as an equinus contracture. We feel that any dorsiflexion with full knee extension less than 10 degrees is possibly pathologic and that dorsiflexion less than 5 degrees is definitely pathologic.

The Silfverskiold test[13] remains the primary method of distinguishing isolated contractures of the gastrocnemius from contractures of the gastrocsoleus complex (Fig. 2–1). The distinction relies on the anatomical fact that the gastrocnemius originates on the distal femur and spans the knee joint, compared to the soleus muscle, which originates on the tibia and only spans the ankle joint. To perform the Silfverskiold test, the ankle is dorsiflexed with the knee in both extension and in 20 to 40 degrees of flexion. The test is considered positive for isolated gastrocnemius contracture if dorsiflexion normalizes with knee flexion but is limited in knee extension (Fig. 2–1). It is important to position the hindfoot in subtalar neutral to slight inversion. This neutral position locks transverse tarsal joint, thus controlling the eversion and abduction that may give a false sense of greater dorsiflexion than is actually present.

While the gastrocnemius contracture release was initially performed primarily in patients with a neurologic disorder such as cerebral palsy, various authors including Hansen, expanded its use to the treatment of conditions not necessarily associated with neurologic disorders.[14-16] These authors and others postulated that the contracted gastrocnemius muscle limits dorsiflexion, which in turn alters normal gait biomechanics. This contracture causes excessive pronation and may evolve into actual peritalar subluxation over time.[8,9]

In 2002, DiGiovanni et al.[12] published a prospective study with a control group that supported the association of gastrocnemius contracture with other common foot disorders like plantar fasciitis, bunions, and midfoot pathology. In addition, Adelman et al.[17] reported in 2008 the use of gastrocnemius recession combined with subtalar arthrodesis and flexor tendon transfer in the successful treatment of Stage II posterior tibialis tendon in dysfunction in 10 patients. EGR is indicated whenever gastrocnemius contracture is impairing normal gait or contributes to other pathologic states (Fig. 2–6).

Endoscopic Gastrocnemius Recession Procedure Setup

The patient can either be placed in a supine or prone position. In general, the supine position is preferred as it allows for performing additional related procedures without intraoperative repositioning. Elevation of the contralateral hip and a small bump under the operative

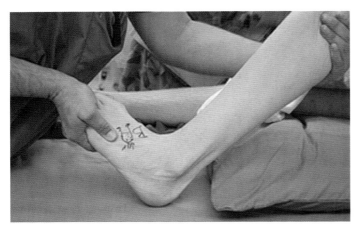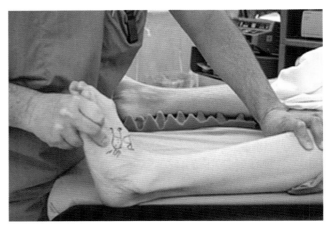

Figure 2–1. The Silfverskiold test distinguishes isolated contractures of the gastrocnemius from the gastrocsoleus complex. It is performed with the foot placed in subtalar neutral and slight inversion, which locks the transverse tarsal joints. The knee is first flexed with ankle dorsiflexion and then compared to passive dorsiflexion with the knee extended. The picture on the right is a positive test with gastrocnemius contracture.

ankle allows for easy manipulation of the endoscope. The medial portal site is located 15 to 17 cm proximal to the insertion of the Achilles tendon.[10] The incisional site is 3 to 4 cm distal to the most distal extent of the gastrocnemius bellies. There is some variance in the distal extension of the muscle bellies beyond the center attachment point of the aponeurosis. In pediatric or small-statured people, the physical examination will determine the ideal location. The muscle bellies of the gastrocnemius muscle are identified and help to determine a point approximately 4 to 6 cm distal to these structures (Fig. 2–2). In obese patients, an ultrasound can help to identify the precise location of the distal extent of these muscles. EGR can be performed using both medial and lateral portals; however, this two-portal technique is not necessary since the medial portal allows for visualization of both the medial and lateral borders of the aponeurosis. A lateral portal is more likely to damage the sural nerve. The approximate location of the sural nerve can be estimated by drawing a line from the center of the popliteal fossa to an area 1 cm behind the lateral malleolus at the level of the ankle.[18]

EGR is routinely performed without the use of a tourniquet. An ankle tourniquet can be applied after the EGR is completed. This helps to limit tourniquet time when concomitant procedures are being performed. After selection of the portal site, a 1- to 2-cm longitudinal incision is drawn. Placement of 0.5% bupivacaine with epinephrine in and around the incision site with a hypodermic needle minimizes bleeding (Fig. 2–3). The

Figure 2–2. The posteromedial portal site is located 15 to 17 cm proximal to the insertion of the Achilles tendon. The muscle bellies can be identified in pediatric patients and the portal site is approximately 4 to 6 cm distal to the bellies. Due to the lack of curvature of the scope, the site needs to be more posterior. Dotted line—inferior border of the medial gastrocnemius, straight line—incision site, curved line—medial malleolus.

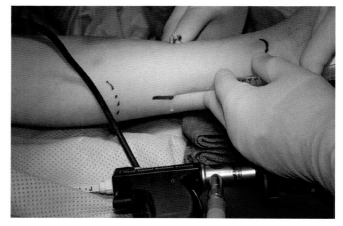

Figure 2–3. Injection before making incision with local anesthetic with epinephrine prevents need for a tourniquet. The posterior fascia is also injected.

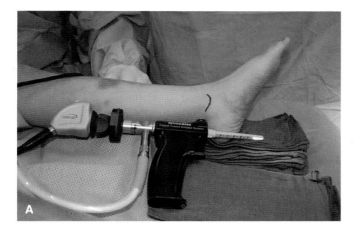

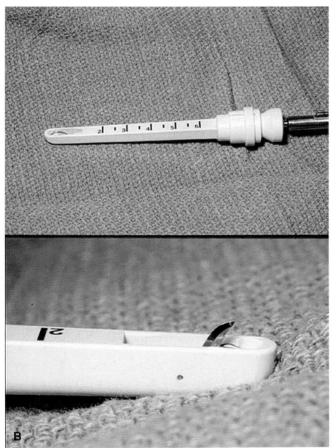

Figure 2–4. **A:** A commercially available endoscopic fascial release device with a pistol-grip triggering device which allows for a single portal approach. It does not have an obturator so a slightly larger incision needs to be made in the deep fascia to allow for the bulky head. **B:** The device has a very minimal blade exposure once actuated, which prevents major damage to the soleus muscle.

posterior aspect of the deep fascia is also injected to provide added hemostasis and analgesia. In obese patients visualization can be obscured and a larger incision may be made. A few commercially available disposable endo-

scopic release kits are available with trigger devices that deploy the blade assembly. They are easily used with a 2.7-mm arthroscope.[19] The sets come with a series of dilators. The amount of exposed blade is quite small minimizing damage and resultant bleeding from the soleus muscle (Fig. 2–4). The endoscope should be covered with a towel to keep it warm until use to prevent fogging of the lens.

OPERATIVE PROCEDURE

A longitudinal incision is made over the portal site to the deep fascia overlying the aponeurosis. A 1-cm longitudinal cut is made into fascia (Fig. 2–5A). With the use of serial dilators the opening in the fascia as well as the interval between the fascia and the Achilles aponeurosis is expanded to allow for the placement of the scope (Fig. 2–5B). If excessive fluid or fat is encountered, this can be cleared using a series of passes with a cotton tip applicator stick. The scope assembly is then inserted (Fig. 2–5C). If the correct scope interval is in question a dimpling test can be performed. This is done by pressing the endoscope directly into the gastrocnemius muscle. When the endoscope is in the correct position the overlying fascia adheres to it and a dimple is noted in the skin (Fig. 2–5D).

Exploration of the aponeurosis is quite simple. The endoscope is used to determine the medial and lateral borders of the aponeurosis. An attempt is made to visualize the sural nerve. If the nerve is not located on the surface of gastrocnemius muscle, the scope is then rotated 180 degrees to visualize the location on the inner surface of the investing fascia. Using this technique to confirm location of the sural nerve, no nerve damage has been experienced. At this point, the assistant dorsiflexes the foot in an inverted position with the knee extended and maintains this position during the rest of the procedure. This puts the gastrocnemius complex under maximum tension (Fig. 2–5E). The endoscope is then placed on the far lateral margin of the aponeurosis and the knife is deployed. With the knife deployed, the scope is withdrawn from lateral to medial while maintaining contact with the gastrocnemius aponeurosis. The assistant holding the foot will note the progressive release of the aponeurosis (Fig. 2–5F) and an increase in the amount of ankle dorsiflexion. The underlying soleus muscle is exposed but minimal bleeding usually occurs. The arthroscope is then readvanced laterally to confirm that complete release has been accomplished. Compared to the open Strayer procedure, there is no extensile incision and no requirement for tourniquet. There is also the potential to minimize anesthesia if the EGR is being done as an isolated procedure. The skin is closed with subcuticular 4-0 absorbable suture and covered with a small transparent dressing. At this point, an ankle tourniquet can be applied if secondary procedures are to be carried out.

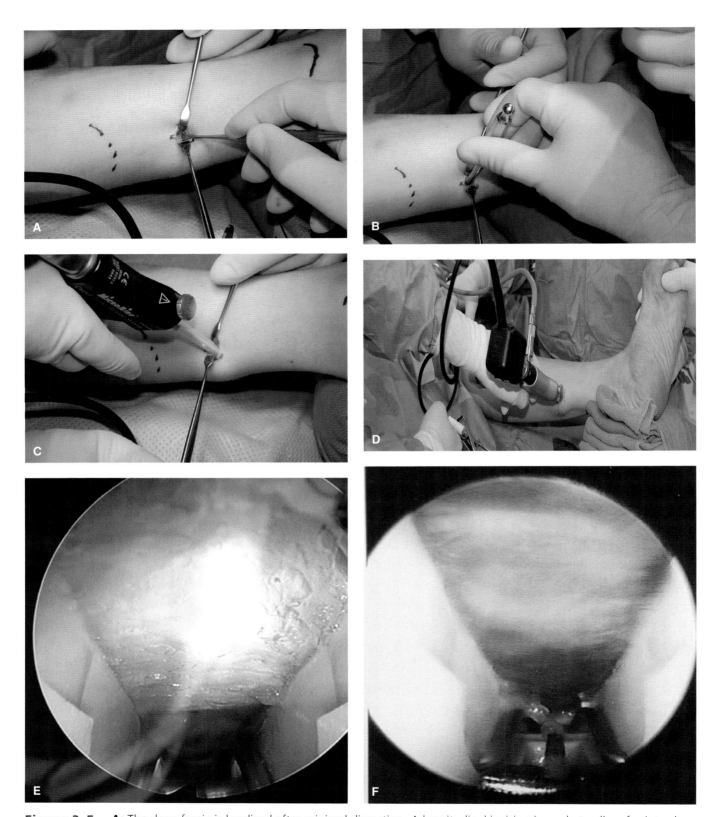

Figure 2–5. **A:** The deep fascia is localized after minimal dissection. A longitudinal incision is made to allow for introduction of the endoscope anterior to the fascia. **B:** The dilator is inserted anterior to the deep fascia to allow for adequate space for the endoscope. **C:** Introduction of the scope. **D:** The dimple test confirms the correct interval for the gastrocnemius recession. It is performed by pressing on the gastrocnemius muscle which is connected to the deep fascia and creates dimpling of the skin. **E:** Endoscopic view of the gastrocnemius aponeurosis. **F:** Appearance of the soleus muscle after division of the gastrocnemius aponeurosis.

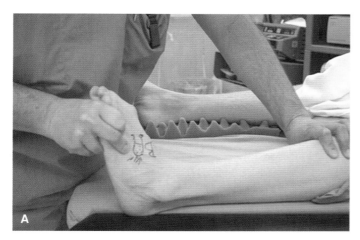 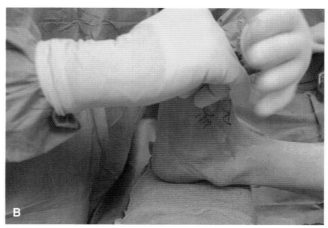

Figure 2–6.   A: Pre-op picture showing the positive Silfverskiold test. **B:** Picture after endoscopic gastrocnemius release.

POSTOPERATIVE MANAGEMENT

Postoperatively an isolated recession is protected with either a short-leg walking cast or boot for a 4-week period. The patient is encouraged to start weight bearing as tolerated and after 2 weeks instructed to start active range motion including dorsiflexion.

COMPLICATIONS

The sural nerve has a variable relationship with the deep fascia[20] and is considered the most at-risk structure during EGR. In 2004, Pinney et al.[16] reported that in 40 cases of open Strayer procedures, the sural nerve was located superficial to the fascia in 17 patients, deep to the fascia in 23 patients and actually attached to the gastrocnemius in 5 patients. Despite this variability, the technique described above resulted in no sural nerve injuries in one study.[7] More recently Shroeder[21] and Phisitkul et al.[22] reported an incidence of sural nerve injury of 5% and 3.1% respectively when EGR was used. Other reported complications include conversions to open procedures in obese patients, delayed healing of incisions, and under corrections in spastic contractures.

There are no real concerns from a cosmetic standpoint with these small incisions.

OUTCOMES OF EGR

The outcomes of EGR reported to date have been encouraging and the complications have been minimal. In the three series noted in Table 2.1, postoperative improvement in dorsiflexion ranged from 18 to 21 degrees. More recently, Adelman et al. reported an average mean improvement of 15 degrees of dorsiflexion in pediatric patients. Shroeder reported improvement of 15.7 degrees[21] and Phisitkul et al., in a large series of 320 patients reported a lesser improvement of 11.8 degrees. These results are at least comparable with the series of Pinney and DiGiovanni who used an open Strayer procedure.[12,23–25]

CONCLUSIONS

EGR is a safe and effective technique for the treatment of gastrocnemius contracture. It has numerous advantages over open procedures including a small cosmetic incision, short operating times, and less risk of overlengthening.

TABLE 2–1. Series of Endoscopic Gastrocnemius Releases with a Summary of Their Results.

Author	# Cases	Portals	Degree Dorsiflexion Improved	Complications
Saxena (2004)[25]	15	12 dual portals, 3 medial portals	21 degrees	3 dysesthesias, 1 skin contracture
DiDomenico (2005)[24]	31	27 dual portals, 4 medial portals	18 degrees	1 hematoma, 3 "weakness"
Trevino (2005)[7]	31	31 single portals	Not documented	2 wrong level, 1 superficial infection

REFERENCES

1. Mueller MJ, Sinacore DR, Hastings MK, et al. Effect of Achilles tendon lengthening on neuropathic plantar ulcers. A randomized clinical trial. *J Bone Joint Surg Am.* 2003;85-A(8):1436–1445.
2. Crenshaw AM. *Campbell's operative orthopaedics.* 8th ed. Philadelphia, PA: Mosby; 1992:2305–2367.
3. Nishimoto GS, Attinger CE, Cooper PS. Lengthening the Achilles tendon for the treatment of diabetic plantar forefoot ulceration. *Surg Clin North Am.* 2003;83(3):707–726.
4. Vulpius OS. Tenotomie der end schnen der mm. gastrocnemius el soleus mittels rutschenlassens nach Vulpius. *Orthopaedische Operationslehre.* Stuttgart: Ferdinard Enke; 1913:29–31. CE: Please check this reference.
5. Strayer LM Jr. Recession of the gastrocnemius; an operation to relieve spastic contracture of the calf muscles. *J Bone Joint Surg Am.* 1950;32-A(3):671–676.
6. Tashjian RZ, Appel AJ, Banerjee R, et al. Endoscopic gastrocnemius recession: Evaluation in a cadaver model. *Foot Ankle Int.* 2003;24(8):607–613.
7. Trevino S, Gibbs M, Panchbhavi V. Evaluation of results of endoscopic gastrocnemius recession. *Foot Ankle Int.* 2005;26(5):359–364.
8. Hansen S. *Functional reconstruction of the foot and ankle.* Philadelphia, PA: Lippincott Williams & Wilkins; 2000.
9. Sgarlato TE, Morgan J, Shane HS, et al. Tendo achillis lengthening and its effect on foot disorders. *J Am Podiatry Assoc.* 1975;65(9):849–871.
10. Barrett SL, Jarvis J. Equinus deformity as a factor in forefoot nerve entrapment: Treatment with endoscopic gastrocnemius recession. *J Am Podiatr Med Assoc.* 2005; 95(5):464–468.
11. Lavery LA, Armstrong DG, Boulton AJ. Ankle equinus deformity and its relationship to high plantar pressure in a large population with diabetes mellitus. *J Am Podiatr Med Assoc.* 2002;92(9):479–482.
12. DiGiovanni CW, Kuo R, Tejwani N, et al. Isolated gastrocnemius tightness. *J Bone Joint Surg Am.* 2002;84-A(6): 962–970.
13. Silverskiold N. Reduction of the uncrossed two-joint muscles of the leg to one-joint muscles in spastic conditions. *Acta Chir Scand.* 1924;56:315–330.
14. Lawrence SJ, Botte MJ. Management of the adult, spastic, equinovarus foot deformity. *Foot Ankle Int.* 1994;15(6): 340–346.
15. Silver CM, Simon SD. Gastrocnemius-muscle recession (Silfverskiold operation) for spastic equinus deformity in cerebral palsy. *J Bone Joint Surg Am.* 1959;41-A:1021–1028.
16. Pinney SJ, Sangeorzan BJ, Hansen ST Jr. Surgical anatomy of the gastrocnemius recession (Strayer procedure). *Foot Ankle Int.* 2004;25(4):247–250.
17. Adelman VR, Szczepanski JA, Adelman RP. Radiographic evaluation of endoscopic gastrocnemius recession, subtalar joint arthroereisis, and flexor tendon transfer for surgical correction of stage II posterior tibial tendon dysfunction: a pilot study. *J Foot Ankle Surg.* 2008;47(5):400–408.
18. Singh S, Naasan A. Use of distally based superficial sural island artery flaps in acute open fractures of the lower leg. *Ann Plast Surg.* 2001;47(5):505–510.
19. Agee JM, Peimer CA, Pyrek JD, et al. Endoscopic carpal tunnel release: A prospective study of complications and surgical experience. *J Hand Surg Am.* 1995;20(2):165–171; discussion 172.
20. Tashjian RA, Banerjee R, DiGiovanni CW, et al. Anatomic study of the gastrocnemius-soleus junction and its relationship to the sural nerve. *Foot Ankle Int.* 2003;24(6):473–476.
21. Shroeder SM. Uniportal endoscopic gastrocnemius recession for treatment of gastrocnemius equinus with a dedicated EGR system with retractable blade. *J Foot Ankle Surg.* 2012;51(6):714–719.
22. Phisitkul P, Rungprai C, Femino JE, et al. Endoscopic gastrocnemius recession for the treatment of isolated gastrocnemius contracture: A prospective study on 320 consecutive patients. *Foot Ankle Int.* 2014;35(8):747–756.
23. Pinney SJ, Hansen ST Jr, Sangeorzan BJ. The effect on ankle dorsiflexion of gastrocnemius recession. *Foot Ankle Int.* 2002;23(1):26–29.
24. DiDomenico LA, Garchar D. Endoscopic gastrocnemius recession for the treatment of gastrocnemius equinus. *J Am Podiatr Med Assoc.* 2005;95(4):410–413.
25. Saxena AW. Endoscopic gastrocnemius recession: Preliminary report on 18 cases. *J Foot Ankle Surg.* 2004;43(5): 302–306.

CHAPTER 3

Tendoscopy

Markus Knupp   V. James Sammarco

INDICATIONS

Surgery for tendon disorders of the posterior foot and ankle are common. Tendons in this area enter a relatively avascular zone as they traverse local fibroosseous tunnels. These avascular zones are also areas of high stress and shear as the tendons undergo marked directional change. Inflammation and synovitis are poorly tolerated due to the tight retinacular structures which direct the tendons and can lead to tears and degenerative conditions of the tendons themselves. Traditional surgical techniques require extensile exposures in this area, and as a result, even simple tenosynovectomy of the ankle tendons can lead to fibrosis, sensory nerve injury, and recurrent symptomatology. Endoscopy of the hindfoot has successfully been used to address articular and periarticular pathologies around the ankle joint and when used for to treat tendons offers the advantage of allowing visualization without disruption of the normal retinacular structures. Endoscopy of tendons and their surrounding structures has been termed tendoscopy. Some tendinopathies can be treated completely endoscopically, but even when open procedures are required, diagnostic tendoscopy can limit the amount of exposure needed. While any tendon can be visualized endoscopically, tendoscopy is particularly useful in addressing the tendons of the tarsal canal and the lateral ankle joint. This chapter will discuss tendoscopic procedures and techniques used for treatment of the peroneal tendons, the posterior tibial tendon, the flexor hallucis longus tendon, and the Achilles tendon. Indications for tendoscopy are diagnostic examination, treatment of tenosynovitis, impingement, degenerative tendon tears, and tendon subluxation.

Peroneal Tendons

Pathologic conditions of the peroneal tendons are common, and MRI may often be ambiguous. We have found tendoscopy to be useful as a diagnostic adjunct in patients with recalcitrant ankle pain localized to the peroneal tendon sheath where definitive diagnosis is lacking. Conditions such as stenosis due to tenosynovitis or an accessory muscle, low lying peroneal muscle bellies, and peroneus quartus tendons can often be treated with tendoscopic debridement alone. Tendoscopic examination facilitates a "mini-open" technique for repair in cases where degeneration is present. Success has also been reported in treating tendon subluxation and dislocation with tendoscopy.[1] Additionally, peroneal tendon disease may be associated with intra-articular pathology and osseous or ligamentous imbalance of the ankle joint.[2] Open or endoscopic tendon debridement, tendon repair,[1,3–5] and groove deepening[6] are indicated if the patients fail to improve with conservative treatment. If necessary, concomitant ankle arthroscopy or ligament stabilization may also be performed.

Posterior Tibial Tendon

Posterior tibial tendonitis can progress to significant degeneration if not recognized and treated early. Patients may present with stage I tenosynovitis where there is inflammation, but an intact and functioning tendon. If untreated, this may progress to dysfunction and rupture of the tendon which in turn may require extensive surgery or bracing to control. While most patients respond to a course of immobilization and physical therapy, some will continue to have pain along the course of the tendon which does not improve. In recalcitrant cases, where inflammation and synovitis persist despite conservative management, tendoscopy has been described to halt disease progression and prevent development of adult acquired flatfoot deformity.[1,7]

Flexor Hallucis Longus Tendon

Certain athletic pursuits such as ballet and other forms of dance pose an increased risk for developing pathology of the flexor hallucis longus tendon. Entrapment often occurs at the posterior ankle as the FHL tendon enters the fibroosseous tunnel system posterior to the talus. Anatomic considerations in this area that predispose to entrapment of the tendon include an enlarged posterolateral process of the talus, os trigonum syndrome, and "bottlenecking" of a flexor hallucis longus muscle belly where hypertrophied muscle fibers impinge and become inflamed when they enter the tendon sheath. The FHL tendon sheath is intimate with the posterior ankle capsule and posteromedial ankle ligaments and as a result is very dense and rigid. Stenosis in this area is poorly tolerated and can lead to attritional tears of the tendon. The sheath often communicates with the ankle and/or subtalar joint and can also be a repository for loose bodies from either joint. In our experience, flexor hallucis longus tendonitis is often associated with a tight flexor retinaculum and thickened tendon sheath that can lead to stenosing tenosynovitis. Symptomatic patients who present with posterior ankle impingement can be treated by endoscopic decompression by FHL myoplasty/synovectomy and retinacular release with or without excision of an os trigonum.[8]

Achilles Tendon

Insertional Achilles tendinopathy is a common condition that often improves with simple eccentric stretching exercises and other physical therapeutic modalities. When symptoms persist despite conservative management, surgical intervention can be considered. Success has been reported with endoscopic decompression for the Achilles insertion by resection of the osseous Haglund deformity and retrocalcaneal bursectomy.[9,10] The ideal candidate for a limited endoscopic procedure is the patient with no significant ossification of the tendon on plain radiographs and minimal tendon degeneration on magnetic resonance imaging.

PATIENT POSITIONING

Peroneal Tendons

The patient is placed in a lateral decubitus position for isolated endoscopy of the peroneal tendons or supine with a sandbag under the buttock of the affected limb if the tendoscopy is combined with an ankle arthroscopy (Fig. 3–1). After exsanguination of the leg, a pneumatic tourniquet is inflated on the thigh.

Posterior Tibial Tendon

The patient is placed in a supine position. A tourniquet is placed on the thigh of the affected leg. If the endoscopy is combined with an ankle arthroscopy, starting with the ankle will allow removing the leg support prior to the tendoscopy and thereby eases the approach to the tendon.

Flexor Hallucis Longus

The patient is placed in a prone position with a thigh tourniquet. A support is placed under the lower leg with the foot at the edge of the operating table allowing the ankle to move freely (Fig. 3–2).

SURGICAL APPROACHES

Peroneal Tendons

Four portals are described for tendoscopy of the peroneal tendon sheath, although often all are not utilized (Fig. 3–3). The first portal established is between the

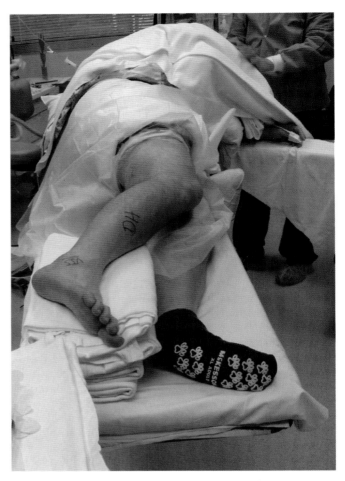

Figure 3–1. Lateral decubitus positioning for tendoscopy of the peroneal tendons.

peroneal tubercle and the tip of the fibula. The tendons are subcutaneous here, and a small nick in the skin with a no. 11 scalpel is all that is needed to allow the tendon sheath to be entered. A blunt trocar is then advanced into

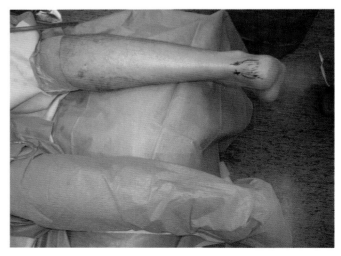

Figure 3–2. Positioning of the patient for hindfoot endoscopy.

the tendon sheath proximally posterior to the fibula, and a 30-degree 2.7-mm (preferred) or 1.9-mm (for patients with a very tight sheath) arthroscope is introduced to allow visualization. The second portal is then established in a similar manner 3 cm proximal to the tip of the fibula. Visualization of an 18-gauge spinal needle which is passed into the tendon sheath as a trial will help verify position and avoid injury to the tendons as the second portal is established (Fig. 3–4). Most lesions can be treated or diagnosed with these two portals alone. Occasionally, synovitis will extend proximally and further debridement will require a more proximal portal. The inferior peroneal retinaculum can be visualized from proximal to distal. If distal synovectomy or release of the inferior peroneal retinaculum is necessary, a portal distal to the peroneal retinaculum may be established. Neurologic structures at risk in this procedure include the superficial peroneal nerve for the more proximal portals, and the sural nerve which crosses the surgical field distal to the lateral malleolus. The course and branching of these nerves is quite variable but the risk of injury can be minimized by using the "nick and spread" technique, where the skin is nicked with a no. 11 scalpel and the subcutaneous tissue and tendon sheath are spread with a small, pointed hemostat.

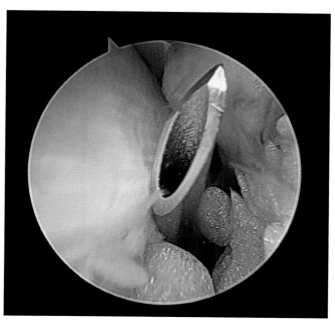

Figure 3–4. After insertion of the arthroscope into the distal portal, the location of the proximal portal is determined under direct visualization using a 18-gauge needle.

Posterior Tibial Tendon

Access to the posterior tibial tendon can be obtained anywhere along the course of the tendon starting proximal of the insertion to the navicular bone to about 5 cm proximal to the posterior edge of the medial malleolus. The most commonly used portals are located about 2.5 cm distal and 3 to 5 cm proximal to the tip of the medial malleolus. For the distal portal a small skin incision portal is made with a no. 11 scalpel blade and the subcutaneous tissue and tendon sheath are spread bluntly with a small hemostat. The endoscope (usually a 2.7-mm, 30-degree arthroscope) is then inserted and the tendon sheath inflated with saline. After inspection of the tendon the second portal is established. Under direct visualization an 18-gauge spinal needle is used to determine the height of the second skin incision. After spreading the subcutaneous tissue bluntly the instruments can be inserted. Particularly the proximal portal carries the risk of damage to the neurovascular bundle. Remaining strictly within the tendon sheath keeps the bundle out of danger.

Flexor Hallucis Longus Tendon

The two portals are created adjacent to the Achilles tendon—one medial and one lateral—at the height of the ankle joint. We recommend confirmation of portal placement under image intensification (Fig. 3–5). First, the lateral portal is created using a no. 11 scalpel blade. The subcutaneous tissue is spread bluntly with a hemostat in the direction of the center of the ankle joint, for example, midline between the tip of the fibula and the

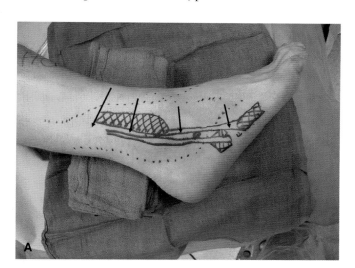

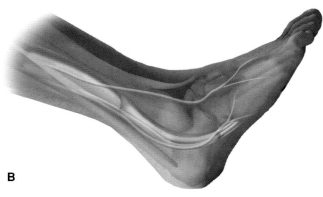

Figure 3–3. **A:** Location of the portals for peroneal tendoscopy. Arrows point to the location where four portals for peroneal tendoscopy should be created. **B:** Surface anatomy.

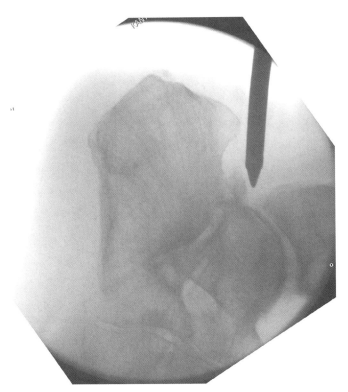

Figure 3–5. Verification of the appropriate height of the trocar for hindfoot endoscopy under image intensification.

tip of the medial malleolus. Thereafter a blunt trocar is used to prepare the portal for the arthroscope. The trocar is advanced until bony resistance of the ankle and the subtalar joint is felt and a 4.5-mm, 30-degree arthroscope introduced. A medial stab incision is made at the same height. Again, a hemostat is used to spread the tissue anterior to the Achilles tendon until the arthroscope is felt. A trocar is then introduced and directed laterally to "meet" the arthroscope anterior to the Achilles tendon. Then the trocar is slid along the arthroscope into the joint. After creation of the second portal a 3-mm shaver is introduced through the second portal in a same manner as the trocar, for example, slid along the arthroscope. Often the joint capsule and the fatty tissue need to be removed to visualize the flexor hallucis longus tendon.

Achilles Tendon

A vertical incision is made at the lateral border of the Achilles tendon. The portal is located at the height of the superior aspect of the calcaneus (Fig. 3–6). The retrocalcaneal space is penetrated by a blunt trocar with the foot in plantar flexion to reduce the tension on the Achilles tendon. In chronically inflamed bursitis the trocar can be used to mobilize the retrocalcaneal bursa thereby creating a work space. Usually a 4.5-mm, 30-degree arthroscope is used which allows for increased fluid flow with lower pressure than the 2.7-mm

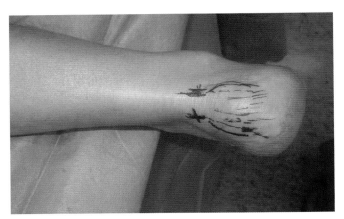

Figure 3–6. Locations of the portals for hindfoot endoscopy are shown by X marks.

arthroscope. After establishing the first portal, an 18-gauge spinal needle is inserted medially to the Achilles tendon, at the same height as the first portal. The second portal is then created under direct visualization using a number 11 scalpel. A hemostat is used to spread the subcutaneous tissue. Thereafter a blunt trocar is used to prepare the portal for the shaver.

SURGICAL PROCEDURES

Peroneal Tendons

A small probe is used to assess the tendons. Inflamed synovium, adhesions, and degenerative areas are debrided with a 3-mm shaver. The posterolateral vinculae that provide blood supply to the tendons should be preserved if possible (Fig. 3–7). However, in case of

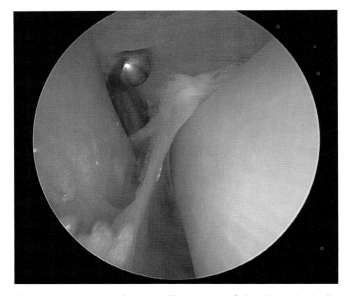

Figure 3–7. Tendoscopic illustration of the physiologically present vinculae between the peroneal tendons.

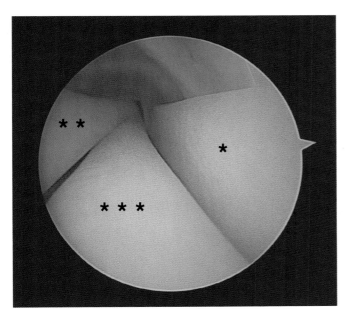

Figure 3–8. Arthroscopic image of a patient with an accessory peroneal tendon (peroneus quartus tendon). *Peroneus brevis tendon; **Peroneus quartus tendon; ***Peroneus longus tendon.

stenosing tenosynovitis due to muscle hypertrophy, a low peroneus brevis muscle belly, or an accessory peroneal tendon (Fig. 3–8), the offending structures can be resected with a shaver (Fig. 3–9). Tendon repair is performed using a "mini-open" technique after identification and localization of the tear (Fig. 3–10).[5] Finally, fibular groove deepening can be performed using a burr and posterior portals.[9]

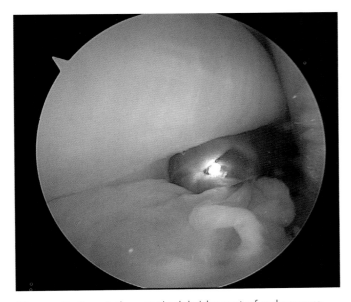

Figure 3–9. Arthroscopic debridement of a degenerative area within the peroneus brevis tendon.

Posterior Tibial Tendon

Debridement of inflamed synovium and degenerated areas of tendon is performed with a 3-mm shaver (Figs. 3–11 and 3–12). For longitudinal ruptures, the site is localized via diaphanoscopy and the tendon repaired through a "mini-open" approach.[1]

Flexor Hallucis Longus Tendon

A 3-mm shaver is used to create a workspace posterior to the ankle joint. For this purpose the adjacent fatty tissue and the joint capsule are partly resected. This usually allows good visualization of the flexor hallucis longus tendon. During the debridement the arthroscope and the shaver are kept strictly lateral to the tendon to avoid damage to the neurovascular bundle. In case of tenosynovitis the flexor retinaculum is released and the tendon debrided (Figs. 3–13 and 3–14).

COMPLICATIONS

The most common complication is neurologic injury, particularly numbness at the incision site.

Peroneal Tendons

Inadequate placement of the distal portal carries the risk for injuries to the sural nerve and penetration of the tendon sheath may lead to damage of the communicating branch of the sural and the superficial peroneal nerve.[3,11]

Posterior Tibial Tendon

Perforation of the tendon sheath can lead damage of the neurovascular bundle.[1,7]

Flexor Hallucis Longus Tendon

Complications in hindfoot arthroscopy are rare[8,12] and include hematoma formation and injury to the tibial nerve. Keeping the arthroscope and the shaver strictly lateral to the flexor hallucis longus tendon minimizes the risk for neurovascular damage.

Achilles Tendon

Complications reported in the literature are limited to areas of hypoesthesia.[9]

REHABILITATION PROTOCOL

The postoperative management is determined by the anomaly found intraoperatively. In a majority of cases

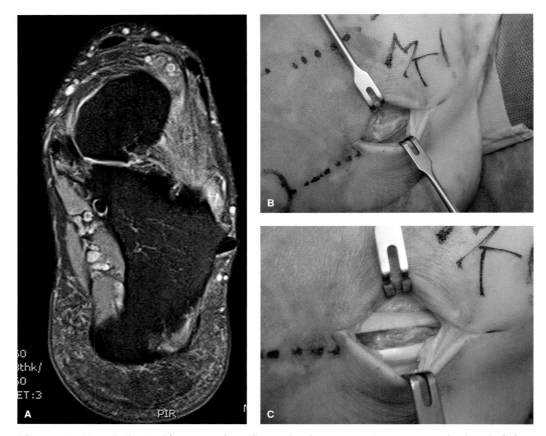

Figure 3–10. Patient with peroneal tendinopathy due to prominent peroneal tubercle **(A)** Coronal MRI of a young athlete presenting with a longitudinal peroneus brevis tendon tear due to a hypertrophic peroneal tubercle. **(B)** After peroneal tendoscopy was performed and demonstrated a limited longitudinal tear of the tendon the area to be repaired was exposed through a small incision the prominence of the peroneal tubercle was reduced. **(C)** Thereafter the tear of the tendon repaired by tubularization.

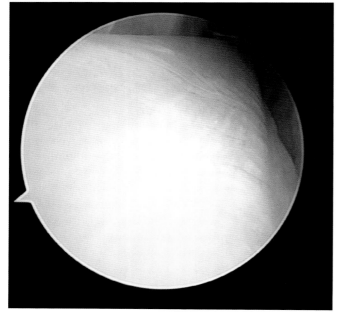

Figure 3–11. Inflammatory changes of a posterior tibial tendon in a patient with tenosynovitis.

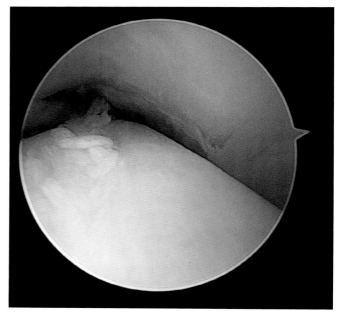

Figure 3–12. Retromalleolar attenuation of a posterior tibial tendon in a patient with a chronic medial pain syndrome.

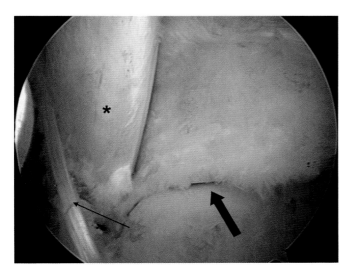

Figure 3–13.   Arthroscopic image of a patient with stenosing tenosynovitis of the flexor hallucis longus tendon after a conservatively treated fracture of the lateral tubercle (*asterisk:* flexor hallucis longus tendon, *arrow:* flexor reti-naculum, *thick arrow:* subtalar joint).

the patients are placed in a removable ankle foot brace allowing for early range of motion exercises and weight bearing as tolerated for about 4 weeks, thereafter they usually are allowed to wear standard shoes.

OUTCOMES

Peroneal Tendon

Scholten et al.[5] reported on 23 patients with a minimum of 2 years follow-up. Eleven patients underwent a "mini-open" tendon reconstruction, ten patients had a tendoscopic synovectomy and in two patients a tendoscopic fibular groove deepening was performed. In these patients no complications and no recurrence of the preoperative pathology was observed.

Posterior Tibial Tendon

Reilingh et al.[1] reported on 33 patients who underwent tendoscopy of the posterior tibial tendon. The procedures were for diagnostic purposes (11 patients), synovectomy (10 patients), and miscellaneous indications in the remaining patients. No complications were observed. Chow et al.[13] reported on tendoscopic synovectomy in six patients presenting with stage I posterior tibial tendon insufficiency who became asymptomatic after the procedure.

FLEXOR HALLUCIS LONGUS TENDON

In our own series 11 patients were treated for recurrent pain of the flexor hallucis longus tendon. One case showed a stenosing tenosynovitis after a conservatively treated fracture of the lateral tubercle (Fig. 3–12). Two cases showed partial tears of the tendon and in eight cases an isolated tenosynovitis was found. After endoscopic debridement one patient (tenosynovitis) stated that the benefit of the procedure was minor, all other patients had a pain-free result (seven patients) or minor residual discomfort (three patients) after 6 months.

ACHILLES TENDON

Scholten et al.[9] reported on 39 cases of Achilles tendinopathy treated endoscopically. After 4.5 years no complications were observed. Four patients had a fair result, six a good result, and 24 an excellent result.

REFERENCES

1. Reilingh M, de Leeuw P, van Sterkenburg M, et al. Tendoscopy of posterior tibial and peroneal tendons. *Tech Foot Ankle Surg.* 2010;9(2):43–47.
2. Molloy R, Tisdel C. Failed treatment of peroneal tendon injuries. *Foot Ankle Clin.* 2003;8(1):115–129, ix.
3. Panchbhavi V Trevino, S. The technique of peroneal tendoscopy and its role in management of peroneal tendon anomalies. *Tech Foot & Ankle Surg.* 2003;2(3):192–198.
4. Sammarco VJ. Peroneal tendoscopy: Indications and techniques. *Sports Med Arthrosc.* 2009;17(2):94–99.
5. Scholten PE, van Dijk CN. Tendoscopy of the peroneal tendons. *Foot Ankle Clin.* 2006;11(2):415–420, vii.
6. De Leeuw P, van Dijk CN, Golano P. A 3-portal endoscopic groove deepening technique for recurrent peroneal

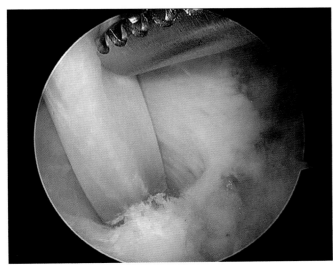

Figure 3–14.   Arthroscopic image of a flexor hallucis longus tendon after removal of the inflamed synovium.

tendon dislocation. *Tech Foot & Ankle Surg.* 2008;7(4):250–256.

7. van Dijk CN, Kort N, Scholten PE. Tendoscopy of the posterior tibial tendon. *Arthroscopy.* 1997;13(6):692–698.

8. van Dijk CN. Hindfoot endoscopy. *Foot Ankle Clin.* 2006;11(2):391–414, vii.

9. Scholten PE, van Dijk CN. Endoscopic calcaneoplasty. *Foot Ankle Clin.* 2006;11(2):439–446, viii.

10. van Dijk CN, van Dyk GE, Scholten PE, et al. Endoscopic calcaneoplasty. *Am J Sports Med.* 2001;29(2):185–189.

11. van Dijk CN, Kort N. Tendoscopy of the peroneal tendons. *Arthroscopy.* 1998;14(5):471–478.

12. Ferkel RD, Small HN, Gittins JE. Complications in foot and ankle arthroscopy. *Clin Orthop Relat Res.* 2001;(391):89–104.

13. Chow HT, Chan KB, Lui TH. Tendoscopic debridement for stage I posterior tibial tendon dysfunction. *Knee Surg Sports Traumatol Arthrosc.* 2005;13(8):695–698.

CHAPTER 4

Limited Incision Achilles Repair— Two Techniques

Bruce Cohen   Emilio Wagner

INTRODUCTION

Achilles tendon ruptures are common in the elite and recreational athlete and most often occur in the noninsertional region of the tendon.[1–3] These injuries typically occur in middle-aged "weekend warriors." The treatment of these injuries has led to much controversy in the literature recently. The previous "gold standard" of open repair has come under much scrutiny due to concerns of significant complication rates including wound healing difficulties and infection.[4–8]

In 1977 Ma and Griffith described a percutaneous approach for acute Achilles tendon repair. This involved sutures passed outside of the tendon sheath percutaneously. While their clinical results were reasonably good they were noted to have a number of patients with sural nerve injury or nerve entrapment as well as tendon reruptures in their initial series.[9] Complications in a randomized trial of minimally invasive Achilles tendon rupture repairs published in 2001 included wound puckering, adhesions, reruptures, and sural nerve paresthesia.[10] Assal et al.[11] in 2002 described the use of a new disposable jig for limited incision repairs that allowed the placement of sutures within the tendon inside the tendon sheath. In this series there were no infections, wound complications, or sural nerve injuries. The authors did report three early reruptures in their series.

The discussion of the most appropriate treatment for the acute Achilles rupture includes nonoperative treatment, standard open Achilles repair, and recently popularized minimal incision techniques.[12,13] Khan in 2005 performed a meta-analysis which included 12 clinical trials and over 800 patients. The rerupture risk was lower in the operative group while the complication rate was significantly higher in the open repair group. The percutaneous group fared better with respect to lower incidence of complications.[14,15] Cetti[16] in 1997 performed a randomized study comparing operative versus nonoperative treatment and found a significant difference in rerupture rates between the two groups. In 2010 Chiodo et al.[17,18] presented the results of the AAOS Clinical Guideline Committee which concluded that nonoperative treatment had lower complication rates and with moderate evidence supporting that the limited incision techniques had advantages over the open technique with respect to wound and overall complication rates. Recent published reports comparing nonoperative management to operative treatment have demonstrated no significant difference between the groups with respect to rerupture but there may be a trend toward better clinical outcomes in the operative group. The rerupture rates have not been shown to be statistically different between the groups but this may be due to the limited power of the studies. The important factor in the nonoperative treatment has been shown to involve early mobilization and weight bearing.[10,12,19–23]

Recent literature evaluating the strength of the limited incision repairs has compared these techniques to standard open repairs. The limited incision repairs were noted to have excellent strength and in some series are superior in strength and load to failure versus standard open techniques.[24–27] Clinical results have not demonstrated any difference in rupture rates between standard repairs and limited incision approaches.[10,20]

Jig (Intrasheath) Technique

Indications

The goals of surgical treatment of Achilles tendon ruptures include the restoration of muscle-tendon integrity, restoring the strength of the repaired tendon, and minimizing the rerupture rate. These all need to be accomplished while avoiding surgical complications. The indications for limited incision repairs take into account the patient's age, medical comorbidities as well as their activity level for sports and recreational activities. This technique is indicated for acute midsubstance ruptures. It is contraindicated in proximal ruptures, insertional ruptures or avulsions, or subacute presentation (greater than 2 to 3 weeks post injury).

Patient Positioning

The patient is positioned prone under general anesthesia with supplemental popliteal block and possible indwelling popliteal catheters for postoperative analgesia. A thigh tourniquet is used and all appropriate pressure points are well padded.

Surgical Approaches

The surgical approach includes a transverse or longitudinal incision at the level of the rerupture. The transverse approach allows better capture of the tendon edges and easier placement of the Achilles jig. The potential downside of this approach is if needed to convert to open repair, although rarely necessary, an S-shaped incision results.

The paratenon is opened and the proximal tendon is grasped with an Allis clamp (Fig. 4–1) and the jig is passed capturing the tendon proximally (Fig. 4–2). The sutures are passed in sequence as per the numbered holes on the jig. It is important to push the tendon down manually as the sutures are passed to maximize the tendon purchase. It is also important to avoid levering with the guide, which may cause the needles to miss the internal arms of the device. The suture technique allows the placement of two transverse sutures followed by two obliquely placed looped sutures. The looped sutures allow the creation of a locked stitch which increases the strength and tendon purchase (Fig. 4–3A,B). A third

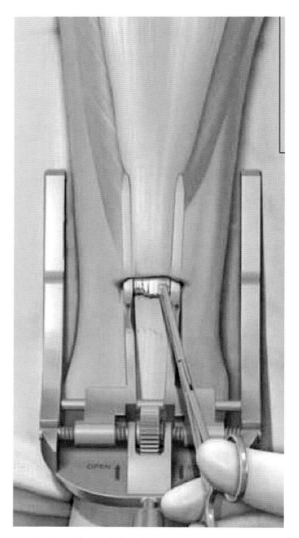

Figure 4–2. The Achilles jig is inserted to capture the tendon.

transverse suture is passed. The guide allows the placement of a second locked suture through the same technique, which we have not found to be necessary. The jig is then withdrawn from the wound leaving the sutures within the tendon sheath (Figs. 4–4A,B and 4–5). Each suture is checked for purchase. If a suture pulls out then the guide is reinserted and that suture is passed again. The identical technique is used for the distal portion of the tendon.

The sutures are then secured with the foot in the plantar flexed position. Sequence of securing sutures is up to surgeon preference (Figs. 4–6A,B and 4–7). The paratenon is then carefully closed followed by a standard skin closure. The incision is dressed and splint in resting equinus is applied.

Complications

Potential complications for this technique are the same as with any operative repair of Achilles tendon rupture.

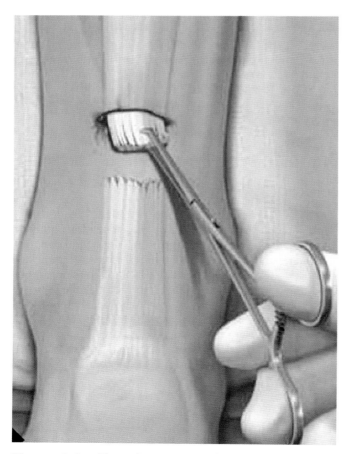

Figure 4–1. Through a transverse incision the proximal end of the tendon is grasped with an Allis clamp.

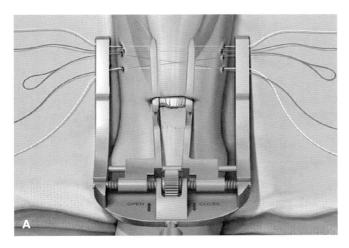

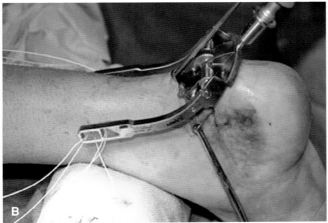

Figure 4–3.   A, B: Sutures are placed as per numbered holes in the jig.

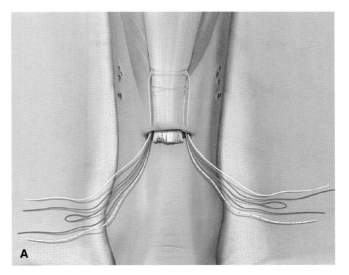

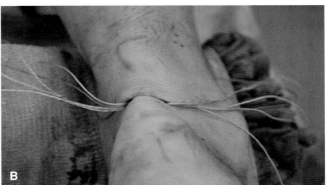

Figure 4–4.   A, B: Jig is removed and sutures are left within the paratenon.

These include infection and wound problems, nerve injury or paresthesias, and reruptures.

Rehabilitation Protocol

The patient is placed in plantar flexion in a splint for 2 weeks. At 2 weeks the sutures are removed and a cast or boot is placed in 10 degrees of plantar flexion. The patient is brought to neutral at 4 weeks postoperatively and full weight bearing is allowed. Supervised physical therapy is initiated at 4 to 6 weeks postoperatively. The boot is discontinued at 8 to 10 weeks. The patient may begin jogging at 12 weeks but no explosive activity allowed until 4 months postoperatively. The patient is released to full activity at 6 months.

Outcome

A retrospective review of 28 patients treated using this technique were followed for greater than 6 months at our institution. The average clinical follow-up was 10.8 months (range 7.0 to 15.8). Twelve patients had 6-month follow-up and 16 had 1-year follow-up. Twenty-six patients were male and two were female. The mean

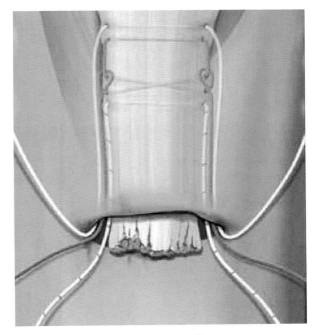

Figure 4–5.   Locked suture is configured and two transverse sutures.

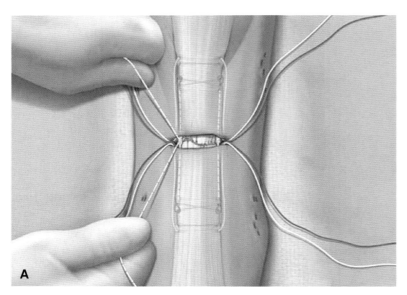
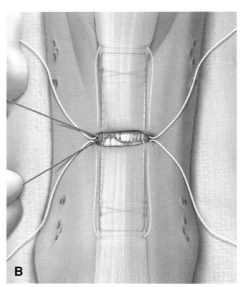

Figure 4–6. **A, B:** Sutures are secured with the foot in plantar flexion.

age was 41.3 years (range 27 to 52 years). The average AOFAS score was 94.6 (range 86 to 100). There were no reruptures in this patient population. There were no clinically detectable sural nerve injuries. There was no wound dehiscence in any patient. One patient had a superficial sterile suture abscess which required removal 5 months postoperatively.[28]

Dresden (Extrasheath) Technique

Indications

The indications for this mini open technique (Dresden Technique) include an acute Achilles tendon rupture less than 10 days from the injury and rupture occurring 2 to 8 cm from the calcaneal insertion of the tendon. The theoretical reason for the maximum 10-day interval from the rupture to be considered for this technique is the

consolidated hematoma formation in the rupture site which would impede a correct apposition of the tendon ends. An ultrasound examination is regularly performed in order to ascertain the level of rupture and the presence of hematoma. A peripheral sensory examination is routinely performed in order to rule out preoperative sural nerve damage.

Surgical Technique

Under regional anesthesia the patient is placed in prone position with both legs in the operative field. No tourniquet is used. The technique was originally described by Amlang and Zwipp.[29,30] A 2-cm paramedial longitudinal incision is performed 3 cm above the proximal end of the

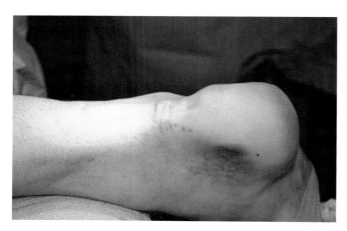

Figure 4–7. Final suture configuration.

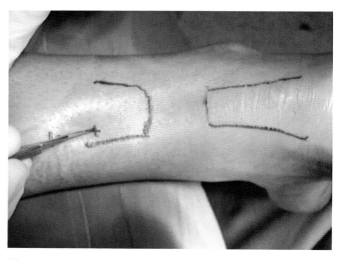

Figure 4–8. A 2-cm paramedial longitudinal incision is performed 3 cm above the proximal end of the ruptured Achilles tendon.

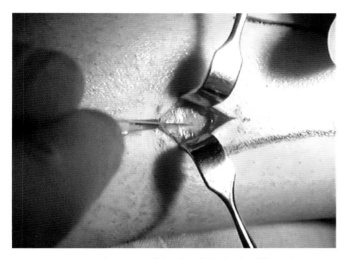

Figure 4–9.   The superficial fascia is incised but the paratenon is not opened and the interval between the fascia and the paratenon is developed.

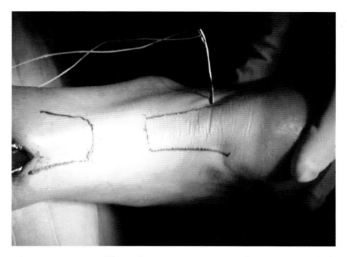

Figure 4–10.   These instruments are used to pass two 2-0 polyblend sutures through the distal end of the Achilles tendon, the second one is placed 1 cm proximal to the first one.

ruptured Achilles tendon (Fig. 4–8). The superficial fascia is incised but the paratenon is not opened and the interval between the fascia and the paratenon is developed (Fig. 4–9). Through this interval, the Dresden instruments are introduced until the calcaneus is reached, one on each side of the tendon. These instruments are used to pass a 2-0 polyblend suture through the distal end of the Achilles tendon (Fig. 4–10). A second one is placed 1 cm proximal to the first one. The instruments are then retrieved proximally through the skin incision (Fig. 4–11A). The grip of the two sutures is tested by pulling them and being able to obtain plantar flexion at the ankle joint (Fig. 4–11B). Then, after direct visualization both threads are sutured to the proximal stump working in the surgical incision already described. The sutures are driven in a criss-cross fashion, grabbing the paratenon

and tendon underneath as one layer, suturing them consecutively, assuring that at least five degrees of additional plantar flexion is achieved compared to the normal physiologic equinus (Fig. 4–12). The fascia and subcutaneous layers are then sutured with no. 0000 absorbable woven suture. A no. 0000 absorbable monofilament is used for the skin closure.

Rehabilitation

The ankle is protected in equinus position in a removable boot without allowing weight bearing for 2 weeks. At the end of the second week weight bearing is allowed as tolerated, with a cam walker and crutches. At the third week full weight bearing is progressively encouraged in the boot and physiotherapy is started. The boot

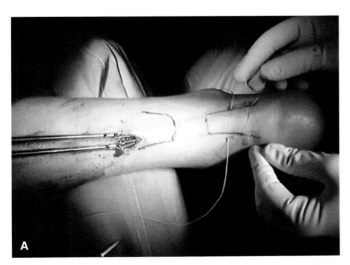

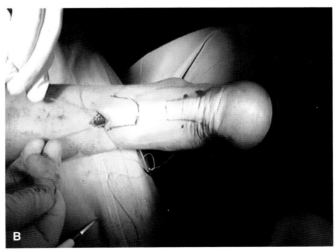

Figure 4–11.   (**A**) The sutures are retrieved through the proximal incision using the Dresden instruments. (**B**) Tensioning of the retrieved sutures demonstrates how well the distal stump is secured as evidenced by the skin folds just above the heel as the ankle is placed into plantar flexion.

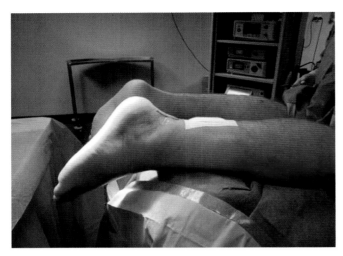

Figure 4–12. Final resting position after securing sutures with the foot in plantar flexion.

is removed at the end of the sixth week and progressive return to daily activities is initiated. Impact sports are allowed after 12 weeks from surgery.

Results

Between May 2007 and October 2010, a retrospective analysis was performed in 21 patients with acute ruptures of the Achilles tendon. All patients were male. The average age was 43 years (range, 35 to 49 years), average follow-up of 24 months, and minimum follow-up of 12 months. The satisfaction rate was 100% (Kenneth-Johnson scale), without pain or restriction in daily activities. The AOFAS score was 99.2 points, (range from 90 to 100), although three patients referred mild ankle instability without loosing points in the AOFAS scale. The time to return to daily activities was 34 days on average. The time to return to sports was 18.6 weeks on average.

No complications regarding soft tissue were reported (i.e., soft tissue infections, wound dehiscence, scar adherence). Reruptures and sural nerve damage were also absent in this series. No loss of joint range of motion was noted, compared to uninjured side.

An isokinetic test was performed on these patients. There was no statistically significant difference between the injured and uninjured side when measuring peak plantar flexion torque or total work at 60 or 120 degrees per second. No difference was noted either when measuring the ratio between the peak torque measured at 60 degrees per second of dorsiflexors and plantar flexors.

DISCUSSION

There is no consensus about the ideal treatment of spontaneous Achilles tendon ruptures.[16,22,31–35] Surgical repair has gained popularity due to an improved return to functional activities and a higher rate of return to previous sports status. Nevertheless, the main drawback of surgical repairs are

soft tissue complications, in fact, a recent systematic review showed complications others than rerupture to be as high as 29%, where wound infections account for 18%. If we accept that the goal of treatment of the acutely ruptured Achilles tendon is to restore the patient to preinjury levels of activity and to avoid major complications, the ideal repair must minimize the risks of infection, sural nerve damage, and at the same time, be strong enough to allow early rehabilitation and avoid tendon rerupture or elongation.[36] This has raised the need for developing less invasive approaches, in the hope of avoiding soft tissue complications, maintaining a high rate of success.

Classic drawbacks ascribed to minimally invasive approaches are a high risk of sural nerve damage, high rerupture rate, and low tensile strength. In relation to sural nerve damage, some series have shown up to 60% of nerve damage, using the Ma and Griffith technique. Contemporary mini open approaches are designed to avoid sural nerve entrapment by eschewing crossing stitches and advancing sutures deep to the sural nerve. In his series, Amlang reported no cases of sural nerve damage and only one case of late infection (1.6%). The rerupture rate observed in open repairs is around 5%, and in patients who received nonoperative treatment it is about 12%.

Another major complaint is that mini open procedures have a greatly diminished tensile strength, with some estimating it to be 50% less than open repairs. We indirectly evaluated the quality of the repair by performing an isokinetic evaluation. Peak torque and total work were compared between the injured and the uninjured tendon. The isokinetic evaluation results showed no statistically significant difference between the injured and uninjured side.

In a controlled laboratory study (data not published) we tested several configurations of Achilles tendon repair techniques in terms of load to failure and gapping using fresh bovine Achilles tendons. The Dresden technique was compared to a single Krackow repair, and to a modified mini open technique which utilized three suture strands crossing the gap. Gapping resistance was significantly greater for the triple technique (246.1 N to initial gapping) versus the Dresden (180 N, $p = 0.012$) and the Krackow repair (101 N, $p < 0.001$). Peak load to failure was significantly greater for the triple strand repair (675 N) versus the Dresden (327.8 N, $p < 0.001$), or Krackow repair (223.6 N, $p < 0.001$). Failure of the tendon was the mechanism of failure for all specimens except for the tendons sutured using the Krackow technique, where the failure occurred at the knot. The triple strand technique significantly increased the tensile strength and gap resistance of bovine tendon repairs, and may allow early postoperative rehabilitation. This data suggests that the mini open technique provides at least a similar strength compared to a classic Krackow repair.

The good results obtained with the Dresden technique may be due at least in part to the fact that it is performed in an interval between the lower leg fascia and the peritenon.

This allows for preservation of the hematoma within the paratenon, with all its growth factors and inflammatory mediators, theoretically promoting a complete and more physiologic restoration of the ruptured tendon. In addition, there is no incision over the rupture site, to cause adhesions or prominent scars that can cause local discomfort.[37–39]

Both of these techniques are easy to perform and to teach. The ease of the procedure, its reproducibility, the avoidance of sural nerve damage, and low cost makes such repairs a very attractive alternative for repairing acute spontaneous rupture of the Achilles tendon.

REFERENCES

1. Samuelson MI, Hecht PJ. Acute Achilles tendon ruptures. *Foot and Ankle Clinics.* 1996;1(2):215–224.
2. Lagergren C, Lindholm A. Vascular distribution in the Achilles tendon. *Acta Chir Scand.* 1956;116:491–495.
3. Mafulli N, Dymond NP, Capasso G. Ultrasonographic findings in subcutaneous rupture of Achilles tendon. *J Sports Med Phys Fitness.* 1989;29:365–368.
4. Bhandari M, Guyatt GH, Siddiqui F, et al. Treatment of acute Achilles ruptures: A systematic overview and meta-analysis. *Clin Orthop Relat Res.* 2002;(400):190–200.
5. Thermann H. Treatment of Achilles tendon ruptures. *Foot and Ankle Clinics.* 1999;4(4):773–787.
6. Beskin JL, Sanders RA, Hunter SC, et al. Surgical repair of Achilles tendon ruptures. *Am J sports Med.* 1987;1:1–8.
7. Kellam JF, Hunter GA, McElwain JP. Review of the operative treatment of Achilles ruptures. *Clin Orthop Relat Res.* 1985;201:80–83.
8. Pajala A, Kangas J, Ohtonen P, et al. Rerupture and deep infection following treatment of total Achilles tendon rupture. *J Bone Joint Surg Am.* 2002;84-A(11):2016–2021.
9. Metz R, Verleisdonk EJ, van der Heijden GJ, et al. Acute Achilles tendon rupture: Minimally invasive surgery versus nonoperative treatment with immediate full weight bearing–a randomized controlled trial. *Am J Sports Med.* 2008;36(9):1688–1694
10. Lim J, Dalal R, Waseem M. Percutaneous vs. open repair of the ruptured Achilles tendon–a prospective randomized controlled study. *Foot Ankle Int.* 2001;22(7):559–568.
11. Assal M, Jung M, Stern R, et al. Limited open repair of Achilles tendon ruptures: A technique with a new instrument and findings of a prospective multicenter study. *J Bone Joint Surg Am.* 2002;84-A(2):161–170.
12. Ingvar J, Tgil M, Eneroth M. Nonoperative treatment of Achilles tendon rupture: 196 consecutive patients with a 7% re-rupture rate. *Acta Orthop.* 2005;76(4):597–601.
13. Lea RB, Smith L. Non-surgical treatment of tendo Achilles rupture. *J Bone Joint Surg Am.* 1972;54(7):1398–1407.
14. Khan RJ, Fick D, Keogh A, et al. Treatment of acute Achilles tendon ruptures: A metaanalysis of randomized, controlled trials. *J Bone Joint Surg Am.* 2005;87(10):2202–2210.
15. Khan RJ, Fick DP, Keogh A, et al. Interventions for treating acute Achilles tendon ruptures. *Cochrane Database Syst Rev.* 2009;(1):CD003674.
16. Cetti R, Christensen SE, Ejsted R, et al. Operative vs nonoperative treatment of Achilles tendon rupture: A prospective randomized study and review of the literature. *Am J Sports Med.* 1993;21:791–799.
17. Chiodo CP, Glazebrook M, Bluman EM, et al. American Academy of Orthopaedic Surgeons clinical practice guideline on treatment of Achilles tendon rupture. *J Bone Joint Surg Am.* 2010;92(14):2466–2468.
18. Chiodo CP, Glazebrook M, Bluman EM, et al. Diagnosis and treatment of acute Achilles tendon rupture. *J Am Acad Orthop Surg.* 2010;18(8):503–510.
19. Suchak AA, Bostick GP, Beaupr LA, et al. The influence of early weight-bearing compared with non-weight-bearing after surgical repair of the Achilles tendon. *J Bone Joint Surg Am.* 2008;90(9):1876–1883.
20. Cretnik A, Kosanovic M, Smrkolj V. Percutaneous versus open repair of the ruptured Achilles tendon: A comparative study. *Am J Sports Med.* 2005;33(9):1369–1379.
21. Twaddle BC, Poon P. Early motion for Achilles tendon ruptures: Is surgery important? A randomized, prospective study. *Am J Sports Med.* 2007;35(12):2033–2038.
22. Haji A, Sahai A, Symes A, et al. Percutaneous versus open tendo achillis repair. *Foot Ankle Int.* 2004;25(4):215–218.
23. Metz R, Verleisdonk EJ, van der Heijden GJ, et al. Acute Achilles tendon rupture: Minimally invasive surgery versus nonoperative treatment with immediate full weight-bearing–a randomized controlled trial. *Am J Sports Med.* 2008;36(9):1688–1694.
24. McKeon BP, Heming JF, Fulkerson J, et al. The Krackow stitch: A biomechanical evaluation of changing the number of loops versus the number of sutures. *Arthroscopy.* 2006;22(1):33–37.
25. Ismail M, Karim A, Shulman R, et al. The Achillon achilles tendon repair: Is it strong enough? *Foot Ankle Int.* 2008;29(8):808–813.
26. Shepard ME, Lindsey DP, Chou LB. Biomechanical comparison of the simple running and cross-stitch epitenon sutures in achilles tendon repairs. *Foot Ankle Int.* 2008;29(5):513–517.
27. Huffard B, O'Loughlin PF, Wright T, et al. Achilles tendon repair: Achillon system vs. Krackow suture: An anatomic in vitro biomechanical study. *Clin Biomech (Bristol, Avon).* 2008;23(9):1158–1164.
28. Metzl J, Garrels K, Cohen B, et al. A retrospective review of a minimally invasive technique of a novel locking device for Achilles tendon repair. Presented at AOFAS annual meeting; June 21, 2012; San Diego, CA.
29. Amlang, MH, Christiani P, Heinz P, et al. The percutaneous suture of the Achilles tendon with the Dresden instrument. *Oper Orthop Traumatol.* 2006;18(4):287–299.
30. Amlang MH, Christiani P, Heinz P, et al. Die perkutane Achillessehnennaht mit dem Dresdner Instrument. *Unfallchirurg.* 2005;108:529–536.
31. Gigante A, Moschini A, Verdenelli A, et al. Open versus percutaneous repair in the treatment of acute Achilles tendon rupture: A randomized prospective study. *Knee Surg Sports Traumatol Arthrosc.* 2008;16:204–209.
32. Longo UG, Ronga M, Maffulli N. Acute ruptures of the achilles tendon. *Sports Med Arthrosc Rev.* 2009;17:127–138.
33. Nistor L. Surgical and non-surgical treatment of Achilles tendon rupture. A prospective randomized study. *J Bone Joint Surg Am.* 1981;63-A:394–399.
34. Wallace R, Traynor I, Kernohan G, et al. . Combined conservative and orthotic management of acute ruptures of

the Achilles tendon. *J Bone Joint Surg Am*. 2004;86:1198–1202.

35. Worth N, Ghosh S, Maffulli N. Management of acute Achilles tendon ruptures in the United Kingdom. *Journal of Orthopaedic Surgery*. 2007;15:311–314.

36. Davies MS, Solan M. Minimal incision techniques for acute Achilles repair. *Foot Ankle Clin N Am*. 2009;14:685–697.

37. Maffulli N. Rupture of the Achilles tendon. *J Bone Joint Surg Am*. 1999;81:1019–1036.

38. Stein SR, Luekens CA. Methods and rationale for closed treatment of Achilles tendon ruptures. *Am J Sports Med*. 1976;4:162–169.

39. Waterston SW, Maffulli N, Ewen SW. Subcutaneous rupture of the Achilles tendon: Basic science and some aspects of clinical practice. *Br J Sports Med*. 1997;31:285–298.

CHAPTER 5

Arthroscopic Lateral Ankle Ligament Reconstruction

Peter Mangone   Jorge Acevedo

INDICATIONS

Lateral ankle sprains are one of the most common reasons for patients to visit an emergency room.[1] Fortunately, patients with residual instability symptoms are often managed successfully with a rehabilitative exercise program and the use of a brace. Of these patients, approximately 20% will go on develop symptomatic chronic recurrent lateral ankle instability that interferes with recreational and daily activities.[2] Traditionally these patients have been surgically treated with an open lateral ankle ligament reconstruction technique, the most common of which is the Brostrom–Gould procedure.[3,4]

Due to the high percentage of pathologic findings discovered during ankle arthroscopy in patients with symptomatic lateral ankle instability,[4–8] its concomitant use at the time of lateral ankle ligament reconstruction has become more frequent. The current use of ankle arthroscopy prior to open stabilization procedures is historically similar to its early use in the knee and shoulder. Initially, the open stabilization procedure was performed after arthroscopic evaluation of the joint. Both of these joints are now stabilized mainly through arthroscopic methods.

Previous reports of arthroscopic assisted ankle stabilization employing staples,[9] secondary incisions for anchor placement,[10,11] or capsular shrinkage techniques[12–14] described moderate early success. More recently, several authors have reported successful arthroscopic lateral ankle ligament reconstruction using bone anchor techniques.[15–17]

Given the historical success of knee and shoulder joint arthroscopic stabilization procedures, along with additional recent success with arthroscopic assisted lateral ankle ligamentous reconstruction, the authors believe arthroscopic lateral ankle ligament reconstruction should be considered for patients with symptomatic chronic lateral ankle instability.

During the patient's preoperative evaluation, it is important to evaluate the patient for any associated injuries, such as osteochondral lesions, peroneal tendon pathology, and syndesmotic instability. Some of these other conditions may be addressed at the time of arthroscopy. On the other hand, some conditions may require the surgeon to proceed with an open ligament reconstruction. All candidates for reconstruction should have a history of symptomatic lateral ankle ligamentous instability with recreational or daily activities. All patients should have clearly documented manual stress testing performed in the office. Although most patients will have increased laxity with anterior drawer and talar tilt testing, some patients will present with functional instability alone. These patients have instability symptoms with activities but do not have significant laxity on physical examination or manual stress testing.[18] Although radiographic stress testing with strict criteria for instability is not required to identify patients with ankle instability,[18,19] it should be considered in every patient given its minimal cost and easily administered adjunct to the physical examination.[20] Osteochondral injuries of the talus or peroneal tendon pathology can usually be treated concomitantly and do not preclude an arthroscopic approach. However, the presence of severe deformity, syndesmotic injury, deltoid ligamentous instability, or severe subtalar instability may necessitate an open approach.

Although this arthroscopic stabilization technique does not repair the calcaneofibular ligament (CFL), recent studies question the need for repair of the CFL.[11,21–23] In a biomechanical evaluation, Lee et al.[21] found no significant difference between the modified Brostrom procedure of a single anterior talofibular ligament (ATFL) and a double ligament (ATFL and CFL) repair. A published clinical study of 30 patients who underwent an open modified Brostrom without CFL reconstruction revealed 28 patients with good to excellent results in terms of functional, clinical, and radiologic assessment.[22] Because of its attachment to the calcaneus at the peroneal tubercle, the inferior extensor retinaculum (IER) most likely augments the stability of the construct. With this in mind, we believe the success of our arthroscopic technique in controlling talar tilt depends on capturing part of the IER during the procedure. Furthermore, Drakos et al.[24] have shown that a minimally invasive arthroscopic technique has equivalent biomechanical strength when compared to the traditional open Brostrom procedure.

SPECIFIC INDICATIONS

The indications for arthroscopic lateral ankle ligament reconstruction are essentially the same as the indications for an open Brostrom–Gould type ligament reconstruction. In

TABLE 5–1. Contraindications for Arthroscopic Lateral Ankle Ligament Reconstruction

1. Significantly increased BMI
2. Collagen disease resulting in joint laxity
3. Previously failed lateral ankle ligament reconstruction
4. Heavy work duty (especially on uneven ground)
5. Severe deformity (e.g., hindfoot varus)
6. Moderate to severe degenerative joint disease
7. Significant peroneal tendon pathology that will require extensive incision for repair

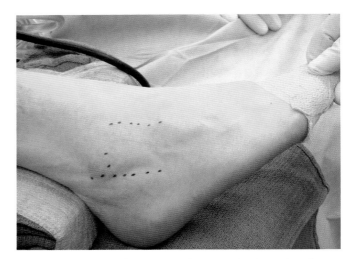

Figure 5–1. "Safe zone": inferior to the lateral malleolus (LM) and between the superior margin of the peroneal tendons (PT) and the lateral branch of the superficial peroneal nerve (SPN).

all cases, patients should undergo an appropriate course of physical therapy focused on peroneal strengthening and proprioception reeducation. If the patient continues to have instability symptoms with normal peroneal motor strength, an arthroscopic lateral ligament reconstruction may be considered. Indications are:

1. Mild to moderate lateral ankle instability affecting daily and recreational activities that has not responded to nonoperative conservative measures. This instability should be documented with stress testing in the office; though stress x-rays are not a necessity.
2. Mild to moderate lateral ankle instability in the presence of an osteochondral lesion which is treated with arthroscopic debridement/drilling.
3. Functional instability recalcitrant to physical therapy.

At this point in time, this procedure is in its relative infancy so we believe understanding when not to perform this procedure is potentially more important than the indications alone. Therefore, we recommend avoiding an arthroscopic lateral ankle ligament reconstruction in the following conditions (Table 5–1).

PATIENT POSITIONING

The patient is placed in supine position on the operating room table and either monitored anesthesia care (MAC) or general anesthesia is performed. If the patient is a candidate for a popliteal block, the block is placed in the preoperative suite. A thigh tourniquet is used to establish a bloodless field. If joint distraction is anticipated, a padded thigh holder is applied. An examination under anesthesia is performed to evaluate the degree of translation with anterior drawer and talar tilt testing. The leg is prepped and draped in usual sterile fashion. Before starting the arthroscopy landmarks are outlined. The "safe zone" lies inferior to the lateral malleolus and between the superior margin of the peroneal tendons and the lateral branch of the superficial peroneal nerve (Fig. 5–1). If distraction is going to be used, a towel roll placed underneath the ankle is usually adequate otherwise slight distraction is placed on the foot and ankle with the external distractor.

SURGICAL APPROACHES

Arthroscopy

The ankle is injected with 30 mL of saline medial to the tibialis anterior tendon and at the level of the ankle joint. The standard anteromedial arthroscopy portal is performed and a 30-degree small joint arthroscope is inserted into the joint. The site for the anterolateral portal is identified by using an 18-gauge needle and visualizing the needle within the joint. The location of the portal should be placed such that the anterior fibula can be accessed for later placement of the bone anchors.

Arthroscopic inspection of the ankle is performed with particular attention to the anterolateral gutter. It is critical to clear all soft tissues from this area to facilitate later visualization of bone anchors and suture shuttling. All necessary ancillary procedures, such as synovectomy, debridement, loose body excision, cheilectomy, or osteochondral drilling, are performed prior to the lateral ligament repair. Final debridement of the lateral and anterolateral gutter is performed such that the fibular tip can be easily probed (Fig. 5–2). This process is accomplished by using the anteromedial portal for arthroscopic viewing while the anterolateral portal functions as a working portal for insertion of instruments used in the debridement.

Arthroscopic Lateral Ligament Reconstruction

- The anteromedial portal is used for arthroscopic viewing throughout the ligament repair.
- The site of the first suture anchor is located 1 cm proximal to the distal tip of the fibula while the drill guide/blunt trocar is introduced through the anterolateral portal and centered over this area

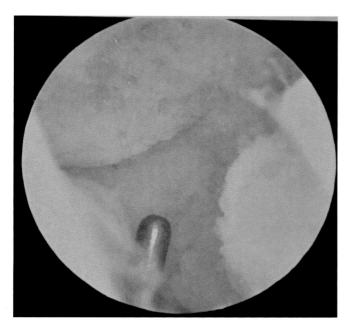

Figure 5–2. Arthroscopic view showing extensive debridement of lateral gutter in order to clearly visualize distal fibula.

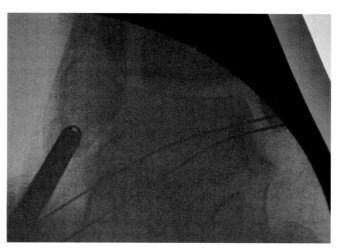

Figure 5–4. Fluoroscopic confirmation of drill guide for distal anchor placement 1 cm proximal to distal fibular tip.

(Fig. 5–3 A,B). A k-wire can be placed through the cannulated trocar in order to confirm appropriate position and depth for anchor. If needed, this location can be confirmed with fluoroscopy (Fig. 5–4).

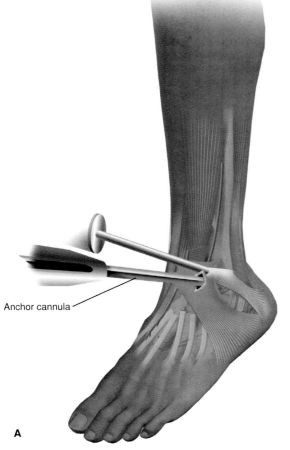

Anchor cannula

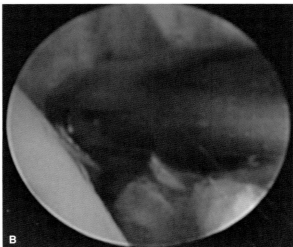

Figure 5–3. **A:** Placement of first suture anchor 1 cm proximal to distal fibular tip. **B:** Arthroscopic view of drill guide placement for first anchor.

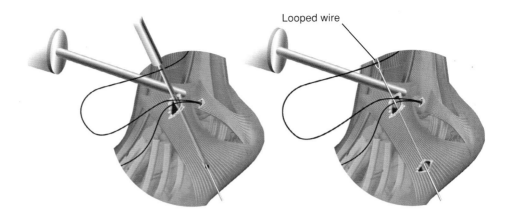

Figure 5–5. View of inside-out technique: withdrawing SutureLasso from anterolateral portal after passing looped wire through capsule, retinaculum, subcutaneous tissue and skin.

- Maintaining the drill guide in place, the anchor is predrilled and inserted through the guide while the sutures limbs are brought out through the anterolateral portal. We prefer 3.0-mm Bio-SutureTak anchors preloaded with zero fiberwire sutures (Arthrex, Naples, FL).
- The surgeon next chooses either an inside-out technique or an outside-in technique which accomplishes the same task of suture shuttling.

Inside-out Technique

- The sharp-tipped curved Micro SutureLasso (Arthrex) is inserted through the anterolateral portal and is brought out of the skin 1.5 cm to 2.0 cm anterior and inferior to the distal part of the lateral malleolus (Fig. 5–5). At this point, the SutureLasso passes through the joint capsule, IER, subcutaneous tissue, and skin but is maintained anterior/dorsal to the peroneal tendons.

- A looped wire is passed through the SutureLasso and the lasso is then removed leaving the loop wire in place.
- One of the suture limbs is passed from the bone anchor out through the skin with the loop wire (Fig. 5–6).
- The Micro SutureLasso is passed again through the anterolateral portal (as described above) 1 cm apart and dorsal to the first pass (Fig. 5–7). Steps 2 and 3 are repeated for the second suture limb. Both suture limbs should run from the distal fibula, through the ankle capsule and IER, and puncture the skin 1.5 to 2 cm from the lateral malleolus.
- Place the second anchor, in a similar manner to the initial anchor, 1 cm proximal to the first anchor and bring the suture limbs out through the anterolateral portal. If needed, this location can be confirmed with fluoroscopy (Fig. 5–8).
- Using the same inside-out technique (steps 1, 2, 3, 4), the two limbs of the second anchor are passed

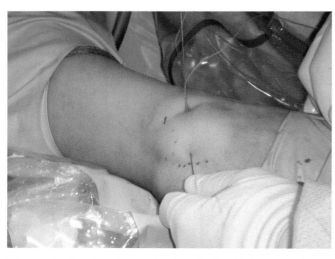

Figure 5–6. Shuttling of suture limb with looped wire from portal through capsule, retinaculum, subcutaneous tissue and skin.

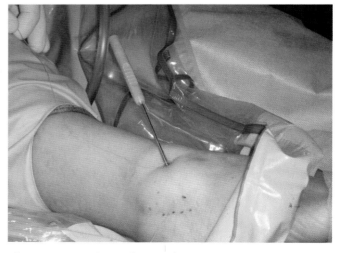

Figure 5–7. Second pass of SutureLasso 1 cm apart from the first pass. First suture limb shown inferior to tip of SutureLasso.

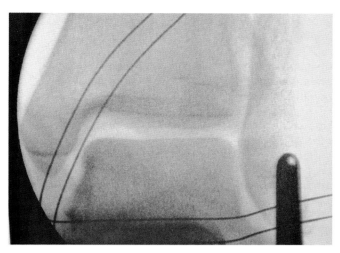

Figure 5–8. Fluoroscopic confirmation of drill guide for second anchor placement 1 cm proximal to location of first anchor.

1 cm apart and slightly anterior/superior to the first set of sutures while penetrating the ATFL and IER.

Outside-in Technique

- The sharp-tipped curved Micro SutureLasso (Arthrex) is inserted 1.5 cm to 2.0 cm anterior and inferior to the distal tip of the lateral malleolus (Fig. 5–9). At this point, the SutureLasso passes through the skin, subcutaneous tissue, IER, and

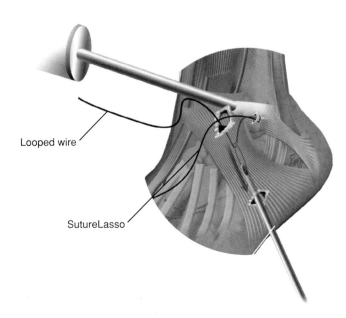

Looped wire

SutureLasso

Figure 5–9. View of outside-in technique: SutureLasso shown piercing skin, subcutaneous tissue, retinaculum, and capsule while exiting through the anterolateral portal.

ankle joint capsule but anterior/dorsal to the peroneal tendons.

- Under direct view with the arthroscope, the SutureLasso is brought up through the joint and out the anterolateral portal.
- A loop wire is passed through the SutureLasso and the first suture limb is placed through the loop and brought out of the skin.
- Steps 2 and 3 are repeated with the second suture limb such that it exits 1 cm anterior to the first suture limb. This is again visualized with the arthroscope to assure the entry point of the suture passer is anterior/dorsal to the first suture limb.
- The second anchor is placed in the distal fibula, as described for the initial anchor, 1 cm proximal to the first anchor. The suture limbs are then brought out through the anterolateral portal. If needed, this location can be confirmed with fluoroscopy.
- Using the same outside-in technique described above (steps 1, 2, 3, 4), the two limbs of the second anchor are passed 1 cm apart and slightly anterior/superior to the first set of sutures penetrating the ATFL and the IER.

Reduction Technique and Fixation

Instruments and Fixation Devices Needed

- 2.7-mm or 4.0-mm 30-degree arthroscope
- Appropriate arthroscopic shavers and tissue ablation device
- External arthroscopic distraction device
- Small (2.5 to 3.5 mm) suture anchors
- Micro SutureLasso device with Nitinol wire (Arthrex)

REDUCTION TECHNIQUE

At this point, both sutures from each individual anchor have been passed through the skin as outlined above. The sutures from the more inferior of the bone anchors should pass through the following tissues in order from deep to superficial:

1. the more inferior anterior ankle capsule,
2. the IER,
3. the subcutaneous tissue,
4. the skin.

The sutures from the more superior bone anchor should pass through the following tissues in order from deep to superficial:

1. the anterior/lateral ankle capsule (the ATFL),
2. the IER (more superiorly/dorsally than the first suture set),
3. the subcutaneous tissue,
4. the skin.

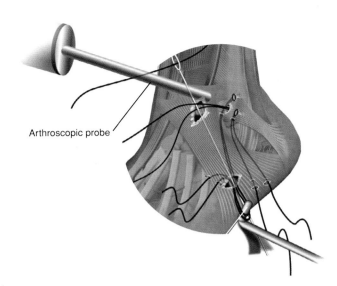

Figure 5–10. Retrieving sutures subcutaneously with probe/hemostat through transverse 1-cm incision.

Between the two sets of exiting sutures, a small 1-cm oblique incision is placed in line with Langer lines. A small curved hook or hemostat is used to pull each suture through this centrally placed incision (making sure each matched pair of sutures remain together) (Fig. 5–10). The subcutaneous tissue is bluntly spread down to the ankle capsule and the IER to decrease the risk of entrapping subcutaneous nerves or causing dimpling of the skin. Before tying the sutures, the lateral gutter is viewed with the arthroscope from the anteromedial portal to verify the lateral gutter is free of loose debris and the sutures are not tangled. If distraction is being used, it is removed and the ankle held by the first assistant in a slightly everted and neutral dorsiflexion/plantarflexion position.

At that point, we recommend the surgeon simulate the tying of the sutures. This is done by crossing the sutures with a single throw and pulling tightly resulting in the lateral tissues tightening down on the anterior fibula. While this is being done, the surgeon should watch the lateral gutter with the arthroscope and make sure there is no tissue entrapped in the joint which could result in an impingement lesion. The arthroscope may be removed at this point; however, it can be held in place by an assistant while the sutures are tied if desired.

With the ankle held in the appropriate position outlined above, the suture limbs are tied tightly down to the capsular/ligamentous tissue planes. The surgeon can tie either set of sutures first depending on preference. The anterior drawer and tilt test are performed. Make sure the suture ends from the tied sutures are not cut down near the knot until after this testing is completed. Assuming satisfactory stability, the lateral ankle area is then revisualized with the arthroscope to verify adequate position of the lateral capsular tissues and insure there

is no tissue in the anterolateral gutter that could create impingement.

If there residual instability present, conversion to an open procedure should be considered. However, two additional techniques can be used to diminish laxity and potentially avoid conversion to the open procedure.

Technique no. 1: The surgeon can see if this can be corrected with the placement of a no. 1 PDS suture through the small 1-cm incision. The suture is passed with its needle (CP2) through additional IER and fibular periosteum. When this suture is tied, it will further advance additional IER tissue to the fibular periosteum. This additional suture has proven adequate to reinforce the repair in several cases such that conversion to an open procedure was not required.

Technique no. 2: A 1- to 2-cm incision can be made posterolateral to the fibular at the metaphyseal/diaphyseal junction. The two sets of sutures tied for the arthroscopic technique are then passed posteriorly and superiorly deep to the subcutaneous tissues but superficial to the ankle capsule/ATFL and the fibular periosteum. These sutures are then brought out of the posterolateral incision site. Two knotless anchors devices (PushLock, Arthrex, Inc.) can be placed in the fibula at this level with one suture from each set placed with each PushLock device creating a suture bridge-type construct deep along the capsule and fibular periosteum. This helps to reinforce the repair and improve stability of the arthroscopic repair.

After the completion of the lateral ankle ligament reconstruction, the arthroscopic portals and the small incision used to tie the sutures are closed with 4-0 nylon suture. Sterile dressings are applied. A well-padded, short posterior splint with sidebars is placed with the ankle in neutral position. The patient is awakened and taken to the recovery room.

COMPLICATIONS

Complications are rare at this point in our experience. The most common complaint has been neuralgia postoperatively in a few patients. It is difficult to know if this is due to nerve irritation from the arthroscopy itself or if this results from the minimally invasive lateral ligament reconstruction. A recent anatomic study by Drakos et al.[25] showed that the technique can be performed through an anatomic safe zone. However, structures at risk for entrapment included the: extensor tendons, peroneus tertius, as well as the common and intermediate branches of the superficial peroneal nerve. Entrapment occurred in these cadaver specimens 16% of the time with all of these being due to the more superior suture.

REHABILITATION PROTOCOL

Given the novel nature of this procedure combined with the fact that the initial technique only used one bone anchor, the initial postoperative rehabilitation protocol was conservative. Patients were immobilized in a short leg non–weight-bearing cast for 4 to 6 weeks. This was followed by a CAM boot, progressive weight bearing, and physical therapy. Finally the patient graduated to a lace-up style ankle gauntlet brace. With additional surgical experience and the advent of our two-anchor technique (both of which have improved our intraoperative stability), the current postoperative rehabilitation protocol is as follows:

- *Day of surgery*—short leg splint placed on the operating room with the ankle in a neutral position to slight eversion. Touchdown weight bearing allowed.
- *7 to 10 days postoperative (visit no. 1)*—short leg cast (or CAM boot) is applied with ankle placed in neutral position (if CAM boot is used no significant ROM exercises are started but patient can remove boot for showering/bathing). Fifty percent weight bearing is allowed at this point. Sutures are removed but this step can be delayed if necessary.
- *3 to 4 weeks postoperative (visit no. 2)*—CAM boot placed and active dorsiflexion/plantarflexion motion allowed by patient TID for 10 to 15 minutes per session. Begin progress from 50% weight bearing to 100% weight bearing in boot.
- *6 weeks postoperative (visit no. 3)*—Begin transition to lace-up style ankle gauntlet brace. Start formal physical therapy to work on active and passive range of motion, TheraBand strengthening, proprioception, and gait training using the ankle brace. Avoid significant passive or active inversion-type stress to the ankle. One hundred percent weight bearing and use brace for all activities. Patient may begin stationary cycling in brace for conditioning.
- *10 to 12 weeks postoperative (visit no. 4)*—Begin transition out of brace for activities of daily living. Continue to use brace for higher impact activities or running. May begin running for conditioning. Begin to incorporate cutting drills in brace for athletes. Continue physical therapy for TheraBand strengthening, proprioception, and gait training.
- *16 to 20 weeks postoperative (visit no. 5)*—Begin competitive athletic drills or heavy duty work for manual laborers. Work toward return to full competitive athletic competition (progress depends on athlete, postoperative course, and type of sport).

We usually recommend the use of a lace-up style ankle gauntlet brace for sports activities and higher level physical activities for 6 to 9 months postoperatively.

OUTCOMES

Recent reports of arthroscopic lateral ankle ligament reconstruction have been promising. Initial series using less advanced techniques reported good early results with a few poor outcomes attributed to prominent hardware (staple).[9,10] In 2009, Corte-Real and Moreira[15] reported the first European study with 28 patients and a 24.5-month follow-up using an arthroscopic assisted approach with one suture anchor. Postoperative AOFAS scores averaged 85.3 and only two patients had recurrent instability. Injury to the superficial peroneal nerve occurred in three cases but only one persisted.

Kim et al.[17] recently published their series of 28 ankles with the use of one suture anchor and two sutures. At a mean follow-up of 15.9 months, AOFAS hindfoot scores improved by greater than 30 points. The authors reported a 17% complication rate including prominent sutures (n = 3), scar sensitivity (n = 4), and superficial infection (n = 1) but no peroneal nerve injuries were identified. Three patients showed laxity on anterior stress radiographs but all were able to return to their preinjury activity level.

In a recent study, the authors reported on a subset of 24 ankles with an average follow-up of 11 months (range 1.5 to 24 months).[16] All patients reported significant improvement in ankle stability as compared to their preoperative symptoms. Four patients were noted to have mildly positive manual stress tests but none required revision surgery. Complications included one persistent peroneal tendonitis requiring debridement and one unrelated neurologic process. In this series, one patient had a self-limiting sural neuritis but no patient developed a superficial peroneal neuritis.

The authors have performed 45 arthroscopic lateral ankle ligament repairs since 2007 and have refined the procedure to improve outcomes. Unlike some of the techniques used in prior studies, the current method avoids the need for ancillary portals and enables the surgeon to use the standard anterior portals. Soft tissue dissection is minimized relative to open techniques. Also, the procedure allows for placement of two anchors and shuttling of the suture limbs separately in order to engage a wider surface area which theoretically improves pull-out strength. Carefully outlining the landmarks and avoiding multiple suture passes prevents inadvertent injury to the superficial peroneal nerve or peroneal tendons. The authors have noted only transient neuritic symptoms most likely related to stretch injury while widening the anterolateral portal. Occasional branches of the sural and superficial peroneal nerves that traverse the area of repair have not posed an issue in regard to entrapment. An integral concept to achieving excellent outcomes lies in the addition of the IER to reinforce the lateral ankle ligament repair. Since the CFL is not repaired with the current technique, the IER plays an important role in providing talar and subtalar inversion stability. Biomechanical and clinical studies comparing open modified Brostrom with single versus double ligament repair further support this concept.[21,22] These studies have shown good to excellent clinical outcomes in a majority of patients and no significant difference in mechanical strength with or without CFL repair.

Future studies will compare the biomechanical strength of the open modified Brostrom versus the arthroscopic lateral ankle ligament reconstruction. We hope to further delineate the anatomical structures in the "safe zone" and establish minimum and maximum distances for the ideal repair.

REFERENCES

1. Lambers K, Ootes D, Ring D. Incidence of patients with lower extremity injuries presenting to US emergency departments by anatomic region, disease category, and age. *Clin Orthop Relat Res.* 2012;470(1):284–290.
2. Karlsson J, Bergsten T, Lansinger O, et al. Lateral instability of the ankle treated by the Evans procedure: A long-term clinical and radiological follow-up. *J Bone Joint Surg Br.* 1988;70:476–480.
3. Brodsky AR, O'Malley MJ, Bohne WH, et al. An analysis of outcome measures following the Brostrom-Gould procedure for chronic lateral ankle instability. *Foot Ankle Int.* 2005;26:816–819.
4. Ferkel RD, Chams RN. Chronic lateral ankle instability: Arthroscopic findings and long-term results. *Foot Ankle Int.* 2007;25:24–31.
5. Komenda GA, Ferkel RD. Arthroscopic findings associated with the unstable ankle. *Foot Ankle Int.* 1999;20:708–713.
6. Hintermann B, Boss A, Schafer D. Arthroscopic findings in patients with chronic ankle instability. *Am J Sports Med.* 2002;30:402–409.
7. Hua Y. Modified Brostrom procedure plus ankle arthroscopy may be effective for ankle instability. *Arthroscopy.* 2010;26:524–528.
8. Cannon LB, Slater HK. The role of ankle arthroscopy and surgical approach in lateral ankle ligament repair. *Foot Ankle Surg.* 2005;11:1–4.
9. Hawkins RB. Arthroscopic stapling repair for chronic lateral instability. *Clin Podiatr Med Surg.* 1987;4:875–883.
10. Kashuk KB, Landsman AS, Werd MB, et al. Arthroscopic lateral ankle stabilization. *Clin Podiatr Med Surg.* 1994; 11:407–423.
11. Nery C, Raduan F, Del Buono A, et al. Arthroscopic-assisted Broström-Gould for chronic ankle instability: A long-term follow-up. *Am J Sports Med.* 2011;39:2381–2388.
12. Maiotti M, Massoni C, Tarantino U. The use of arthroscopic thermal shrinkage to treat chronic lateral ankle instability in young athletes. *Arthroscopy.* 2005;21:751–757.
13. Berlet GC, Saar WE, Ryan A, et al. Thermal-assisted capsular modification for functional ankle instability. *Foot Ankle Clin.* 2002;7:567–576.
14. de Vries JS, Krips R, Blankevoort L, et al. Arthroscopic capsular shrinkage for chronic ankle instability with thermal radiofrequency: Prospective multicenter trial. *Orthopedics.* 2008;31:655.
15. Corte-Real NM, Moreira RM. Arthroscopic repair of lateral ankle instability. *Foot Ankle Int.* 2009;30:213–217.
16. Acevedo JL, Mangone PG. Arthroscopic lateral ankle ligament reconstruction. *Tech Foot & Ankle.* 2011;10(3):111–116.
17. Kim ES, Lee KT, Park JS, et al. Arthroscopic anterior talofibular ligament repair for chronic ankle instability with a suture anchor technique. *Orthopedics.* 2011;34(4):273.
18. Tropp H, Ekstrand J, Gillquist J. Stabilometry in functional ankle instability of the ankle and its value in predicting injury. *Med Sci Sports Exerc.* 2002;16:64–66.
19. Colville MR. Reconstruction of the lateral ankle ligaments. *J Bone Joint Surg Am.* 1994;76-A:1092–1102.
20. Raatikainen T, Putkonen M, Puranen J. Arthrography, clinical examination, and stress radiograph in the diagnosis of acute injury to the lateral ligaments of the ankle. *Am J Sports Med.* 1992;20:2–6.
21. Lee KT, Lee JI, Sung KS, et al. Biomechanical evaluation against calcaneofibular ligament repair in the Brostrom procedure: A cadaveric study. *Knee Surg Sports Traumatol Arthrosc.* 2008;16:781–786.
22. Lee KT, Park YU, Kim JB, et al. Long term results after modified Brostrom procedure without calcaneofibular ligament reconstruction. *Foot Ankle Int.* 2011;32(2):153–157.
23. Okuda R, Kinoshita M, Morikawa J, et al. Reconstruction for chronic lateral ankle instability using the Palmaris longus tendon: Is reconstruction of the calcaneofibular ligament necessary? *Foot Ankle Int.* 1999;20:714–720.
24. Drakos MC, Behrens SB, Paller D, et al. A biomechanical comparison of an open vs. arthroscopic approach for the treatment of lateral ankle instability. *Arthroscopy.* 2011;27(5 Suppl):e60–e61.
25. Drakos MC, Behrens SB, Mulcahey MK, et al. Anatomic Safe Zone for Placement of Suture Anchors in Arthroscopic Repairs for Chronic Ankle Instability. (Abstract) Presentation, AOFAS 27th Annual Summer Meeting. July, 2011.

CHAPTER 6

Tendon Harvesting

Vinod K. Panchbhavi

INDICATIONS

Tendons are often harvested and used to replace or reinforce a dysfunctional or diseased tendon.[1–6] The conditions in which tendon transfer techniques are frequently utilized in the leg include posterior tibial tendon and Achilles tendon disorders. The posterior tibial tendon in early stages is amenable to debridement and repair. In later stages repair alone may not be sufficient requiring a tendon transfer to reinforce or replace the diseased tendon. Similarly tendon transfer is utilized in reconstructive procedures for management of a chronic tear or degenerative condition in the Achilles tendon. End-to-end repair is possible for Achilles tendon defects less than 2 cm and V-Y advancement of the Achilles tendon can bridge defects ranging 2 to 6 cm long but in gaps over 6 cm long, adjacent tendons can be transferred to the calcaneus to provide plantar flexion at ankle.[6]

Flexor digitorum longus (FDL) tendon in the vicinity is transferred to the navicular bone to reconstruct the posterior tibial tendon, and flexor hallucis longus (FHL) tendon is transferred to the calcaneus to reconstruct Achilles tendon. The tendon to be transferred is harvested as distal as necessary to provide adequate length for rerouting and attachment at the different site.

The surgical technique to harvest FDL tendon was described by Mann and Thompson.[1] They advocated a medial-based approach and a dissection that proceeded along the FDL tendon in the deeper layers from the medial border of the foot toward the midfoot laterally.

A similar open approach was reported by Wapner et al.[2] for harvesting the FHL tendon. This approach required an incision placed on the medial border of the midfoot, extending from the navicular tuberosity to the head of the first metatarsal when FHL was used for reconstruction of chronic tears of the Achilles tendon.

These open medial approaches to harvesting the FDL and FHL, however, require an incision that extends along almost the entire medial border of the foot and an extensive, deep, and difficult dissection. The dissection starts from the incision and is carried across the midfoot in the vicinity of blood vessels and nerves almost to the midfoot to reach the tendons in the depth of the surgical exposure. There is a risk for injury to the medial and lateral plantar neurovascular structures.[3–5] A longer incision and exposure is required because of an indirect approach to the point of division of the tendon.

The following percutaneous techniques can be used instead of open surgical approach to harvest the FHL and FDL tendons through small incisions placed directly overlying the tendon in the midfoot and forefoot.

MINIMALLY INVASIVE HARVEST OF THE FDL

Patient Positioning

The FDL tendon for posterior tibial tendon reconstruction is harvested with the patient in the supine position. A single dose of an antibiotic is administered intravenously for prophylaxis against infection. A thigh tourniquet is applied in preference to a calf tourniquet. A calf tourniquet can tether muscle bellies and interfere with the determination of appropriate musculotendinous length and tension in the tendon transferred.

Surgical Approach

A skin marker is used to mark the incision site on the location where the FDL starts dividing into individual slips for the lesser toes. This location can be determined on the sole of the foot using the coordinates previously described by Panchbhavi et al.[7] The FDL division can be located topographically on the plantar surface of the foot, approximately midway between the back of the heel and the base of the second toe and at this midpoint, about two-thirds of the width medially from the lateral border of the foot.

A metallic ruler is held parallel to the plantar surface of the foot and a longitudinal line is drawn from the posterior center of the heel to the proximal flexor crease at the base of the second toe and the midpoint marked. Another line is drawn at this midpoint perpendicular to the longitudinal line. A point two-thirds of the distance away from the lateral border of the foot on this second line is the location of the FDL division. A 2 cm longitudinal skin marking at this second point is used for limited incision access to the FDL. A no. 15 blade is used to incise the skin, vertically in a skin crease if one is available close to the planned incision site. The skin incision is about 2 cm long, extended proximally if necessary. The plantar fascia is incised in the line of skin incision.

Harvest Technique

The vertically oriented fibers of the aponeurosis are separated to expose the flexor digitorum brevis muscle. The dissection is carried out in the same plane as the incision separating the muscle fibers to expose the FDL tendon. The lateral branch of the medial plantar nerve passes along the medial border of the flexor digitorum brevis and therefore could be at risk. Therefore, it is important to make the plantar incision long enough to allow adequate visualization.

The identity of the tendon is verified by applying a pulling tension on the tendon through the proximal wound in the hindfoot and assessing transmission of the tension distally to the tendon identified in the midfoot and at the same time observing maximal flexion either in lesser toes or the great toe.

The tendon is then cut sharply in the midfoot and the cut end pulled proximally through the wound in the hindfoot region. If there is resistance, and if the great toe flexes, a slip between the FDL and FHL tendons exists. Passive plantar flexion of the foot and the toes as well as pulling distally on the cut end of FDL allows visualization of the interconnecting slip. After this interconnecting band is cut, the resistance is no longer felt and the FDL tendon can then be pulled proximally for routing into the navicular bone (Figs. 6–1–6–13).

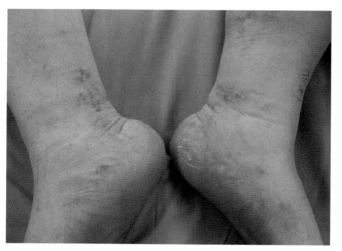

Figure 6–1. A patient with PTT dysfunction showing diffuse swelling over the medial aspect of the left ankle.

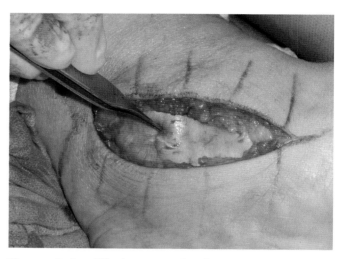

Figure 6–3. Effusion emanating from opening made in the PTT sheath.

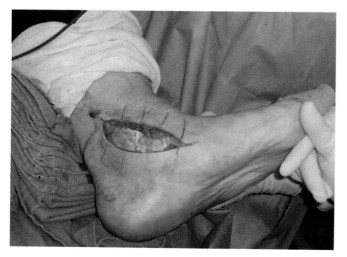

Figure 6–2. Intraoperative picture showing the PTT sheath exposed.

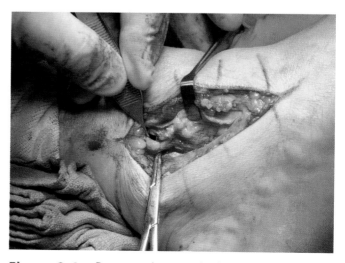

Figure 6–4. Degenerative tears in the PTT.

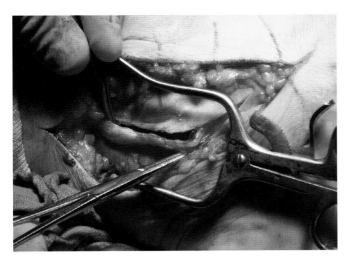

Figure 6–5.   Exposure of the entire PTT.

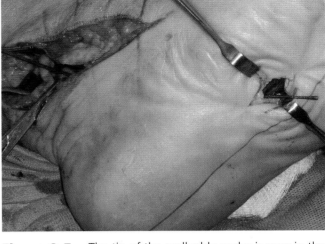

Figure 6–7.   The tip of the malleable probe is seen in the plantar exposure.

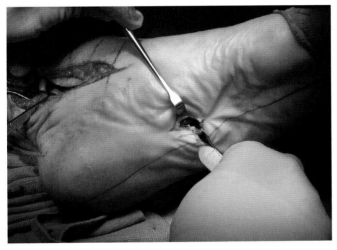

Figure 6–6.   A malleable probe introduced in hindfoot within the PTT sheath.

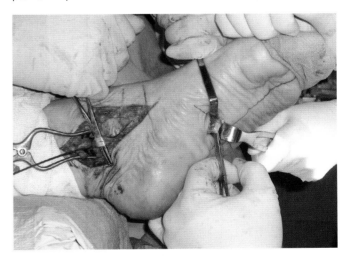

Figure 6–8.   The FDL tendon brought out into the plantar wound and the tendon continuity confirmed by a hemostat under the FDL tendon in the proximal wound applying tension.

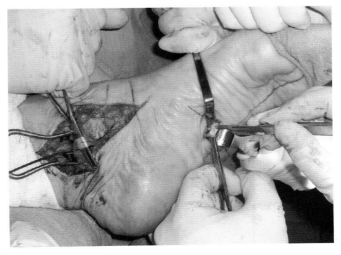

Figure 6–9.   The FDL tendon being cut.

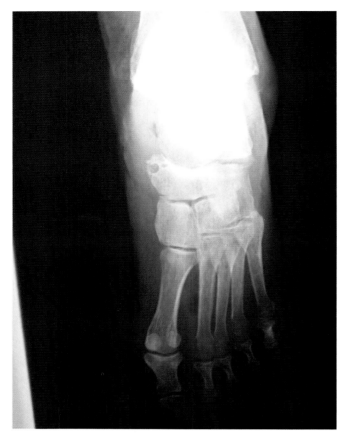

Figure 6–10. A bone tunnel in the navicular bone prepared for routing the FDL.

MINIMALLY INVASIVE HARVEST OF THE FHL

Patient Positioning

The FHL tendon for Achilles tendon reconstruction is harvested with the patient in the prone position. A thigh

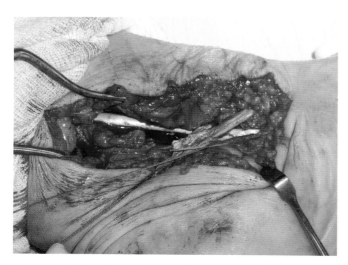

Figure 6–11. The FDL routed and sutured back on itself.

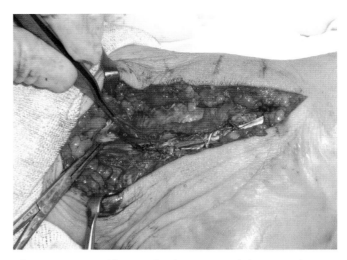

Figure 6–12. The proximal remnant of the posterior tibial tendon sutured to the transferred FDL.

tourniquet is applied before the patient is turned prone on the operative table. A calf tourniquet is not used as noted above. Both lower extremities are prepared to a level above the knee and draped in a sterile fashion. Draping the nonoperative extremity within the sterile field allows direct comparison of the tension imparted to the repaired tendon with that in the intact tendon. A single dose of an antibiotic is administered intravenously for prophylaxis against infection.

Surgical Approach

The Achilles tendon is approached through a posterior central longitudinal incision. The incision is carried deeper into the tendon sheath, thus creating full thickness flaps. The tendon sheath is incised in line with the incision and reflected off the tendon. Scar tissue in between

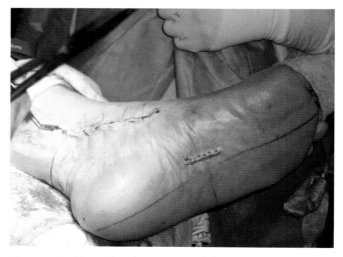

Figure 6–13. The plantar wound for minimally invasive harvest of the FDL sutured.

the ends of the tendon is excised. If the gap between the cut ends of the tendon is greater than 6 cm harvesting the FHL tendon is undertaken as follows.

Through the gap in the Achilles tendon the fascia over the posterior compartment is incised vertically to expose the FHL muscle and tendon. A Penrose drain is looped round the tendon. Tension placed upon the FHL tendon in the hindfoot can be felt in the midfoot and also observed as flexion of great toe.

Technique

The olive tip of a malleable probe or sound is introduced within the sheath of the FHL tendon and gently passed without resistance distally toward the midfoot. The tip is then palpated in the midfoot. A longitudinal incision 3 cm in length is centered over the palpable probe tip in the plantar aspect of the midfoot. The incision is deepened to expose the plantar fascia. The fibers of the plantar fascia are then separated to expose flexor hallucis brevis (FHB) muscle. The fibers of the FHB are separated to expose the FHL tendon and the tendon slip that it sends to that branch of the FDL which goes to the second toe. Deep-bladed retractors are necessary to retract the wound edges and visualize the tendon.

A tendon hook or Penrose drain can be passed under the FHL tendon to bring it more superficially into the wound. Similarly, the FDL tendon and the intertendinous slip can be drawn more superficially into the wound. This allows confirmation of their identity, clearance of adjacent neurovascular structures, and more easy release of intertendinous connections. These all allow more safe performance of the tenotomy.

The identity of the FHL tendon in the midfoot can be confirmed by pulling the tendon in the hindfoot and confirming plantar flexion of the great toe. The tendon can be cut at this level if the length of the graft is deemed adequate for repair. The cut distal stump of the FHL tendon may be tenodesed to the FDL tendon holding all toes and the ankle in a neutral position.

When a longer portion of the FHL tendon is required, the FHL tendon is not cut in the midfoot but more distally at the base of the great toe. A transverse incision 1 cm in length is made in the proximal flexion crease at the base of the great toe. The incision is carried down to the level of the FHL tendon. This tendon is then exposed through its sheath and a Penrose drain passed to loop around it. The tendon is cut at the base of the great toe. The FHL can then be pulled into the midfoot. Pulling distally on the cut end of FHL brings the interconnecting slip between the FHL and FDL tendons into visibility.

After this interconnecting slip is cut, the FHL tendon can be pulled through the wound in the hindfoot and transferred to the calcaneus through a transverse tunnel, and the remaining length used to bridge the gap and reconstruct the Achilles tendon (Figs. 6–14–6–25).

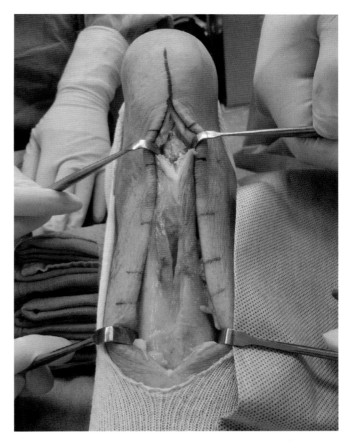

Figure 6–14. Chronic degeneration in the Achilles tendon exposed through its sheath.

Complications

Possible complications related to the technique of minimally invasive percutaneous harvesting of the FHL or the FDL tendons include wound infection, wound dehiscence, painful or hypersensitive plantar scar, medial or lateral plantar nerve or vessel injury, poor function due to weakness in plantar flexion of the great toe.

To avoid wound complications neurovascular status and condition of soft tissues in the leg and the foot should be evaluated and surgery performed only in those with adequate circulation. Patients should be counseled regarding possible weakness in plantar flexion in the toes. The FHL and FDL frequently have interconnections in the midfoot. The presence of these interconnections can be determined preoperatively. Flexing of the lesser toes when the great toe is being actively flexed or vice versa is indicative of the presence of an interconnecting band between the FDL and FHL tendons. A likely deficit in great toe flexion power and its effect on athletic activity should be mentioned when reconstruction of the ruptured Achilles tendon is contemplated using the FHL tendon or an alternative technique preferred.

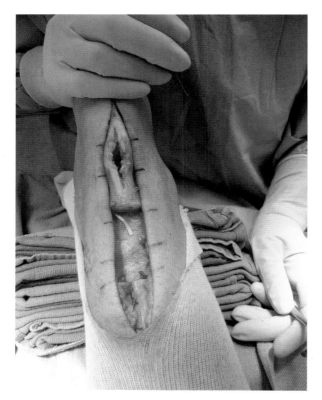

Figure 6–15. Excision of the degenerated parts of the Achilles tendon.

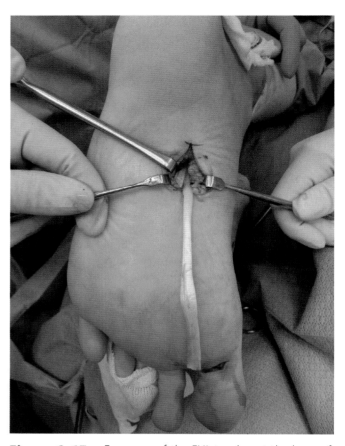

Figure 6–17. Exposure of the FHL tendon at the base of the great toe.

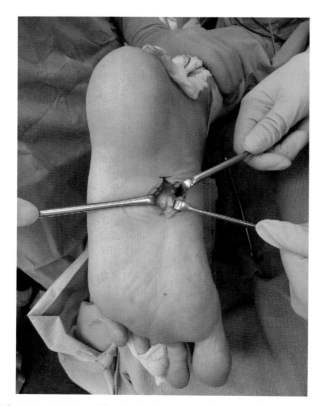

Figure 6–16. Direct plantar surgical approach to expose the FHL tendon in the midfoot.

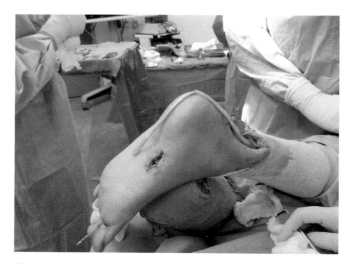

Figure 6–18. The FHL tendon harvested and brought out through the hindfoot.

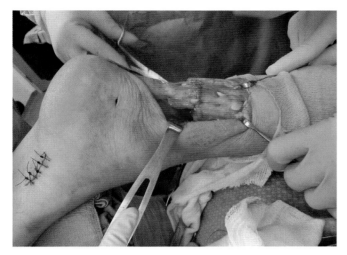

Figure 6–19. The harvested FHL tendon used for reconstruction of the Achilles tendon.

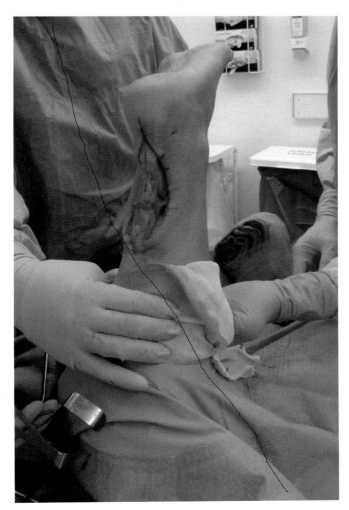

Figure 6–20. The restoration of the plantar flexion tension.

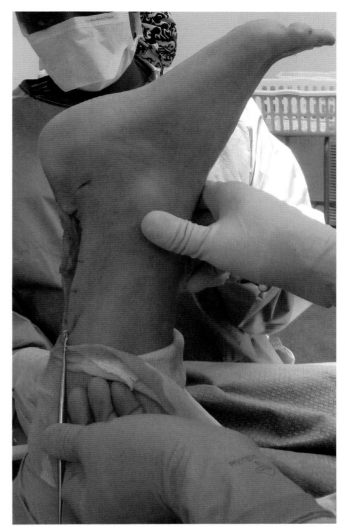

Figure 6–21. The restoration of the plantar flexion tension view from the side.

Rehabilitation

The postoperative management following the tendon transfer is tailored by the needs of the concomitant procedures. The limb is rested in a splint to accommodate any swelling and the wounds checked at 1 week. A cast replaces the splint and the tendon transfer is protected for further 5 weeks.

A rehabilitation program for strengthening, gait training, and ankle range-of-motion exercises is gradually initiated at 6 weeks and return to full activities is usually allowed by 12 weeks.

Outcomes

Panchbhavi et al.[7] harvested the FDL using the percutaneous technique described above in a cadaver study to test the feasibility and safety of this minimally invasive technique. Measurements were obtained to define

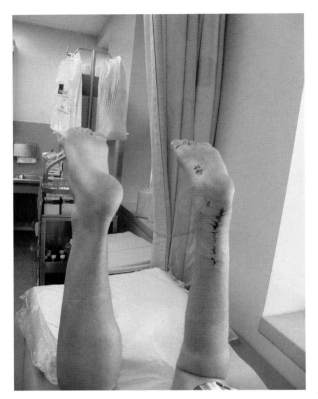

Figure 6–22. Postoperative follow-up showing the wound at 2 weeks.

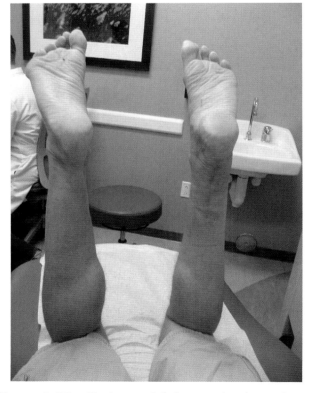

Figure 6–23. Twelve-week follow-up showing active plantar flexion.

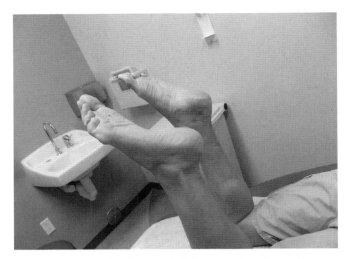

Figure 6–24. Twelve-week follow-up showing active plantar flexion from the back. Weaker plantar flexion in the great toe on the operated side.

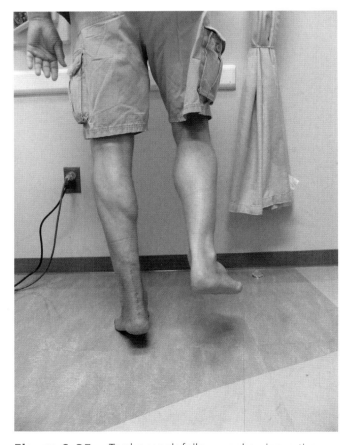

Figure 6–25. Twelve-week follow-up showing active single toe raise on the operated side.

the location of the division of the FDL tendon in relation to the plantar surface of the foot and the adjacent neurovascular structures. In all of the 83 feet studied, it was possible to harvest the FDL using this technique. In 11 feet (13.25%), a connecting band to the FHL required division. No damage was apparent to the adjacent neurovascular structures on subsequent dissection to expose the underlying layers in the feet. The FDL division was located topographically on the plantar surface of the foot, approximately midway between the back of the heel and the base of the second toe. The incision should be centered at this midpoint, about two-thirds of the width medially from the lateral border of the foot.

They concluded that the FDL tendon can be harvested in the hindfoot after its division through a small plantar incision in the midfoot and that surface anatomy guides placement of the plantar incision over the FDL division.

The author has been using the percutaneous techniques for tendon transfer described here since 2007. The FDL tendon was harvested in 19 cases and the FHL was harvested in 15 cases. A connecting band between the FDL and FHL tendons required cutting in 31 of the 34 cases. In all cases the tendons could be successfully harvested through the plantar incision itself and the length of the harvested tendon was found to be adequate for the primary purpose. There were no instances of intraoperative nerve injury or harvest of a wrong tendon. Postoperatively, one patient had hyperesthesia in the midfoot that lasted for 3 months and had resolved completely by her 6-month checkup.

REFERENCES

1. Mann RA, Thompson FM. Rupture of the posterior tibial tendon causing flat foot. Surgical treatment. *J Bone Joint Surg Am.* 1985;67(4):556–561.
2. Wapner KL, Pavlock GS, Hecht PJ, et al. Repair of chronic Achilles tendon rupture with flexor hallucis longus tendon transfer. *Foot Ankle.* 1993;14(8):443–449.
3. Herbst SA, Miller SD. Transection of the medial plantar nerve and hallux cock-up deformity after flexor hallucis longus tendon transfer for Achilles tendinitis: Case report. *Foot Ankle Int.* 2006;27(8):639–641.
4. Sullivan RJ, Gladwell HA, Aronow MS, et al. An in vitro study comparing the use of suture anchors and drill hole fixation for flexor digitorum longus transfer to the navicular. *Foot Ankle Int.* 2006;27(5):363–366.
5. Wapner KL, Hecht PJ, Shea JR, et al. Anatomy of second muscular layer of the foot: Considerations for tendon selection in transfer for Achilles and posterior tibial tendon reconstruction. *Foot Ankle Int.* 1994;15(8):420–423.
6. Panchbhavi VK. Chronic Achilles tendon repair with flexor hallucis longus tendon harvested using a minimally invasive technique. *Tech Foot Ankle Surg.* 2007;6(2):123–129.
7. Panchbhavi VK, Yang J, Vallurupalli S. Minimally invasive method of harvesting the flexor digitorum longus tendon: A cadaver study. *Foot Ankle Int.* 2008;29(1):42–48.

CHAPTER 7

Extracorporeal Shock Wave Therapy in the Foot and Ankle

John P. Furia   Eric M. Bluman

INTRODUCTION

Extracorporeal shock wave therapy (ESWT) is an effective treatment for both bony and soft tissue disorders. ESWT was initially utilized in musculoskeletal application as a treatment for bone pathologies.[1,2] Investigators antidotally noted that when lithotriptor-type devices were utilized to treat nephrolithiasis, posttreatment radiographs revealed an osteoblastic response in the area of the treated tissues.[1] This prompted other investigators to utilize ESWT as a treatment for delayed healing of bone.[3–7]

Initial investigators utilized ESWT to treat delayed and established nonunions of fractures.[3–5] Anecdotal experience was quite positive and this prompted other investigators to utilize ESWT as a treatment for soft tissue conditions.[8–36]

Presently, ESWT is used to treat both bone and soft tissue conditions. Bony conditions include delayed and established fracture nonunions, medial tibial stress syndrome, avascular necrosis, as well as stress fractures.[1–7,37–44] Soft tissue conditions include plantar fasciopathy, lateral epicondylitis, greater trochanteric pain syndrome, calcific tendinopathy of the shoulder, as well as patellar tendinopathy.[8–36]

In addition to the above indications, ESWT has been shown to be a safe and highly effective treatment for both insertional and noninsertional Achilles tendinopathy[11,12,14–20] and plantar fasciitis.[45–47] There are now numerous trials that support the use of this technology for these indications.[11,12,14–20]

The aim of this chapter is to explain the rationale, justify the use, and elaborate on the clinical results of using ESWT as a treatment for Achilles tendinopathy and plantar fasciitis. After a brief discussion of some of the basic principles and biologic effects associated with shock wave therapy, the remainder of the chapter will focus on how ESWT is currently used in clinical practice to treat Achilles tendinopathy and plantar fasciitis.

SWT BASIC PRINCIPLES

What Is a Shock Wave?

A shock wave is an acoustic sound wave, characterized by a high peak pressure (up to 500 bar), a fast initial time of less than 10 ns, a short life cycle (less than 10 ms), and a broad frequency spectrum (16 to 20 MHz).[48–50] Just as an opera singer can break a glass when she sings a high note or a jet can break windows when accelerating past the sound barrier, sound waves can transmit significant quantities of energy. For clinical use, the energy of multiple sound waves can be coupled, focused, targeted and applied to tissues in order to produce a biologic response.

How Do You Make Shock Waves?

Shock waves are produced using commercially available shock wave–generating devices. These devices are a by-product of lithotripsy technology. Several have been

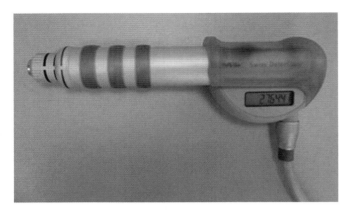

Figure 7–1. Handpiece for a radial shock wave machine. The tip through which the shock wave is transmitted to the patient is oriented to the left.

approved by the Federal Drug Administration and are available in the United States.[48–50] There are many others available in other parts of the world.

There are several methods of shock wave production. Electrohydraulic devices use a spark plug to generate the shock waves. Electromagnetic devices use a coil to generate the shock waves. Piezoelectric systems use a crystal to generate the shock waves. Finally, radial devices use pressure to generate a shock wave (Fig. 7–1).

Focused verses Radial Shock Waves

Shock wave devices produce shock waves in either a focused or radial manner. The differences are as follows:

Focused devices are transmitted to a relatively small area (the "focus") and can be targeted in such a way so that the maximal energy is delivered well below the level of the skin. These devices are often utilized when the area of intended treatment is deep, such as a bone. The depth of penetration can be manipulated by varying the intensity of these treatments allowing the clinician to treat relatively deep structures as well as more superficial structures.

In contrast, "radial" shock waves are produced by smaller, less expensive devices. These devices are usually office-based and somewhat portable. Radial devices transfer their maximal energy superficially at or just below the level of the skin. Shock waves impact the tissue and then are distributed radially and treat an area more broad than a focused device.

Of note, the biologic response produced by both radial and focused devices is similar.[51] Specifically, the physical parameters of a shock wave are the same regardless of the method of production.[51]

Effects of Shock Waves on Treated Tissue

Shock waves can have both a direct and indirect effect on treated tissues. Energy from a shock wave produces tensile forces. The tensile forces produce a biologic response, that is, growth factor release, inflammatory factor inhibition, and enhanced neovascularity in the treated tissues. These responses are the direct effects of shock wave therapy.

Shock waves also have an indirect effect on treated tissues. Indirect effects can be likened to a "grenade." One of the well-recognized physical phenomena associated with the application of shock waves is the production of so-called cavitation bubbles. These small bubbles are a source of tremendous potential energy. Cavitation bubbles when produced in treated tissues expand, contract, collide, and ultimately collapse, thereby releasing additional energy and generating additional shock waves.[49] These additional waves, and the energy associated with these waves, account for the so-called "indirect" effect of shock wave therapy, and enhance the biologic response.

Parameters

The biologic response associated with shock wave therapy is often parameter-specific. Much like altering a recipe for a cake, altering a shock wave therapy protocol can yield unexpected, and often unwanted results. Indeed, alteration of critical treatment parameters usually produces poor results.

When proven protocols are followed, shock wave therapy is extremely safe. Significant deviation from a protocol, however, can have deleterious effects. As an example, investigators using animal models have shown that very excessive amounts of shock wave therapy can produce irreversible damage to treated tissues.[52] For these reasons it is imperative to understand just how shock wave parameters can be adjusted to produce a desired response.

Energy Levels, High versus Low

There are no universal guidelines as to what represents a high-energy treatment and what represents a low-energy treatment. In general, a high-energy treatment (>0.2 mJ/mm^2) usually consists of one or two treatment sessions, each of which is typically performed in an operating room or ambulatory surgical center with the use of some form of anesthesia. High-energy treatments tend to be painful. They are typically used when treating deeper structures and for this reason are often times performed in a more controlled environment.

In contrast, low-energy treatments typically have energy flux density ranging from 0.05 to 0.2 mJ/mm^2. In general, low-energy shock wave therapy is applied in a greater number of sessions, usually between one and four sessions. Low-energy treatments are generally used for more superficial structures, require minimal or no anesthesia and are often used for treating tendinopathy, fasciopathy, and more superficially located bones. In regard to efficacy, there is minimal comparative data, and what little exists, is conflicting.

PARAMETERS
Number of Treatments

One of the most obvious parameters that can be manipulated is the number of treatment sessions. ESWT can be delivered in a single session or over multiple sessions. In general, high-energy SWT is applied in one session or two sessions usually 1 week or 1 month apart. Low-energy SWT is usually applied in one treatment session, or more commonly, over multiple sessions at weekly, bimonthly, or monthly intervals.

Number of Shocks

A second easily manipulated parameter is the number of shocks. The number of shocks per treatment session is variable but usually ranges between 1,000 and 4,000 shocks per session.

Frequency of Delivery

Shock waves are usually delivered at a frequency between 60 and 240 shocks per minute. Many clinicians begin a treatment session at a low frequency and then ramp up the frequency over the remaining sessions.

Interval of Time

Finally, the interval of time between treatments can also vary. The time interval tends to be protocol specific. In the United States single treatment sessions are quite common. In Europe and other parts of the world, weekly, bimonthly, and monthly treatments are more common.

BIOLOGIC RESPONSE TO ESWT

There are numerous histologic, biochemical, and immunologic studies that have helped clarify the mechanism of action of shock wave therapy.[52–64] Numerous studies have shown that shock wave therapy enhances neovascularity, accelerates growth factor release, produces a selected neural inhibition, inhibits molecules that promote inflammation, and stimulates osteogenic stem cell recruitment.[53–64] Taken together, the net effect of these biologic responses is anabolic. What follows is a brief review of some of these trials.

Shock wave therapy enhances angiogenesis.[57,58] Wang et al.[58] reported their results using low-energy shock wave therapy on neovascularization at the tendon/bone junction in rabbits. Bone/tendon junctions treated with low-energy ESWT had a significantly increased number of neovessels and angiogenesis-related markers such as endothelial nitric oxide synthase, vascular endothelial growth factor, and proliferating cell nuclear antigen, than did untreated controls.[58] These markers have then shown to be increased with angiogenesis.[58]

Shock wave therapy enhances growth factor release.[64] Chen et al. demonstrated that low-energy shock wave therapy stimulated healing of collagenase-induced Achilles tendinopathy in a rat model by enhancing the function of transforming growth factor beta I (TGF-β1) and insulin-like growth factor-I (IGF-I).[64] Both TGF-β1 and IGF-I can have anabolic effects on pathologic tissues.[64]

Shock wave therapy has both central and peripheral effects on neurologic function.[53] Maier et al. used an animal model to demonstrate that shock wave therapy resulted in a significant decrease in substance P, approximately 6 weeks following treatment. In the periphery, shock wave therapy leads to a selective dysfunction of various sensory fibers while preserving the larger motor neurons.[53]

In addition, shock wave therapy has been shown to liberate various neuropeptides such as calcitonin gene-related peptide (CGRP).[62] There is some data to suggest that higher concentrations of CGRP results in a local "neurogenic inflammation" which prevents sensory nerve reinnervation in the area of treatment.[62] Some have proposed that it is this inhibition of reinnervation that contributes to the long-term pain reduction following ESWT.[62]

In summary, shock wave therapy appears to produce its effects on diseased tendons by upregulating various proteins and enzymes critical for angiogenesis, as well as selectively inhibiting various afferent nerve fibers important in pain transmission. Growth factors that have an anabolic effect on tissues are increased after shock wave therapy. Future studies will investigate the role gene expression plays in the healing process.

CLINICAL APPLICATIONS OF SWT
Indications and Contraindications

Indications for shock wave therapy as a treatment for tendinopathy or plantar fasciitis include a failure of traditional nonoperative therapies or chronicity of symptoms, usually defined as a period from 3 to 6 months. Absolute contraindications include active infection, unresolved fracture, malignancy, skeletal immaturity, pregnancy, as well as advanced peripheral neuropathy. Relative contraindications include poor generalized health, as well as untreated or poorly controlled systemic inflammatory arthropathy.

PROCEDURE

Both high-energy and low-energy SWT can be used to treat Achilles tendinopathy[11–20] or plantar fasciitis.[45–47] High-energy treatments are performed in either the operating room or ambulatory surgical center setting and usually require IV sedation with or without a regional block or a general anesthetic. Low-energy treatments are typically

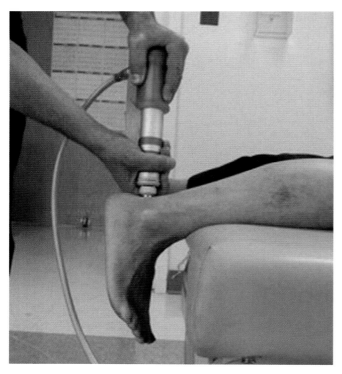

Figure 7–2. Radial shock waves being given to a patient at the midsubstance of the Achilles tendon in the treatment of Achilles tendinopathy.

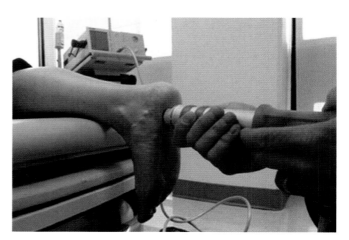

Figure 7–3. Radial shock waves being given to a patient at the medial origin of the plantar fascia in the treatment of plantar fasciitis. The control module and the compressor of the machine are seen in the background.

performed in the office setting in one or multiple sessions. Low-energy treatments rarely require anesthesia.

The procedure is similar for both high- and low-energy treatments. Patients are positioned in either a lateral decubitus or prone position for treatment of Achilles tendinopathy. The area of intended treatment is prepared with an ultrasound gel. The targeting device is positioned in such a way that the administered shock waves are directly over the area of intended treatment.

Shock waves are delivered in either a lateral to medial direction, tangential to the Achilles tendon, or posterior to anterior, in line with the Achilles tendon fibers (Fig. 7–2). For the plantar fascia energy is delivered at the origin of the fascia. This can be done with the patient either in a supine or prone position (Fig. 7–3). The shock waves are aimed at the center of maximal tenderness. The targeting device is then moved proximally, distally, and as well as circumferentially to treat surrounding tissues. The area of intended treatment is usually approximately 2 to 4 cm in length and 2 cm in width.

Application of shock waves is a dynamic process. For treatment of the Achilles tendon the ankle is repetitively dorsiflexed, plantar flexed, inverted, and everted throughout the procedure to insure that the entire pathologic area receives treatment. The plantar fascia is tensioned through the windlass effect of dorsiflexing of the toes. To verify that the depth of penetration was adequate, the examiner can usually feel vibrations along the margins of the treated tissues.

POSTTREATMENT CARE

Posttreatment protocols vary from center to center. In most cases, patients are allowed unrestricted range of motion, may be weight bearing as tolerated, and do not require any immobilization. Patients who work in a sedentary occupation can usually return to work that same day or within 24 hours of the treatment. Low impact activities such as cycling, swimming, weight training, and rowing can be resumed immediately. Return to higher impact activities such as running is made on a case-by-case basis and usually is within 4 to 6 weeks or treatment.

COMPLICATIONS

Worldwide there have been millions of patients treated with shock wave therapy for musculoskeletal problems. Some have reported transient and minor local effects such as skin rash, petechiae, superficial limited hematoma, swelling, and local pain as complications. However, these are expected and in some cases universal effects of the treatment that do not have any chronicity. We are aware of only two individual complications resulting substantial morbidity directly attributable to this treatment. The first is osteonecrosis of a humeral head after treatment of a calcific tendonitis[65] and the other is an osseous stress reaction of the calcaneus.[66] Given the number of treatments that have been administered we consider the effective complication rate nearly nonexistent.

CLINICAL RESULTS

Achilles Tendinopathy

Lohrer et al.[15] in a small uncontrolled clinical trial reported significant pain reduction, and increased functionality in a cohort of individuals with Achilles tendinopathy who were treated with radial shock wave therapy. There were no significant complications and patients were generally satisfied with their outcomes.

In a small controlled trial consisting of 39 patients, Peers reported his experience using a low-energy protocol for the treatment of patients with chronic Achilles tendinopathy.[17] Twelve weeks following initiation of the study, the 20 treated patients had significantly improved visual analog scores (VAS) when compared with the untreated control group. A success rate of 77% was reported.[17]

Perlick et al.[16] compared ESWT with surgery as a treatment for both insertional and noninsertional Achilles tendinopathy. At 1 year following treatment, there was a statistically significant reduction in the VAS in both groups.[16]

Fridman et al.[19] reported their experience using a high-energy device to treat 23 patients with chronic insertional and noninsertional Achilles tendinopathy. They noted 80% of the entire cohort were improved and indicated that they would endure another procedure.[19]

The results from these early trials stimulated more rigorous investigation.[20] Rasmussen et al.[20] performed a double-blind, placebo-controlled trial in which patients with chronic Achilles tendinopathy were randomized to receive either active ESWT or sham ESWT as a supplement to eccentric strengthening and stretching. At short-term follow-up (12 weeks), the American Foot and Ankle Society (AOFAS) Score was significantly increased in both the placebo and intervention group.[20] The authors concluded that ESWT was as effective as eccentric strengthening and stretching and that it was an effective supplemental procedure to treat this chronic condition.[20]

Using a more strict inclusion criteria, Furia evaluated the effects of high-energy ESWT on a consecutive series of patients with chronic insertional Achilles tendinopathy who had failed traditional conservative measures.[12] Thirty-five patients with chronic insertional Achilles tendinopathy were treated with single-dose high-energy ESWT. Thirty-three patients with chronic insertional Achilles tendinopathy were not treated with ESWT but instead were treated with additional forms of nonoperative therapy. One month, 3 months, and 12 months following treatment, the mean VAS for the ESWT groups were significantly greater than those of the control groups. Chi-square analysis revealed the number of patients with excellent or good functional scores was greater in the ESWT group than in the control group.[12]

A subsequent randomized control trial performed by Rompe et al.[18] compared eccentric loading with shock wave therapy as a treatment for chronic insertional Achilles tendinopathy. Fifty patients with chronic recalcitrant insertional Achilles tendinopathy who had failed treatment with traditional nonoperative measures received either an eccentric strengthening program or repetitive low-energy shock wave therapy. Outcome criteria included the Victorian Institute of Sport Assessment-Achilles score.

At 4 months from baseline, the mean VISA-A score had increased in both groups. The mean pain rating decreased in both groups. For all outcome measures, the group that received the shock wave therapy showed significantly more favorable improvement than did the group treated with eccentric loading. Of note, the favorable results after shock wave therapy at 4 months were stable up to 1-year follow-up.[18]

Plantar Fasciitis

Recently Golwitzer et al. conducted a double-blind randomized placebo-controlled study in which subjects were randomized to focused ESWT (0.25 mJ/mm^2) or placebo intervention, with three sessions of 2,000 impulses in weekly intervals. Primary outcomes were both the percentage change of heel pain on the visual analog scale composite score (pain during first steps in the morning, pain with daily activities, and pain with a force meter) and the Roles and Maudsley score at 12 weeks after the last intervention compared with the scores at baseline. Almost 250 patients were available for follow-up at 12 weeks post treatment. There was a highly significant difference in the reduction of heel pain as measured by the VAS pain scale in the ESWT group (69.2%) compared with the placebo therapy group (34.5%). ESWT was also significantly superior to the placebo therapy for the Roles and Maudsley score ($p = 0.0006$, one-sided).

Another study compared the results obtained with high-energy shock wave therapy and those with endoscopic partial plantar fascial release.[67] At 12 months following the completion of treatment reduction in pain as well as the AOFAS ankle hindfoot score did not show any significant differences.

A randomized, placebo-controlled study looked at not only pain reduction as an outcome measure but also the ultrasonographically measured thickness of the plantar fascial origin.[68] In the study the treatment group received 4,000 shock waves/session at 0.2 mJ/mm flux in three sessions at weekly intervals. The control group received no energy through the use of a sham applicator. Results were obtained at baseline and 12 weeks after the completion of the treatments. The plantar fascia thickness was significantly reduced in the ESWT group while that of the control group was slightly increased in the sham group. Both groups showed significant pain improvement over the course of the study though pain scores were significantly more reduced in the ESWT than the control group.

It is clear from the above studies that ESWT has therapeutic effect in the treatment of plantar fasciitis. However it seems that combining ESWT with physiotherapy leads to a more beneficial effect in those refractory to other nonoperative treatments. Rompe et al.[68] conducted a study with the control group receiving RSWT alone and the experimental group receiving RSWT and plantar fascial specific physiotherapy. The results showed that those in the experimental group had not only significantly better outcome scores but also a greater proportion of individuals satisfied with the treatment.

CONCLUSION

ESWT is a safe and effective treatment for chronic Achilles tendinopathy and refractory plantar fasciitis. The procedure "burns no bridges" and can be performed in patients who have failed to respond to traditional nonoperative measures or who have failed surgical procedures. The procedure is well tolerated, easy to perform, and associated with speedy return to work and sport. Further improvements in shock wave generators as well as advances in orthobiologics should result in wider applications of this promising technology.

REFERENCES

1. Graff J, Pastor J, Richter KD. Effect of high-energy shock waves on bony tissue. *Urol Res.* 1988;16:252–8.
2. Valchanou VD, Michailov P. High energy shock waves in the treatment of delayed and nonunion of fractures. *Int Orthop.* 1991;15(3):181–184.
3. Schaden W, Fischer A, Sailler A. Extracorporeal shock wave therapy of nonunion or delayed osseous union. *Clin Orthop Relat Res.* 2001;387:90–94.
4. Wang CJ, Chen HS, Chen CE, et al. Treatment of nonunions of long bone fractures with shock waves. *Clin Orthop Relat Res.* 2001;387:95–101.
5. Rompe JD, Rosendahl T, Schollner C, et al. High-energy extracorporeal shock wave treatment of nonunions. *Clin Orthop Relat Res.* 2001;387:102–111.
6. Cachio A, Giordano L, Colafarina O, et al. Extracorporeal shock-wave therapy compared with surgery for hypertrophic long-bone nonunions. *J Bone Joint Surg Am.* 2009;91:2589–2597.
7. Haupt G. Use of extracorporeal shock wave therapy in the treatment of pseudarthrosis, tendinopathy, and other orthopedic diseases. *Urology.* 1997;158:4–11.
8. Buch M, Knorr U, Fleming L, et al. Shock wave therapy for the treatment of chronic plantar fasciitis. *Orthopade.* 2002;31(7):637–644.
9. Caccio A, Rompe J, Furia JP, et al. Shockwave therapy for the treatment of chronic proximal hamstring tendinopathy in professional athletes. *Am J Sports Med.* 2011;39:146–153.
10. Furia JP, Rompe JD, Maffulli N. Low energy extracorporeal shock wave therapy as a treatment for greater trochanteric pain syndrome. *Am Journal of Sports Med.* 2009;37:1806–1813.
11. Furia JP. High energy extracorporeal shock wave therapy as a treatment for chronic noninsertional Achilles tendinopathy. *Am Journal of Sports Med.* 2008;36:502–508.
12. Furia JP. High energy ESWT as a treatment for chronic insertional Achilles Tendinopathy. *Am Journal of Sports Med.* 2006;34:733–740.
13. Furia JP. Safety and efficacy of extracorporeal shock wave therapy for chronic lateral epicondylitis. *Am J Orthop (Belle Mead NJ).* 2005;24:13–19.
14. Lakshmanan P, O'Doherty D. Chronic achilles tendinopathy: Treatment with extracorporeal shock waves. *Foot Ankle Surg.* 2004;10:125–130.
15. Lohrer H, Scholl J, Arentz S. Achilles tendinopathy and patellar tendinopathy. Results of radial shockwave therapy in patients with unsuccessfully treated tendinoses. *Sportverletz Sportschaden.* 2002;16:108–114.
16. Perlick L, Schiffmann R, Kraft CN. Extracorporeal shock wave treatment of the Achilles tendinitis: Experimental and preliminary clinical results. *Z Orthop Ihre Grenzgeb.* 2002;140:275–280.
17. Peers K. *Extracorporeal shock wave therapy in chronic Achilles and patellar tendinopathy.* Leuven: Leuven University Press; 2003:61–75.
18. Rompe JD, Nafe B, Furia JP, et al. Eccentric loading, shock wave treatment, or a wait-and-see policy for tendinopathy of the main body of tendo Achillis: A randomized controlled trial. *Am J Sports Med.* 2007;35:374–383.
19. Fridman R, Cain D, Weil L Jr, et al. Extracorporeal shock wave therapy for the treatment of Achilles tendinopathy: A prospective study. *J Am Podatr Med Assoc.* 2008;98:466–468.
20. Rasmussen S, Christensen M, Mathiesen I et al. Shockwave therapy for chronic Achilles tendinopathy-A double blind, randomized clinical trial of efficacy. *Acta Orthopaedica.* 2008;79:249–256.
21. Gerdesmeyer L, Wagenpfeil S, Haake M, et al. Extracorporeal shock wave therapy for the treatment of chronic calcifying tendonitis of the rotator cuff: A randomized controlled trial. *JAMA.* 2003;290:2573–2580.
22. Kudo P, Dainty K, Clarefield M, et al. Randomized, placebo-controlled, double-blind clinical trial evaluating the treatment of plantar fasciitis with an extracorporeal shock wave therapy (ESWT) treatment device: A North American confirmatory study. *J Orthop Res.* 2006:24:115–123.
23. Lohrer H, Natuck T, Dorn-Lange NV, et al. Comparison of radial versus focused extracorporeal shock waves in plantar fasciitis using functional measures. *Foot and Ankle Intl.* 2010;31:1–9.
24. Ogden JA, Alvarez RG, Levitt RL, et al. Electrohydraulic high-energy shock-wave treatment for chronic plantar fasciitis. *J Bone Joint Surg Am.* 2004;86A:2216–2228.
25. Ogden JA, Alvarez RG, Levitt R, et al. Shock wave therapy for chronic plantar fasciitis. *Clin Orthop Relat Res.* 2001;387:47–59.
26. Rompe JD, Furia J, Maffulli N. Eccentric loading compared with shock wave treatment for chronic insertional Achilles tendinopathy. *J Bone Joint Surg Am.* 2008;90:52–61.
27. Rompe JD, Furia JP, Weil L, et al. Shock wave therapy for chronic plantar fasciopathy. *Br Med Bull.* 2007;24:1–26.
28. Rompe JD, Nafe B, Furia J, et al. Eccentric loading, shock wave treatment or a wait-and-see policy for tendinopathy of the main body of the tendo Achilles: A randomized controlled trial. *Am J Sports Med.* 2007;35:374–383.
29. Rompe JD, Meurer A, Nafe B, et al. Repetitive low-energy shock wave application without local anesthesia is more efficient than repetitive low-energy shock wave application with local anesthesia in the treatment of chronic plantar fasciitis. *J Orthop Res.* 2005;23:931–41.
30. Rompe JD, Decking J, Schoellner C, et al. Repetitive low-energy shock wave treatment for chronic lateral epicondylitis in tennis players. *Am Journal of Sports Med.* 2004;32:734–743.
31. Rompe JD, Schoellner C, Nafe B. Evaluation of low energy extracorporeal shock wave treatment for treatment of chronic plantar fasciitis. *J Bone Joint Surg Am.* 2002;84:335–341.
32. Theodore GH, Buch M, Amendola A, et al. Extracorporeal shock wave therapy for the treatment of plantar fasciitis. *Foot and Ankle Int.* 2004;25:290–297.

33. Wang CJ, Yang KD, Wang FS. Shock wave therapy for calcific tendonitis of the shoulder. *Am Journal of Sports Med.* 2003;31:425–430.

34. Peers KH, Lysens RJ, Brys P, et al. Cross-sectional outcome analysis of athletes with chronic patellar tendinopathy treated surgically and by extracorporeal shock wave therapy. *Clin J Sports Med.* 2003;13:79–83.

35. Vulpiani MC, Vetrano M, Savoia V, et al. Jumper's knee treatment with extracorporeal shock wave therapy: A long-term follow-up observational study. *J Sports Med Phys Fitness.* 2007;47:323–328.

36. Wang CJ, Ko JY, Chan YS, et al. Extracorporeal shockwave for chronic patellar tendinopathy. *Am J Sports Med.* 2007;35:972–978.

37. Xu ZH, Jiang Q, Chen DY, et al. Extracorporeal shock wave treatment in nonunions of long bone fractures. *Int Orthop.* 2009;33:789–793.

38. Birnbaum K, Wirtz DC, Siebert CH, et al. Use of extracorporeal shock-wave therapy (ESWT) in the treatment of non-unions. A review of the literature. *Arch Or-thop Trauma Surg.* 2002;122(6):324–330.

39. Biedermann R, Martin A, Handle G, et al. Extracorporeal shock waves in the treatment of nonunions. *J Trauma.* 2003; 54(5):936–942.

40. Taki M, Iwata O, Shiono M, et al. Extracorporeal shock wave therapy for resistant stress fractures in athletes. *Am J Sports Med.* 2007;35:1188–1192.

41. Moretti B, Notarnicola A, Garofalo R, et al. Shock waves in the treatment of stress fractures. *Ultrasound Med Biol.* 2009;35:1042–1049.

42. Wang CJ, Wang FS, Huang CC, et al. Treatment for osteonecrosis of the femoral head: Comparison of extracorporeal shock waves with core decompression and bone-grafting. *J Bone Joint Surg Am.* 2005;87:2380–2387.

43. Wang CJ, Wang FS, Yand KD, et al. Treatment of osteonecrosis of the hip: Comparison of extracorporeal shockwave with shockwave and alendronate. *Arch Orthop Trauma Surg.* 2008;128:901–908.

44. Wang CJ, Wang FS, Ko JY, et al. Extracorporeal shockwave therapy shows regeneration in hip necrosis. *Rheumatology.* 2008;47:542–546.

45. Gollwitzer H, Saxena A, DiDomenico LA, et al. Clinically relevant effectiveness of focused extracorporeal shock wave therapy in the treatment of chronic plantar fasciitis: A randomized, controlled multicenter study. *J Bone Joint Surg Am.* 2015;97:701–708.

46. Vahdatpour B, Sajadieh S, Bateni V, et al. Extracorporeal shock wave therapy in patients with plantar fasciitis. A randomized, placebo-controlled trial with ultrasonographic and subjective outcome assessments. *Int Orthop.* 2012;36:2147–2156.

47. Ibrahim MI, Donatelli RA, Schmitz C, et al. Chronic plantar fasciitis treated with two sessions of radial extracorporeal shock wave therapy. *Foot Ankle Int.* 2010;31(5):391–397.

48. Ogden JA, Toth-Kischkat A, Schultheiss R. Principles of shock wave therapy. *Clin Orthop Relat Res.* 2001;387:8–17.

49. Gerdesmeyer L, Henne M, Gobel M, et al. Physical principles and generation of shockwaves. In: Gerdsmeyer L, ed. *Extracorporeal shock wave therapy: technologies, basics, clinical results.* Towson, MD: Data Trace Media; 2007:11–20.

50. Sems A, Dimeff R, Iannotti JP. Extracorporeal shock wave therapy in the treatment of chronic tendinopathies. *J Am Acad Orthop Surg.* 2006;14:195–204.

51. Lohrer H, Natuck T, Dorn-Lange NV, et al. Comparison of radial versus focused extracorporeal shock waves in plantar fasciitis using functional measures. *Foot Ankle Int.* 2010;31:1–9.

52. Rompe JD, Kirkpatrick CJ, Kullmer K, et al. Dose-related effects of shock waves on rabbit tendo Achillis. A sonographic and histological study. *J Bone Joint Surg Br.* 1998;80:546–552.

53. Maier M, Averbeck B, Milz S, et al. Substance P and prostaglandin E2 release after shock wave application to the rabbit femur. *Clin Orthop Relat Res.* 2003;406:237–245.

54. Martini L, Giavaresi G, Fini M, et al. Effect of extracorporeal shock wave therapy on osteoblastlike cells. *Clin Orthop Relat Res.* 2003;413:269–280.

55. Wang FS, Yang KD, Chen RF, et al. Extracorporeal shock wave promotes growth and differentiation of bone-marrow stromal cells towards osteoprogenitors associated with induction of TGF-beta1. *J Bone Joint Surg Br.* 2002;84(3):457–461.

56. Wang FS, Yang KD, Kuo YR, et al. Temporal and spatial expression of bone morphogenetic proteins in extracorporeal shock wave-promoted healing of segmental defect. *Bone.* 2003;32(4):387–396.

57. Wang CJ, Wang FS, Yang KD, et al. Shock wave therapy induces neovascularization at the tendon-bone junction. A study in rabbits. *J Orthop Res.* 2003;21: 984–989.

58. Wang CJ, Wang FS, Yang KD, et al. The effect of shock wave treatment at the tendon-bone interface-an histomorphological and biomechanical study in rabbits. *J Orthop Res.* 2005;23:274–280.

59. Takahashi N, Wada Y, Ohtori S, et al. Application of shock waves to rat skin decreases calcitonin gene-related peptide immunoreactivity in dorsal root ganglion neurons. *Auton Neurosci.* 2003;107:81–84.

60. Takahashi N, Ohtori S, Saisu T, et al. Second application of low-energy shock waves has a cumulative effect on free nerve endings. *Clin Orthop Relat Res.* 2006;443:315–319.

61. Martini L, Fini M, Giavaresi G, et al. Primary osteoblasts response to shock wave therapy using different parameters. *Artif Cells Blood Substit Immobil Biotechnol.* 2003; 31(4):449–466.

62. Ohtori S, Inoue G, Mannoji C. Shock wave application to rat skin induces degeneration and reinnervation of sensory nerve fibres. *Neurosci Lett.* 2002;315:57–60.

63. Murata R, Ohtori S, Ochiai N. Extracorporeal shockwaves induce the expression of ATF3 and GAP-43 in rat dorsal root ganglion neurons. *Auton Neurosci.* 2006;128:96–100.

64. Chen YJ, Wang CJ, Yang KD. Extracorporeal shock waves promote healing of collagenase-induced Achilles tendinitis and increase TGF-beta1 and IGF-I expression. *J Orthop Res.* 2004;22:854–861.

65. Durst HB, Blatter G, Kuster MS. Osteonecrosis of the humeral head after extracorporeal shock wave lithotripsy. *J Bone Joint Surg Br.* 2002;84:744–746.

66. Erduran M, Akseki D, Ulusal AE. A complication due to shock wave therapy resembling calcaneal stress fracture. *Foot Ankle Int.* 2013;34:599–602.

67. Radwan YA, Mansour AM, Badawy WS. Resistant plantar fasciopathy: Shock wave versus endoscopic plantar fascial release. *Int Orthop.* 2012;36:2147–2156.

68. Rompe JD, Furia J, Cacchio A, et al. Radial shock wave treatment alone is less efficient than radial shock wave treatment combined with tissue-specific plantar fascia-stretching in patients with chronic plantar heel pain. *Int J Surg.* 2015;pii: S1743-9191(15)00209-5.

CHAPTER 8

Endoscopic Plantar Fascia Release

Jeremy J. Miles   Michael J. Shereff

ANATOMY

The plantar fascia is composed of sheets of dense collagen bundles located between the skin and superficial muscle layer of the plantar foot. It functions to provide static and dynamic support to the longitudinal arch of the foot. This aponeurosis shares an origin off the anteromedial plantar aspect of the calcaneal tuberosity with the flexor digitorum brevis (deep) and abductor hallucis (medial). Thereafter, the fascia divides into several fibrous slips which insert on the plantar plates of the metatarsophalangeal joints, bases of the proximal phalanges, and the flexor tendon sheaths.

Biomechanically it acts to provide support to the arch of the foot both dynamically and statically. Plantar fascial tension is generated from it being wound around the metatarsal heads to generate a windlass mechanism. Metatarsophalangeal joint dorsiflexion during toe off tensions the plantar fascia, which aids to lock the transverse tarsal joint and provide the stable lever arm needed for efficient gait. Cadaveric studies have shown that transection of the plantar fascia leads to a loss of longitudinal arch height during terminal stance. Plantar fascia transection also alters pressure distribution of the forefoot, thereby increasing the load on the second metatarsal.[1,2]

PLANTAR FASCIITIS OVERVIEW

Plantar fasciitis is thought to be the most common cause of plantar heel pain. Other pathologies on the list of differential diagnoses include heel fat pad atrophy, calcaneal stress fractures, and compression neuropathy of the first branch of the lateral plantar nerve. Epidemiologically, men and women are affected equally. Risk factors for developing the disorder include obesity, heel cord tightness, prolonged weight bearing, and repeated trauma on hard surfaces (e.g., road running). The pathogenesis is thought to be repetitive microtears and chronic inflammation of the plantar fascia at its origin.[3]

Classically, patients give a history of "start-up pain" localized to the medial plantar heel. The pain is worse with the first few steps after getting out of bed or after sitting for a protracted period. At rest, the foot is relaxed in plantar flexion with the metatarsophalangeal joints in slight flexion, resulting in minimal tension on the plantar fascia. When arising from a non-weightbearing position, tension is applied to the plantar fascia leading to microtears and resultant pain. Each time the patient arises after a prolonged time off their feet this process recurs resulting in a chronic nonhealing pathology. Additionally, activity-related plantar fasciitis is often increased with repetitive loading of the heel and toes, especially when performed on hard surfaces.

Physical examination reveals a point of maximal tenderness at the proximal medial origin of the plantar fascia. The trigger point is usually just distal to the area where the soft skin of the medial hindfoot transitions to the thicker, tougher plantar skin on the medial heel. A classic history in conjunction with this finding is generally sufficient to make the clinical diagnosis of plantar fasciitis. Additional workup is rarely necessary for acute plantar fasciitis.

Recalcitrant plantar fasciitis nonresponsive to conservative intervention merits further workup. Routine radiographs are used as a primary investigation of the affected extremity and can be useful to rule out other etiologies of heel pain. Radiographs are also used to assess for predisposing anatomical deformity, or to identify calcification at the origin of the plantar fascia. However, it should be noted that one study looking at radiographs of a random sample of patients encountered a heel spur in 13% of subjects while only one-third of the spurs detected were symptomatic.[4] Ultrasound has been shown to be useful in identifying plantar fasciitis when the proximal plantar fascia thickness measures greater than 4 to 5 mm.[5,6] Ultrasound may also be helpful in following treatment as subjective improvement from conservative therapy has been correlated with thinning of the plantar fascia.[7] Magnetic resonance imaging (MRI) has also been demonstrated to be useful to measure the plantar fascia thickness, intra- or perifascial edema, fascial tears, and calcaneal edema suggestive of enthesopathy.[8,9] The improved soft tissue detail appreciated with MRI can be used to help rule out more rare soft tissue disorders such as a tumor or abscess.

INDICATIONS

After the clinical diagnosis of plantar fasciitis is made, multimodal conservative treatment is warranted. Generally, first-line treatment consists of plantar fascia, heel cord, and hamstring stretching, which the patient should perform daily.[10,11] Patients are advised to wear soft rubber wedge sole shoes to act as a shock absorbing cushion and decrease forces to the heel. Soft, flexible inserts with a well to float the heel thereby decrease pressure on the fascial origin and an arch support to diminish the excursion of the plantar fascia during stance phase of gait are recommended. Activities are recommended within the limits of discomfort. Patients are instructed to follow-up at 4- to 6-week intervals for repeat evaluation.

If a patient returns to clinic with persistent symptoms, the nonsteroidal anti-inflammatory agent may need to be changed. We feel night splints may be helpful, despite their mixed outcomes in randomized studies.[12,13] The use of a plantar fascia strap is another option that some patients may find beneficial.

At the third appointment, custom orthotics designed with soft heel flotation and arch support to decrease plantar fascia stretch while standing may be beneficial.[14,15] These may work better than over-the-counter orthotics as they take into account a patient's individual anatomy and not simply shoe size. A corticosteroid injection is offered, which can provide relief of varying degrees and duration. Supervised stretching protocols with physical therapy and massage therapy are also prescribed. Physical therapy modalities are of potential benefit and iontophoresis provides another method for localized corticosteroid delivery. Autologous platelet-rich plasma may provide patients with some benefit. However the lack of supporting clinical evidence and the hesitancy of insurance companies to reimburse for the treatment may prohibit general use.

High-energy extracorporeal shock-wave therapy has been shown to improve symptoms in over 80% of patients with chronic plantar fasciitis and can be offered to patients.[16,17] Low-energy or radial shock-wave therapy has also been shown to be effective in recalcitrant cases of plantar fasciitis.[18] However, despite good evidence showing their efficacy neither of these treatments are currently reimbursed by insurance. If nonoperative regimens fail to provide relief, the patient is considered to have refractory plantar fasciitis and more invasive measures are indicated.

Plantar fascia release by either open or endoscopic technique is the most commonly utilized treatment for plantar fasciitis refractory to nonsurgical methods. Plantar fascia release has two principle indications. The first and most common indication is chronic recurrent plantar fasciitis pain that has failed conservative measures. The second indication is persistent pain status post traumatic plantar fascia partial tear to complete the release of the medial band of the plantar fascia. Endoscopic plantar fascia release has the benefit of a shorter recovery period and fewer complications compared to the more widely used open release.[3,19,20]

Contraindications to endoscopic plantar fascia release are few. General medical conditions which preclude anesthesia and surgery are the most common contraindication. Prior endoscopic plantar fascia release is also a contraindication as revision surgery, if required, should be performed by open technique. Endoscopic plantar fascia

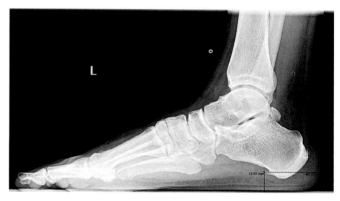

Figure 8–1. Lateral weight-bearing foot radiograph with measurements from the plantar fascia origin to the skin edges.

release should not be performed in patients with compromised skin at the portal sites. Also, neurologic or vascular dysfunction of the peripheral distal extremity that may compromise wound healing are contraindications.

PATIENT POSITIONING AND OPERATIVE TECHNIQUE

Patients scheduled for surgery should all have a lateral radiograph of the foot or ankle which allows full visualization of the overlying soft tissue (Fig. 8–1). From these images, the insertion of the plantar fascia is identified and the distance from the posterior heel skin edge and the plantar skin edge to the insertion of the plantar fascia on the calcaneus is measured. This measurement maybe used for portal placement.

In the operating room, the patient is placed supine with a bump under the operative calf to elevate the heel (Fig. 8–2). Regional block with intravenous sedation is sufficient for the procedure, however, general anesthesia

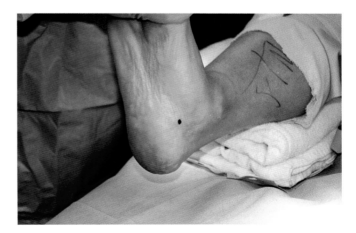

Figure 8–2. Extremity positioning with draping and tourniquet.

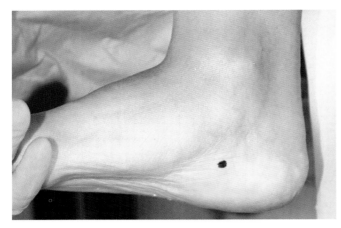

Figure 8–3. Skin mark on medial skin over the plantar fascia origin using the measurements obtained from the preoperative radiograph.

may be required in some cases. After prepping and draping, a 4-in Esmarch tourniquet is applied and secured in the supramalleolar region of the leg. The anterior portion of the calcaneal tuberosity is palpated medially and the skin is marked using the radiographic measurements obtained preoperatively from the plantar and posterior heel skin (Fig. 8–3). A small (<1 cm) vertical puncture wound is then made with a 15 blade. The subcutaneous tissue is dissected using a hemostat to the level of the plantar fascia, completing the exposure for the endoscopic release.

An endoscopic plantar fascia release system with procedure-specific instruments should be used such as the EPF system (Instratek, Houston, Texas) or the ECTRA II system (Smith & Nephew, Andover, Massachusetts). The tissue elevator is inserted into the medial incision and used to palpate the plantar fascia, verifying the inferior margins of the aponeurosis (Fig. 8–4A,B). The elevator is withdrawn and the blunt obturator and trocar are then passed through the medial puncture wound (Fig. 8–5A,B), just plantar to the plantar fascia, until the lateral skin is tented. A vertical puncture wound is then made over the trocar and the cannula is advanced through the lateral skin so that the medial and lateral ends of the trocar are external. The obturator is removed leaving the trocar in place.

Next, the 4.0-mm arthroscope is inserted into the trocar from the medial side and the entire width of the plantar fascia is visualized from medial to lateral (Fig. 8–6A,B). Under scope visualization, the medial, middle, and lateral one-thirds of the plantar fascia are distinguished. Most instrument sets have custom trocars with gradations for normal plantar fascia widths to help aid in measuring the medial third. Next with scope visualization medially, the probe is inserted into the lateral opening of the cannula and used to inspect the medial margin of the plantar fascia (Fig. 8–7A,B). Once the full extent of the medial plantar fascia is appreciated, the probe is exchanged for the hook

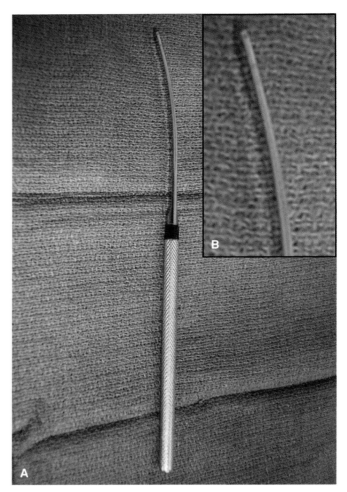

Figure 8–4. The tissue elevator is used to palpate the inferior border of the plantar fascia. **A:** Entire instrument. **B:** Detail of the tip used to separate tissue layers.

blade (Fig. 8–8A) and positioned along the medial border of the plantar fascia. The superficial fibers of the medial band are cut with the hook blade, incising only the medial one-third. The hook blade is then retracted and exchanged for the triangle blade (Fig. 8–8C), which is used to cut the deep fibers of the medial one-third of the plantar fascia. At this point, the short flexor muscles are visible through the scope assuring complete release (Fig. 8–9). The portion of incised fascia is then verified with the scope and aided by the sleeve markings to ensure adequacy of the incised fascia. All instruments and the sleeve are then removed. The incisions are sutured with no. 00 absorbable sutures and a soft, sterile compressive dressing is applied (Fig. 8–10).

POSTOPERATIVE CARE

Postoperatively, patients are instructed to elevate and ice the operative extremity. Patients are kept nonweight bearing until the first office visit, 1 week postoperatively. At 7 to 10 days postoperatively, patients are seen in clinic to remove the dressing and examine the surgical incisions.

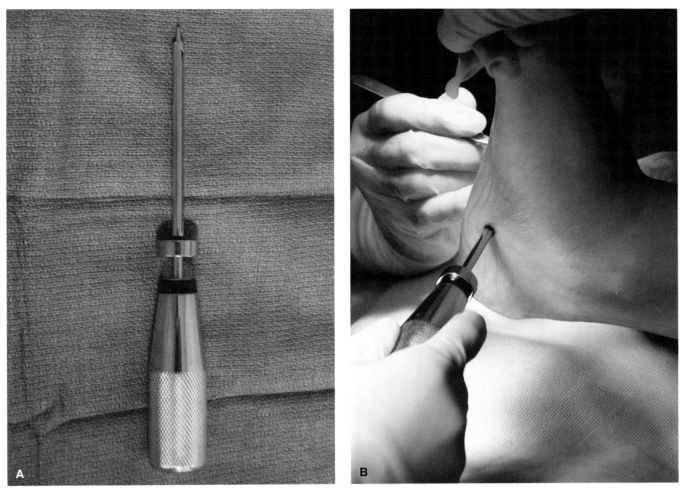

Figure 8–5.   A: Blunt obturator and trocar. **B:** Medial insertion of the trocar that is used to make the lateral skin incision.

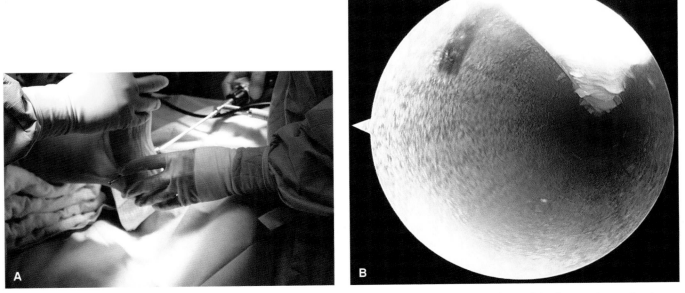

Figure 8–6.   A: Insertion of the endoscope into the medial trocar opening. **B:** Endoscopic view of the intact plantar fascia.

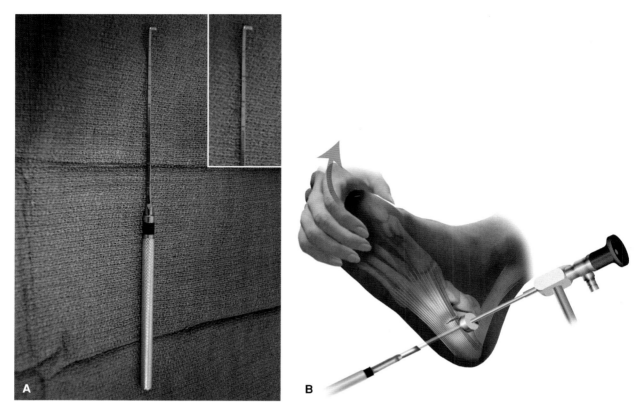

Figure 8–7. **A:** Plantar fascia probe. **B:** Insertion of the plantar fascia probe to inspect the medial plantar fascia under endoscopic visualization.

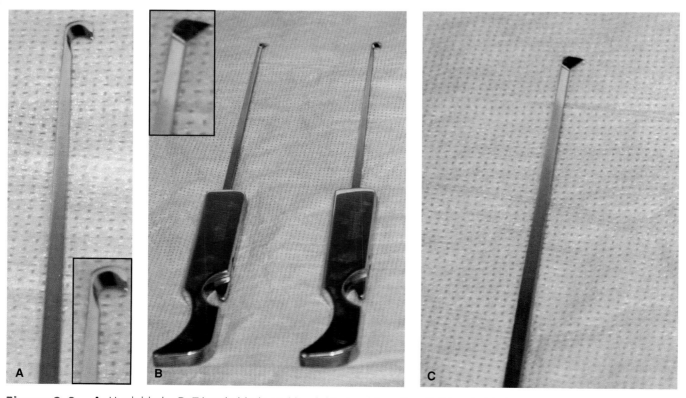

Figure 8–8. **A:** Hook blade. **B:** Triangle blade and hook blade on handles. **C:** Triangle blade.

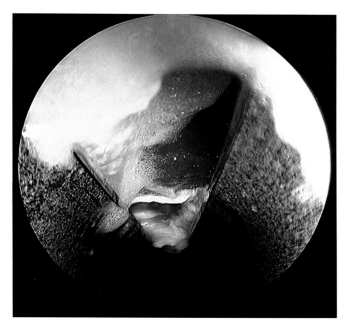

Figure 8–9. Endoscopic view of incised plantar fascia with short flexor muscle fibers visible.

At this point, patients are progressed to gradual weight bearing with crutches using the following protocol: 1 week nonweight bearing, 2 weeks partial weight bearing, 1 week full weight bearing with crutches, and then a cane or no ambulatory aids. Patients are advised to elevate the operative leg while sitting for the first 4 weeks postoperatively and thereafter to elevate as pain and swelling direct. Ice may be helpful. Throughout the postoperative period, nonsteroidal anti-inflammatory medications are used as needed for pain. Patients are seen back in clinic approximately 1 month postoperatively and at that point are progressed to activity and shoe wear as tolerated. However, patients are encouraged to continue to wear wide, soft rubber sole shoes that are soft and flexible with an arch support.

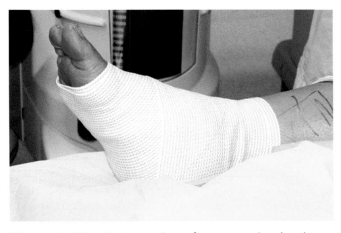

Figure 8–10. Postoperative soft, compressive dressing.

TECHNICAL PITFALLS

Potential intraoperative complications of plantar fascia release are relatively few. Inadvertent release of the lateral band of the plantar fascia causing complete plantar fascia release is the most common operative error. Complete release may lead to loss of the height of the medial longitudinal arch. Similarly, incomplete release of the medial band of the plantar fascia can lead to continued symptoms postoperatively. Injury to the lateral plantar nerve can occur, but is avoided by using careful blunt dissection of the subcutaneous tissues after skin incision for portal placement.

COMPLICATIONS AND OUTCOMES

The largest case series of endoscopic plantar fascia releases included 652 patients in a multi-surgeon study that found 97% of the patients undergoing endoscopic release reported the operation was successful in relieving heel pain.[21] Barrett et al. reported an 8% postoperative complication rate with lateral column pain accounting for over half of these complications while only one superficial wound infection was recorded.

Two studies directly compared open to endoscopic plantar fascia release. In a case series including results from 25 surgeons, Kinley and associates compared the results of 66 endoscopic plantar fasciotomies to 26 open releases with heel spur excision.[3] They found that 80% of all patients had complete pain relief regardless of technique, but patients returned to full activity 4 weeks earlier and had 45% less pain in the endoscopically released group. Tomczak and Haverstock[20] conducted a retrospective review that compared 34 cases of endoscopic plantar fasciotomy to 34 cases of open fasciotomy with calcaneal spur resection and noted quicker return to work in those who underwent endoscopic release.

Few single-surgeon, retrospective, consecutive studies have been published on patients undergoing endoscopic plantar fascia release after failed conservative therapy for plantar fasciitis. O'Malley et al. reported results on 20 feet with 22 months of average follow-up. Eighteen of 20 feet had improvement in symptoms and 9 of 20 experienced complete relief.[22] The most common complication in this series, observed in three patients, was postoperative foot pain not localized to the heel. Boyle and Slater described 17 patients undergoing endoscopic release with 82% of subjects reporting minimal or no residual pain and the other 18% having lateral foot pain postoperatively.[23] In a single-surgeon retrospective series of 22 cases with 8.5 months of average follow-up, Hogan et al.[24] had a 97% satisfaction rate overall with all patients reporting at least 50% improvement in pain. They had no surgical complications, but two patients reported subjective loss of longitudinal arch compared to their nonoperative side. In Ferkel's series of 19 feet in 16 patients with 1-year minimum follow-up, patients obtained a 33% improvement in

AOFAS ankle–hindfoot scores postoperatively with pain improvement noted in 84%.[25] No wound or lateral column pain complications were reported, but one patient in this series developed complex regional pain syndrome that required pain management referral.

TECHNIQUE VARIATIONS

Although most of the published studies utilize the biportal approach, variations on the procedure have been described. A uniportal approach was originally described by Barret and Day in a series of six patients,[26] but was abandoned for the biportal approach. However, the uniportal approach has been revisited by Saxena,[27] which utilizes only the medial side of the original approach with specialized equipment to mount the probing and cutting instruments directly to the endoscope as well as depth gauges to measure the extent of fascial release. These instruments are now commercially available (Uniportal EPF System, Wright Medical, Arlington, Tennessee). In this single-surgeon series of 29 feet in 26 patients, significant improvement postoperatively in the mean plantar fascia score was found with 76% of feet having a good or excellent result while BMI >27 was associated with poor outcomes. Four feet had continued symptoms that resolved after corticosteroid injection and three obese patients developed pseudohernias at the incision not requiring treatment.

In a recently published series of 10 feet, a deep fascial approach was used with conventional 2.7-mm arthroscope, shaver, and burr equipment.[28] This technique has the benefit of using more readily available, less-specialized equipment and the ability to excise a calcaneal spur or calcaneal periostitis when present. However, it has the drawback of requiring excision of the fatty tissue superficial to the flexor digitorum brevis muscle in order to obtain an adequate field of view. Nonetheless, all patients in this series returned to full athletic activities and had nearly 50% improvement in their AOFAS ankle and hindfoot score 2 years after the operation.

If entrapment of the first branch of the lateral plantar nerve is suspected, a concomitant release of the abductor hallucis deep fascia should also be performed. The portal openings for this procedure are located 16 mm inferior and 23 mm posterior to the tip of the medial malleolus for the proximal site and just distal to the medial calcaneal tubercle at the inferior edge of the deep fascia of the abductor hallucis muscle for the distal portal site.[29] The deep abductor fascia release can be performed reliably using this technique with visualization of the nerve deep to the portal tract when accurately placed.

REFERENCES

1. Sharkey NA, Ferris L, Donahue SW, et al. Biomechanical consequences of the plantar fascial release or rupture during gait: Part I – disruptions in the longitudinal arch conformation. *Foot Ankle Int.* 1998;19:812–820.

2. Sharkey NA, Donahue SW, Ferris L. Biomechanical consequences of the plantar fascial release or rupture during gait: Part II – alterations in forefoot loading. *Foot Ankle Int.* 1999;20:89–96.

3. Kinley S, Frascone S, Calderone D, et al. Endoscopic plantar fasciotomy versus traditional heel spur surgery: A prospective study. *J Foot Ankle Surg.* 1993;32:595–603.

4. Shama SS, Kominsky SJ, Lemont H. Prevalence of non-painful heel spur and its relation to postural foot position. *J Am Podiatry Assoc.* 1983;73:122–123.

5. McMillan AM, Landorf KB, Barrett JT, et al. Diagnostic imaging for chronic plantar heel pain: A systematic review and meta-analysis. *J Foot Ankle Res.* 2009;13:32.

6. Wearing SC, Smeathers JE, Urry SR, et al. Plantar enthesopathy: Thickening of the enthesis is correlated with energy dissipation of the plantar fat pad during walking. *Am J Sports Med.* 2010;38:2522–2527.

7. Fabrikant JM, Park TS. Plantar fasciitis (fasciosis) treatment outcome study: Plantar fascia thickness measured by ultrasound and correlated with patient self-reported improvement. *Foot (Edinb).* 2011;21:79–83.

8. Berkowitz JF, Kier R, Rudicel S. Plantar fasciitis: MR imaging. *Radiology.* 1991;179:665–667.

9. Chimutengwende-Gordon M, O'Donnell P, Singh D. Magnetic resonance imaging in plantar heel pain. *Foot Ankle Int.* 2010;10:865–870.

10. DiGiovanni BF, Nawoczenski DA, Malay DP, et al. Plantar fascia-specific stretching exercise improves outcomes in patients with chronic plantar fasciitis: A prospective clinical trial with two-year follow-up. *J Bone Joint Surg Am.* 2006;88A:1775–1781.

11. Rompe JD, Cacchio A, Weil L Jr, et al. Plantar fascia-specific stretching versus radial shock-wave therapy as initial treatment of plantar fasciopathy. *J Bone Joint Surg Am.* 2010;92A:2514–2522.

12. Powell M, Post WR, Keener J, et al. Effective treatment of chronic plantar fasciitis with dorsiflexion night splints: A crossover prospective randomized outcome study. *Foot Ankle Int.* 1998;19:10–18.

13. Probe RA, Baca M, Adams R, et al. Night splint treatment for plantar fasciitis, a prospective randomized study. *Clin Orthop Relat Res.* 1999;368:190–195.

14. Gross MT, Byers JM, Krafft JL, et al. The impact of custom semirigid foot orthotics on pain and disability for individuals with plantar fasciitis. *J Orthop Sports Phys Therapy.* 2002;32:149–157.

15. Seligman DA, Dawson DR. Customized heel pads and soft orthotics to treat heel pain and plantar fasciitis. *Arch Phys Med Rehabil.* 2003;84:1564–1567.

16. Metzner G, Dohnalek C, Aigner E. High-energy extracorporeal shock-wave therapy (ESWT) for the treatment of chronic plantar fasciitis. *Foot Ankle Int.* 2010;31:790–796.

17. Lee GP, Ogden JA, Cross GL. Effect of extracorporeal shock waves on calcaneal bone spurs. *Foot Ankle Int.* 2003;24:927–930.

18. Gerdesmeyer L, Frey C, Vester J, et al. Radial extracorporeal shock wave therapy is safe and effective in the treatment of chronic recalcitrant plantar fasciitis: Results of a confirmatory randomized placebo-controlled multicenter study. *Am J Sports Med.* 2008;36:2100–2109.

19. Barrett SL, Day SV, Brown MG. Endoscopic plantar fasciotomy: Preliminary study with cadaveric specimens. *J Foot Surg.* 1991;30:170–172.

20. Tomczak RL, Haverstock BD. A retrospective comparison of endoscopic plantar fasciotomy to open plantar fasciotomy with heel spur resection for chronic plantar fasciitis/heel spur syndrome. *J Foot Ankle Surg.* 1995;34:305–311.

21. Barrett SL, Day SV, Pignetti TT, et al. Endoscopic plantar fasciotomy: A multi-surgeon prospective analysis of 652 cases. *J Foot Ankle Surg.* 1995;34:400–406.

22. O'Malley MJ, Page A, Cook R. Endoscopic plantar fasciotomy for chronic heel pain. *Foot Ankle Int.* 2000;21:505–510.

23. Boyle RA, Slater GL. Endoscopic plantar fascia release: A case series. *Foot Ankle Int.* 2003;24:176–179.

24. Hogan KA, Webb D, Shereff M. Endoscopic plantar fascia release. *Foot Ankle Int.* 2004;25:875–881.

25. Bazaz R, Ferkel RD. Results of endoscopic plantar fascia release. *Foot Ankle Int.* 2007;28:549–556.

26. Barrett SL, Day SV. Endoscopic plantar fasciotomy for chronic plantar fasciitis/heel spur syndrome: Surgical technique–early clinical results. *J Foot Surg.* 1991;30:568–570.

27. Saxena A. Uniportal endoscopic plantar fasciotomy: A prospective study on athletic patients. *Foot Ankle Int.* 2004;25:882–889.

28. Komatsu F, Takao M, Innami K, et al. Endoscopic surgery for plantar fasciitis: Application of a deep-fascial approach. *Arthroscopy.* 2011;27:1105–1109.

29. Chan LK, Lui TH, Chan KB. Anatomy of the portal tract for endoscopic decompression of the first branch of the lateral plantar nerve. *Arthroscopy.* 2008;24:1284–1288.

Endoscopic Compartment Release for Chronic Exertional Compartment Syndrome

Jeremy T. Smith   Eric M. Bluman

INDICATIONS

Compartment syndrome is defined as an elevated pressure within a closed muscular compartment that limits vascular perfusion to the contents of that compartment. This ischemia can lead to pain and tissue injury. Compartment syndrome can occur both in the acute and chronic settings. Acute compartment syndrome, which often results from trauma, is characterized by a progressive rapid onset and often requires urgent compartment release. Chronic compartment syndrome, in contrast, is typically recurrent and results from exercise-induced muscle swelling. This swelling can increase the compartment volume by as much as 20% of the resting muscle volume with strenuous exercise.[1] This is referred to as chronic exertional compartment syndrome (CECS).

The most common sites affected by CECS are the leg, thigh, and forearm. The leg has four fibroosseous compartments: anterior compartment (tibialis anterior muscle, extensor hallucis longus muscle, extensor digitorum longus muscle, deep peroneal nerve, anterior tibial artery), lateral compartment (peroneal muscles, superficial peroneal nerve [SPN]), superficial posterior compartment (gastrocnemius and soleus muscles, sural nerve), and deep posterior compartment (tibialis posterior muscle, flexor digitorum longus muscle, flexor hallucis longus muscle, posterior tibial nerve, posterior tibial artery). CECS most commonly affects the anterior and deep posterior compartments of the leg,[2] with bilateral symptoms reported in 37% to 82% of patients.[3–6]

The diagnosis of CECS is made by history, examination, and compartmental pressure measurement. Patients with CECS typically report aching discomfort that occurs with exercise. With persistent exertion, the pain often reaches a level that requires the individual to stop activities. Numbness or tingling can accompany this discomfort as the structures within the compartment experience transient ischemia. Most patients report resolution of symptoms with rest. In the office, the examination may be quite unremarkable unless the patient is asked to replicate the provocative exertion by jogging or running stairs, for example. With exertion, a fullness of the muscle compartment may be present and be accompanied by a decrease in distal sensation. Foot drop on the affected side(s) may also be observed. When concern for CECS exists, invasive compartment pressure measurement is helpful to confirm the diagnosis and determine which compartment(s) is involved. Pressure measurement in each compartment is often taken at rest, 1 minute post exercise, and 5 minutes post exercise. The type of exercise performed may vary and should provoke the patient's symptoms. The criteria for CECS typically used is a resting pressure ≥15 mm Hg, and/or a pressure 1 minute after exercise ≥30 mm Hg, and/or a pressure 5 minutes after exercise ≥20 mm Hg.[7]

Nonsurgical management of CECS typically requires activity modification such that compartment pressures do not reach a critical level. Many athletes are not willing to accept this and surgical compartment release offers an alternative. Fasciotomy has been shown to be effective in relieving pain and allowing return to activities.[6,8–10] Fasciotomy has been described with different techniques, including open techniques, mini-open techniques, and endoscopic techniques.[1,3,4,6,8–10] An interest in smaller incisions has been brought about by a theoretical decreased risk of wound problems and an interest in improved cosmesis. Some of the smaller incision techniques limit visualization and therefore risk nerve injury. Endoscopic fasciotomy offers an alternative to open procedures and can improve visualization through limited incisions while reducing the risk of wound complications and improving cosmesis.

PATIENT POSITIONING

The patient is placed supine on the operating room table and a thigh tourniquet is applied. A peripheral nerve block is used for the majority of patients. Folded blankets are placed under the ipsilateral hip and buttock as necessary to internally rotate the operative extremity. Both extremities are prepped if bilateral extremity compartment release is to be performed (Fig. 9–1).

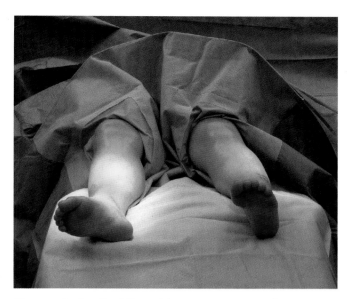

Figure 9–1.   For bilateral leg compartment release, both extremities are prepped into the field using a double extremity drape.

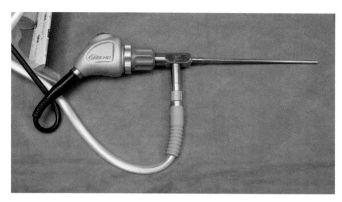

Figure 9–2.   A 30-degree 4-mm arthroscope is utilized for endoscopic compartment release.

SURGICAL TECHNIQUE

Esmarch exsanguination of the limb is performed and the thigh tourniquet is inflated. To release the anterior and lateral compartments, a 2 cm incision is made at the proximal leg between Gerdy tubercle and the fibular head overlying the intermuscular septum. Dissection is carried down to the level of the deep fascia. A second 2 cm incision is made 12 to 15 cm above the ankle joint along the intermuscular septum, in the region where the SPN exits the crural fascia. A Cobb elevator is inserted through the proximal incision into the plane between the deep fascia and the overlying tissue. This elevator is passed distally to create a working space superficial to the deep fascia, enabling access to both the anterior and lateral compartment fascia. The Cobb is similarly used to free up the deep fascia through the distal incision, with care taken to avoid the SPN. Optimally the SPN is directly visualized at the level of the distal incision.

An endoscopic compartment release is then performed using a 30-degree 4-mm arthroscope (Fig. 9–2). The arthroscope is passed proximally through the distal incision to the level of the proximal incision, shifting slightly anteriorly to clearly visualize the anterior compartment fascia. Through the proximal incision a small cut is made in the fascia of the anterior compartment with a knife. Long Metzenbaum scissors are then used to cut the fascia from proximally to distally under direct endoscopic visualization (Fig. 9–3). The scissors are followed with the endoscope as the fascia is cut (Fig. 9–4). Complete release of the fascia is confirmed by endoscopic visualization (Fig. 9–5). Near the distal extent of the incision, care is again taken to avoid injury to the SPN, which can often be visualized (Fig. 9–6). For lateral compartment release,

the scope is passed again to the level of the proximal incision and the lateral compartment is released using a similar technique. At times, fat tethered to the deep fascia can limit the view. In this situation, the Cobb elevator is again used to clear off the deep fascia. Overlying

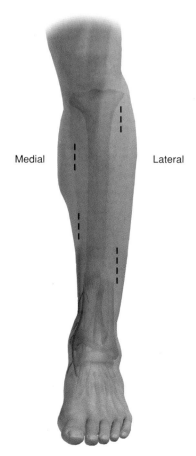

Medial   Lateral

Figure 9–3.   Illustration depicting the arthroscope inserted from distal to proximal to allow visualization of the long Metzenbaum scissors which have been inserted into the proximal incision.

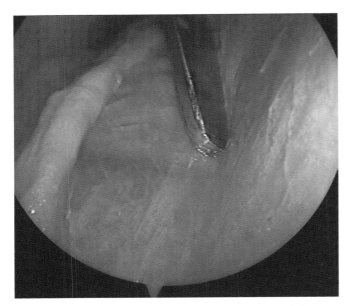

Figure 9–4. Through the arthroscope the tips of the scissors are visualized cutting the fascia.

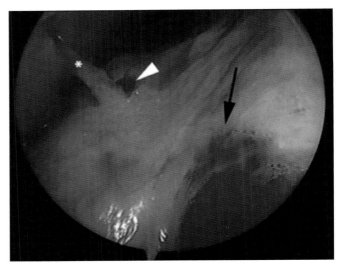

Figure 9–6. The superficial peroneal nerve (*asterisk*) can be visualized as it travels through the meatus (*arrowhead*) in the crural fascia. The apex of the cut fascia of the lateral compartment is shown (*arrow*).

integument that inhibits visualization can be elevated with towel clamps placed through the skin.

The posterior compartments are also accessed and released endoscopically. Two 2 cm incisions are made just posterior to the medial border of the tibia, at a level determined by dividing the leg into thirds and placing the incisions ⅓ and ⅔ down the length of the leg (Fig. 9–7). The Cobb elevator is used to free the fascia from adherent soft tissue both proximally and distally. Towel clips may be used to elevate the overhanging soft tissue and increase the working cavity. The fascia of the superficial posterior compartment is released longitudinally under

endoscopic visualization. This permits access to the deep posterior compartment, which is released off of the posterior border of the tibia using the long Metzenbaum scissors.

Wittstein et al.[9] have described a technique of endoscopic lower extremity compartment release using a balloon dilator. This technique is similar to our described technique although the anterior and lateral compartments are released through a single proximal incision. A balloon dilator is passed distally and inflated to create a cavity overlying the deep fascia. The balloon is then removed and the release performed endoscopically. The posterior compartments are accessed through a small incision just medial to the tibial crest also with balloon dilation with maintenance of the cavity using towel clips.

Our preference is to close the incisions in layers with a monofilament subdermal suture and then nylon for the skin. A soft sterile dressing is applied with mild compression over the incisions and a tall walking boot is applied.

COMPLICATIONS

Complications of fasciotomy for CECS may include nerve injury (specifically SPN), hemorrhage, deep venous thrombosis, wound infection, and recurrence of symptoms. Although no comparative studies exist, one potential advantage of endoscopic fasciotomy is improved visualization and therefore decreased risk of nerve injury. At this time, only one study exists reporting the outcomes and complications of this technique.[9] Of 14 legs, no nerve injuries occurred. Two patients developed a postoperative hematoma.

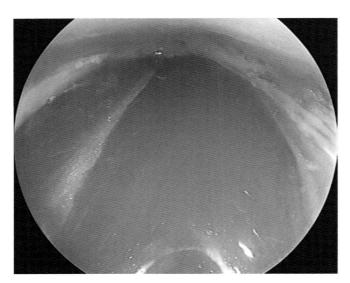

Figure 9–5. Complete release of the fascia should be confirmed endoscopically. The muscle here is seen free of overlying fascia.

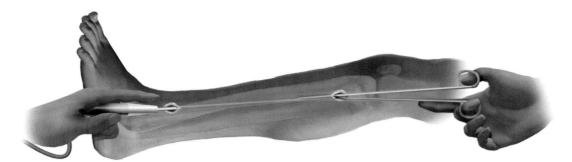

Figure 9–7. Illustration depicting the placement of portals for release of the superficial and deep posterior compartments.

REHABILITATION PROTOCOL

A tall walking boot is used for several weeks for patient comfort. Elevation of the leg postoperatively is encouraged. Although crutches are provided, patients may weight bear as tolerated. Patients typically use the crutches for the first 2 weeks for comfort. Sutures are removed 2 weeks postoperatively. Patients are encouraged to begin exercise on a stationary bicycle at roughly 3 weeks. A return to unrestricted athletics is typically possible by 6 weeks.

OUTCOMES

Wittstein et al.[9] reported the outcomes of an endoscopic fasciotomy technique using a balloon dissector in nine patients (14 legs). Mean duration of follow-up was

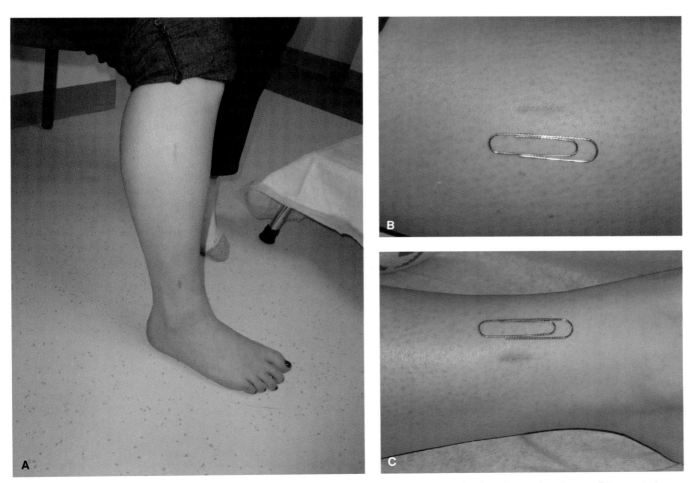

Figure 9–8. **A:** Image of the healed incisions on the lateral leg in a patient who had endoscopic release of the anterior and lateral compartments of the leg. Close-ups of the **(B)** proximal and **(C)** distal incisions with paper clip shown for scale.

3.75 years. Compartment release ranged from a single compartment to release of all four compartments. Of the nine patients, eight were able to return to full athletics (five at an intercollegiate level). The average time to return to preoperative athletic level was 4.7 months. There were no neurovascular injuries reported and no recurrence of symptoms (Fig. 9–8).

REFERENCES

1. Fronek J, Mubarak SJ, Hargens AR, et al. Management of chronic exertional anterior compartment syndrome of the lower extremity. *Clin Orthop Relat Res.* 1987;(220):217–227.
2. Martens MA, Moeyersoons JP. Acute and recurrent effort-related compartment syndrome in sports. *Sports Med.* 1990;9:62–68.
3. Detmer DE, Sharpe K, Sufit RL, et al. Chronic compartment syndrome: Diagnosis, management, and outcomes. *Am J Sports Med.* 1985;13:162–170.
4. Schepsis AA, Martini D, Corbett M. Surgical management of exertional compartment syndrome of the lower leg. Long-term followup. *Am J Sports Med.* 1993;21:811–817.
5. Schepsis AA, Gill SS, Foster TA. Fasciotomy for exertional anterior compartment syndrome: Is lateral compartment release necessary? *Am J Sports Med.* 1999;27:430–435.
6. Styf JR, Korner LM. Chronic anterior-compartment syndrome of the leg. Results of treatment by fasciotomy. *J Bone Joint Surg Am.* 1986;68:1338–1347.
7. Pedowitz RA, Hargens AR, Mubarak SJ, et al. Modified criteria for the objective diagnosis of chronic compartment syndrome of the leg. *Am J Sports Med.* 1990;18:35–40.
8. Rorabeck CH, Fowler PJ, Nott L. The results of fasciotomy in the management of chronic exertional compartment syndrome. *Am J Sports Med.* 1988;16:224–227.
9. Wittstein J, Moorman CT, 3rd, Levin LS. Endoscopic compartment release for chronic exertional compartment syndrome: Surgical technique and results. *Am J Sports Med.* 2010;38:1661–1666.
10. Raikin SM, Rapuri VR, Vitanzo P. Bilateral simultaneous fasciotomy for chronic exertional compartment syndrome. *Foot Ankle Int.* 2005;26:1007–1011.

CHAPTER 10

Mini-Open Ankle Arthrodesis

Christopher P. Chiodo   Eric M. Bluman

INDICATIONS

Tibiotalar arthrodesis is indicated for symptomatic ankle arthritis that sufficiently interferes with activities of daily living and has not responded to several months of nonoperative therapy. Potential nonoperative interventions include anti-inflammatory medications, bracing, and cortisone injections. In older and less active individuals, arthroplasty may be considered. However, for most younger and higher-demand patients with advanced disease, arthrodesis remains the surgical treatment of choice. When considering less-invasive procedures deformity should be minimal, especially with an attempted arthroscopic procedure.

Absolute contraindications for less-invasive arthrodesis include active infection, advanced deformity that necessitates fibular osteotomy and/or flat bone cuts, as well as inability to comply with the postoperative regimen. Relative contraindications include moderate deformity, the presence of advanced cystic disease, and nicotine dependence. In some patients with a compromised soft tissue envelope a less-invasive technique may be tolerated where a traditional open procedure would not.

PATIENT POSITIONING

For the mini-arthrotomy technique, the patient is positioned supine. The ipsilateral hip is bumped if necessary such that the toes point toward the ceiling and both sides of the ankle are accessible. It is also helpful to elevate the operative leg on a foam wedge or stack of blankets (Fig. 10–1). This facilitates access to the ankle as well as facilitating intraoperative imaging. Intraoperative

fluoroscopy is necessary to guide and confirm proper fixation and alignment.

Regional anesthesia, specifically a long-acting popliteal and saphenous nerve block, is advantageous and used whenever possible. This allows the majority of procedures to be performed on an outpatient basis.

SURGICAL APPROACH AND TECHNIQUES

With the arthroscopic technique, standard anteromedial and anterolateral arthroscopy portals are utilized, just adjacent to the anterior tibial and peroneus quartius tendons, respectively. One portal is used for visualization while the other is used as a working portal. An accessory posterolateral portal, located in the interval between the Achilles and peroneal tendons, can also be used if necessary. Cartilage is removed with arthroscopic instruments and then the subchondral bone is prepared with a burr.

With the mini-arthrotomy technique, two longitudinal incisions, approximately 2 to 3 cm in length, are utilized (Fig. 10–2). The locations of these anterior incisions approximate those of the standard anterolateral and anteromedial ankle arthroscopy portals. The roles of these portals alternate during the surgery. One incision is used as a distraction portal while the other is used as a working portal (Fig. 10–3).

The first incision is centered over the joint line just medial to the anterior tibial tendon. The anterior joint is exposed and anterior osteophytes are resected. A Cobb elevator is then used to release the capsule anteriorly. Any scar tissue or synovium that may impede visualization is

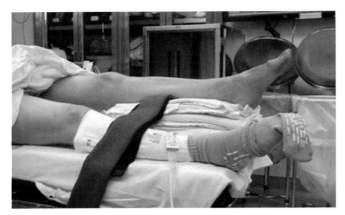

Figure 10–1. Patient positioning for the mini-arthrotomy technique.

removed. The lateral incision is made next and is positioned just lateral to the peroneus tertius tendon. Great care should be taken to protect the superficial peroneal nerve with subcutaneous dissection. These steps are all critical to adequately visualize the joint and ensure that it is actually "exposed" and not simply "approached."

A lamina spreader is inserted through the medial incision to distract the joint while a small Weitlaner retractor is placed laterally. The lateral aspect of the joint is then prepared according to the surgeon's preference. If a burr is used to perforate the subchondral bone, thermal necrosis may be minimized by copious irrigation and keeping the burr speed at or below 20,000 revolutions per minute.

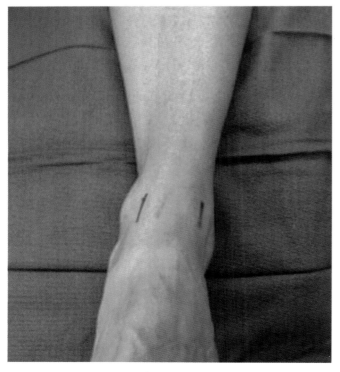

Figure 10–2. Incisions for the mini-arthrotomy technique.

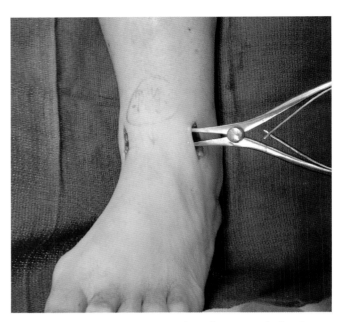

Figure 10–3. Distraction and working portals for the mini-arthrotomy technique. (From Bluman EM, Chiodo CP. Tibiotalar arthrodesis. *Semin Arthro.* 2010;21:240–246, Elsevier with permission.)

After preparing the articular surface, the deeper bone is drilled with a 2-mm bit. This allows bleeding and hematoma formation within the joint. A drill is preferred to a Kirschner wire because the flutes remove bone, rather than simply impacting it.

The instruments are alternated from one portal to another. The lamina spreader is placed laterally while the medial side of the joint is prepared as described above.

After preparation of the articular surfaces is complete, the joint is reduced. The talus is positioned in neutral dorsiflexion/plantarflexion, neutral to slight valgus, and slight external rotation to match the contralateral limb. Varus should be avoided. Also, careful attention must be paid to "dunking" the talus, that is, dorsiflexing it to neutral while also translating it posteriorly while maintaining neutral sagittal alignment. This decreases the lever arm effect of the foot thereby facilitating more efficient ambulation and, in the authors' opinion, may minimize the likelihood of developing arthritic change at the talonavicular joint.

Any residual voids in the joint, especially posteriorly, are filled with bone graft. Allograft, autograft, or a combination of the two, are all acceptable. Autograft, and in particular iliac crest graft or aspirate, should be considered in those patents at higher risk for nonunion (e.g., diabetics or those with prior trauma associated with soft tissue stripping). Biologic adjuvants may also be considered, especially when risk factors for nonunion are present.

Fixation is inserted percutaneously under fluoroscopic guidance and typically entails two or three large diameter (6.5 to 7.0 mm) cannulated screws. After provisional

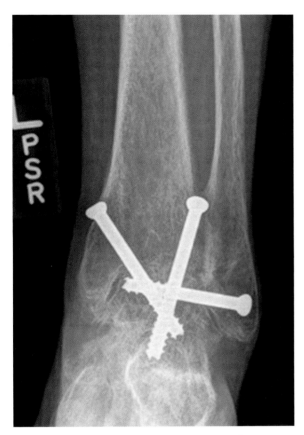

Figure 10–4. Typical percutaneous screw fixation.

fixation is obtained an initial "home-run" screw is inserted from proximal and posterolateral to distal and anteromedial. Proximally, it enters the posterior tibia in the region of the metaphyseal–diaphyseal junction. Distally, it runs within the talar neck. This screw is then augmented with one or two more screws inserted from proximal to distal. Finally, this construct may be augmented by an additional screw that runs from lateral to medial securing the distal fibula to the talus. This creates a rigid "box" construct (Fig. 10–4).

At the end of the case, there should be rigid fixation of well-perfused, well-aligned, and well-apposed bone.

REHABILITATION PROTOCOL

The incisions are closed in layers and a dry sterile compression dressing applied followed by a plaster splint. The patient is instructed to be nonweight bearing.

Consultation with a physical therapist is obtained, often preoperatively, to maximize safety and compliance with regard to nonweight bearing ambulation with crutches. At approximately 2 weeks postoperatively the sutures are removed and a short-leg, non–weight-bearing cast is applied. At 6 weeks postoperatively the cast is changed or, alternatively, switched to a CAM boot. The patient is kept nonweight bearing for another 3 to 6 weeks, based on the quality of bone and fixation, as well as anticipated compliance. Thereafter, weight bearing is progressed in a boot or shoe with a rocker bottom sole.

OUTCOME

Several authors have examined the clinical results of minimally invasive ankle arthrodesis. The mini-arthrotomy technique has been as successful as arthroscopically performed ankle arthrodesis.[1,2] Pioneering this technique, Myerson et al. demonstrated a 96% fusion rate in 32 patients at a mean of 8 weeks postoperatively. One patient had a non-union and two others had a delayed union. These authors also performed a cadaveric dye study demonstrating that this technique preserved the peroneal arterial circulation when compared to an open procedure.

COMPLICATIONS

Complications associated with minimally invasive ankle fusion are uncommon. The limited incisions used with this technique minimize the risks of wound healing problems and infection. Nonunion is also minimized by the minimal nature of the incisions as bony perfusion is nominally disrupted. The superficial peroneal nerve is at risk with the lateral incision and should be protected. The morbidity associated with injury to this structure should not be discounted, especially in the young, non-neuropathic patient.

REFERENCES

1. Miller SD, Paremain GP, Myerson MS. The miniarthrotomy technique of ankle arthrodesis: A cadaver study of operative vascular compromise and early clinical results. *Orthopedics*. 1996;19(5):425–430.
2. Paremain GD, Miller SD, Myerson MS. Ankle arthrodesis: Results after the miniarthrotomy technique. *Foot Ankle Int*. 1996;17(5):247–252.

CHAPTER 11

Arthroscopic Ankle Fusion Methods

Timothy C. Fitzgibbons   David J. Inda

INDICATIONS

Multiple open surgical techniques have been described for ankle arthrodesis. In the 1980s, advancements in arthroscopic instrumentation and techniques made arthroscopic ankle arthrodesis (AAA) feasible.

The early experience with AAA was fraught with many complications and discouraged many from doing the procedure. In 1996, our published complication rate using a skeletal pin distraction technique was 55%.[1] Almost all complications were due to the use of external distraction. After we discontinued using the external distraction, the complication rate significantly decreased. Other authors in the 1990s reported similar improved results.[2–14]

More recent reports in the literature have been quite favorable.[15–34] Ferkel in 2005 documented a 97% fusion rate with minimal complications.[19] Rinson, Robinson, and Allen in 2005 published a 92.4% fusion rate, shorter time to fusion and minor complications.[35] As noted above, our more recent experience has been similar.

This chapter describes our technique of arthroscopic ankle fusion that has evolved over a 20-year period. The general indications for arthroscopic ankle fusion are the same as for open ankle fusion: most commonly degenerative or inflammatory arthritis with loss of articular cartilage.

Critics have questioned the technique of arthroscopic ankle fusion claiming that it takes considerable time and effort to learn the procedure. Most studies demonstrate the fusion rates of open and arthroscopic techniques to be about the same.[36–41]

The advantages of AAA in our opinion are the following:

1. Maintenance of the inherent stability of the ankle makes it easier for positioning of the ankle in the optimum position at the time of screw insertion.
2. The technique preserves the fibula and medial malleolus for possible future total ankle arthroplasty.
3. There is decreased morbidity for the patient, especially less pain and fewer wound complications.

The disadvantages of AAA have been that it does not allow for the correction of significant deformities. However, we and others have found that with the addition of supplemental procedures such as calcaneal osteotomies, tendo Achilles lengthening, and dorsiflexion producing first metatarsal osteotomies the indications can be broadened to a larger population of patients (Table 11–1).

We feel that this procedure should be chosen if the surgeon is an experienced ankle arthroscopist and comfortable with this approach.

PATIENT POSITIONING AND EQUIPMENT

The patient is positioned on a regular operating table with a bump under the affected hip and padding of the other leg in anticipation of flexing the foot of the bed at the time of screw insertion.

We forego pin-based distraction techniques in favor of no distraction or simple noninvasive distraction using a foot strap apparatus (Fig. 11–1).

We place a high-thigh tourniquet on the patient's thigh, but it is not always inflated. The use of preoperative 0.25% Marcaine with epinephrine and adequate distention is usually adequate for intra-articular hemostasis without tourniquet inflation, but the tourniquet is available if visualization is not adequate. An infusion pump is used to facilitate adequate distention.

A sterile, padded Mayo stand is prepared. This is used at the end of the procedure in placing the screws and has been found to be quite helpful (Fig. 11–2).

Although a small joint arthroscopy set can be used, we have found that using the 4-mm 30-degree large joint arthroscope is better. Because there is no concern for "scuffing" the articular surface in these cases, a large arthroscope not only gives better visualization and better distension but also allows for better fragment evacuation.

The use of large joint shavers and burrs is also recommended. We use the 5-mm aggressive resectors, 4- or 5-mm round burrs and occasionally a 5-mm egg burr. In

TABLE 11–1. Arthroscopic Ankle Fusion

Advantages

1. Maintains inherent stability of the ankle
2. Preserves malleoli
3. Decreased morbidity

Disadvantages

1. Learning curve for the surgeon
2. Does not allow for correction of deformity—although addition of supplemental procedures does allow for expansion of indications

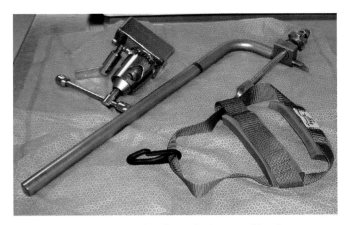

Figure 11–1. Example of a soft tissue ankle distractor used occasionally in arthroscopic ankle fusion.

the recent years, however, we have found that use of an aggressive resector only in combination with various size curettes is adequate. The use of these burrs can create large holes or furrows that are detrimental to maintaining optimally congruent fusion surfaces.

Other instruments include curved curettes, osteotomes, an inflow cannula, and large joint grasping tools (Fig. 11–3).

We routinely insert bone graft at the fusion site before inserting our fixation. Our protocol is to obtain bone marrow aspirate from the ipsilateral iliac crest using an 11-gauge bone marrow aspiration needle with a heparinized syringe. This is then mixed with demineralized

bone matrix powder and is injected into the joint prior to placement of fixation (Fig. 11–4). For this reason the iliac crest is prepped out.

SURGICAL APPROACHES

Standard anterior ankle arthroscopy is utilized. The anatomic landmarks have been well described by Ferkel and others. We do not use posterior arthroscopic portals. However, when placing our fixation, as will be described in the next section, we utilize a direct posterior Achilles tendon approach. Going directly through the Achilles tendon in the midline prevents trauma to the tibial nerve and other structures (Fig. 11–5).

It should be noted as the procedure progresses, these incisions can be enlarged, sometimes approaching a "mini-open" procedure. The enlarged portals allow insertion of standard (nonarthroscopic) osteotomes for feathering and preparation of the surfaces of the distal tibia and proximal talus.

SURGICAL TECHNIQUE

STEP ONE: Insertion of the arthroscope and instrumentation.

A no. 15 scalpel is used to incise the skin to establish standard anterior-lateral and anterior-medial portals. A mosquito forceps is utilized to carefully dissect down to the capsule while avoiding injury to the cutaneous nerves.

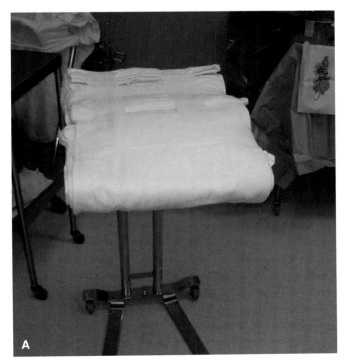
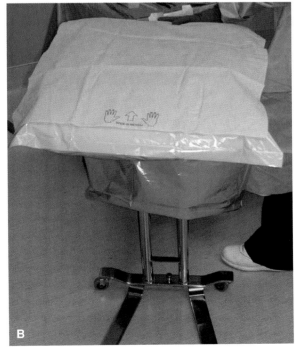

Figure 11–2. **A:** Padded Mayo stand used at time of home run and other screw insertion. **B:** Padded Mayo stand covered with a sterile drape.

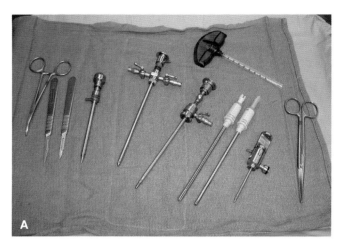
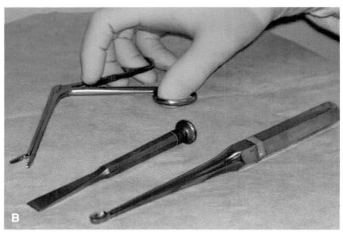

Figure 11–3. **A:** Equipment for an arthroscopic ankle fusion: note both large and small arthroscopic cannulae but large aggressive resectors. Also pictured, 11-gauge iliac crest bone marrow aspiration needle. **B:** Curette, osteotome, and rasping forceps.

A larger arthroscope with a blunt trocar is inserted either anteromedially or anterolaterally. Once initial visualization is obtained the other incision is made. The same dissection technique is used. The blunt trocar from the arthroscope is used to make a small capsulotomy followed by insertion of a large joint aggressive resector.

STEP TWO: Subtotal synovectomy and excision of soft tissues to obtain visualization.

At this point, depending on the severity of the arthritic change, visualization can be difficult. There are some cases where the surgeon will need to "burrow" into the joint to obtain exposure. Soft tissue distraction can be helpful as noted above, but taking time to resect excess soft tissues, proliferative synovium, and in some cases articular surface fragments is necessary to obtain proper visualization. In these cases, dramatic improvement in visualization is obtained. This part of the procedure is usually very minimal, but there are some cases where it can take a number of minutes. An oscillating full radius resector with suction is used to clean out the joint.

STEP THREE: Removal of the remaining cartilage from the articular surfaces.

In patients with a large amount of cartilage denudation this step can be done quite quickly but can take longer

Figure 11–4. Example of demineralized bone matrix—mixed with iliac crest bone marrow aspirate and injected into the ankle joint before inserting fixation.

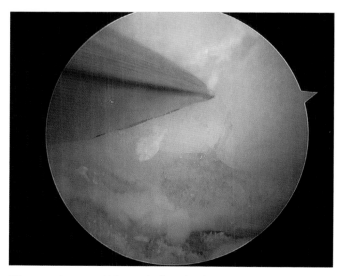

Figure 11–5. When placing the home run screw go directly through the center of the Achilles tendon. This prevents trauma to the posterior tibial nerve and other structures.

with greater amounts of intact cartilage. We use the large joint aggressive resector on continuous high speed or various sized curettes to accomplish this part of the procedure. Although various types of burrs are available, we have found that it is easy to excavate larger holes than are necessary and feel that the control and visualization with a large curette or the aggressive resector is better. Again, the curettes used are standard curettes, not the small joint curettes designed for arthroscopic débridement of an OCD lesion. During this part of the procedure, a so-called "snow storm" or "whiteout" can occur from cartilage and subchondral bone fragments becoming suspended in the arthroscopy fluid. Periodically the surgeon needs to clear the fluid with suction or the large cannula alone.

Any surface area that will fuse together will improve the fusion mass. As such, it is very important that the articular cartilage from both sides of the medial gutter be removed. On the fibular side, only occasionally will a fibulotalar fusion occur. We, however, routinely remove the cartilage from that gutter also, although it is not as crucial. Although a satisfactory tibiotalar arthrodesis can occur if not all of the articular cartilage is removed, it is recommended to try to remove as much or all of the articular cartilage on both sides of the joint as best as possible.

STEP FOUR: "Feathering" of the joint surface.

This is one of the most important parts of the procedure. If the surgeon simply removes the articular cartilage leaving hard, eburnated bone, no matter how much fixation or bone graft is inserted, many of these patients will not achieve satisfactory arthrodesis. We have found that an aggressive feathering of these surfaces is crucial to a successful and expedient arthrodesis. It is at this point that the anterior-medial and anterior-lateral incisions may be enlarged. Under direct visualization, osteotomes from a standard orthopedic instrument tray are used (Fig. 11–6A). Straight or curved osteotomes can be used. Effective penetration of the osteotome can be as much as 5 mm from the subchondral bone surface. The feathering process can be supplemented with the use of the threaded guide pin from the cannulated screw set that will be used for eventual fixation, especially in those areas that are somewhat difficult to get to. In the gutters, final use of a curette aggressively is sometimes adequate. After completion, the surgeon should see soft cancellous surfaces on both sides of the joint (Fig. 11–6B).

STEP FIVE: Bone grafting.

After joint preparation but before hardware insertion it is our standard to insert biologics to help facilitate arthrodesis. In most cases this consists of bone marrow aspirated from the ipsilateral iliac crest. The crest is prepped out as part of the original prepping and draping. An 11-gauge aspiration needle is inserted into the ilium through a small skin incision. Using careful manual pressure or a small mallet, the needle is advanced into the iliac crest between the two tables of bone. Using a heparinized syringe, bone marrow is aspirated in 2½-cc aliquots.

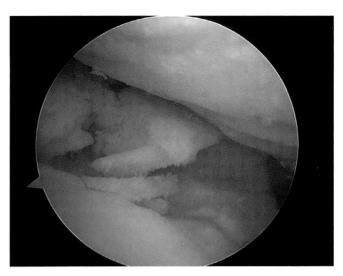

Figure 11–6.   A: Example of "feathering" using a small osteotome. **B:** Appearance of the ankle joint after aggressive feathering.

The aspiration needle is rotated 90 degrees between each aspiration. This bone marrow then is mixed with demineralized bone matrix powder. It is important that the final mixture of the bone marrow and the demineralized bone matrix results in a slurry-like consistency, as it is easier to inject into the joint. The mixture then is injected into the joint usually through the arthroscopic cannula. The blunt trocar can be used to smooth out the bone graft if necessary. The arthroscope is usually left in one of the portals when the bone graft is injected to document proper positioning. At this point, the arthroscopic portion of the procedure is concluded.

STEP SIX: Tendo Achilles lengthening.

We routinely perform a tendo Achilles lengthening using the Hoke triple incision technique to maximizing dorsiflexion. If the surgeon feels more comfortable performing a gastrocnemius recession, it can also be performed, but in our experience, the Hoke is easier and more expedient (Fig. 11–7).

STEP SEVEN: Insertion of internal fixation.

As originally described by Hansen et al., our standard fixation has been the use of percutaneously inserted, partially threaded, cannulated screws with the initial screw being the "home run" screw placed from posterior through the Achilles tendon, into the tibia, and subsequently into the talar neck.[42] This initial screw is meant to draw the talus back into the tibia thereby "ducking" the talus posteriorly under the tibia as well as providing compression and fixation. Placing this posterior screw is more challenging with the patient in a supine position. Just before placing the guide wire we have the circulating nurse remove the bump from the ipsilateral buttock. We then drop the end of the operative table making it vertical. Great care is taken by the nurses to make sure the contralateral leg is well padded and protected. The

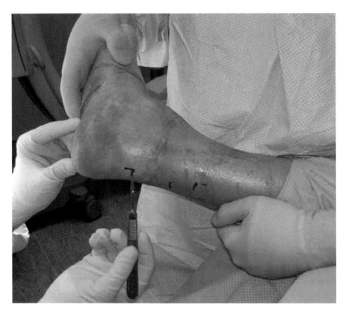

Figure 11–7. Example of Achilles tendon lengthening using the Hoke 3 incision technique.

padded Mayo stand that has been previously draped is brought in. The surgical foot is placed on the radiolucent padded Mayo stand, and because of the bump under the buttock has been removed the leg will now very easily externally rotate. With the contralateral knee flexed, this allows the surgeon to sit in a chair in front of the non-operative knee and have direct access to the posterior aspect of the operative ankle. With the assistant holding the ankle at 90 degrees and correcting any varus or valgus that may have been present, the surgeon can then place the cannulated screw guide pin percutaneously through the central portion of the Achilles tendon and subsequently through the tibia.

In most cases, the fluoroscopy unit is brought in from the nonoperative side. In the arthroscopic ankle fusion technique, we prefer to bring the fluoroscopy unit in from the ipsilateral side. The fluoroscope beam oriented vertically with respect to the floor will result in a lateral view on the fluoroscopic image because the leg is so externally rotated.

Over the years, we have used various sized partially threaded cannulated cancellous screws with the maximum size being 7.3 mm. Recently in an effort to get more than one home run screw in, we downsized to either the 7.0-mm screws or even 6.5 mm diameters. Stainless steel or titanium screws may be used.

The cannulated screw guide pin, again, is placed directly through the center of the Achilles tendon through the posterior aspect of the tibia and ultimately into the talar neck (see Fig. 11.18). With this approach, it is very easy to be too lateral in the talar neck, so the surgeon must take care to try to direct the guide pin centrally in the talar neck to be sure there is good purchase. Once the initial guide pin is placed under fluoroscopic guidance, the

Mayo stand must be removed temporarily, and the knee flexed to approximately 80 degrees to allow an antero-posterior fluoroscopic image of the talus and the navicular area to visualize the guide pin being in the talar neck. This can be somewhat difficult, and care must be taken to prevent the pin from perforating the drapes, as it extends out from the posterior leg. Once the guide pin is found to be well positioned, a screw can be inserted percutaneously.

In our initial procedures, we placed one home run screw, one screw from the medial malleolus and one from the lateral malleolus. We now insert more than one home run screw as it is the screw that gives the best fixation in many cases. The guide pins can all be placed before the insertion of any screws.

Once the home run screws are inserted, the foot can be brought from external rotation to a position where the toes point to the ceiling. This sometimes requires an assistant rotating the extremity through the hip. The leg is again placed on the padded Mayo stand. The fluoroscopy unit can be brought in underneath the Mayo stand, and an excellent AP view of the ankle can be obtained. A screw is then inserted from the medial malleolus into the talus, and, if possible, a screw is placed through the fibula into the talus. Since you may have as many as three home run screws in the talar neck, the screws coming from medial and lateral have to be placed more posteriorly. Care is taken to not penetrate the subtalar joint. Most of the time, these screws are short, and the fixation is not as good as the home run screws, but they contribute to the construct stability (Figs. 11–8, 11–9A,B, 11–10A,B). A screw can also be placed from the lateral distal tibia into the talus (Fig. 11–11A,B).

Previously placed hardware can be used to improve construct stability. For example, if a lateral fibular plate is present from a previous fracture the distal screws can be removed and replaced with longer screws that allow fixation of the fibula to the talus (Fig. 11–12). The use of headless screws has also been described.[43] Yoshimura et al.[44] recently published their study of fixation methods and concluded three parallel screws from the medial tibia to the talus produced the fastest union (Fig. 11–13).

STEP EIGHT: Supplemental procedures.

As noted above, one of the contraindications for arthroscopic ankle fusion has been excess deformity. We have found these indications can be expanded if supplemental procedures are done. If a medial or lateral displacement calcaneal osteotomy or a dorsiflexion first metatarsal osteotomy are necessary, it is usually at this time that we perform those procedures (Fig. 11–14A,B).

TRICKS AND TIPS

A few tips to help you:

1. If you become "lost" during the procedure – especially during removal of the cartilage from the gutters – LOOK AWAY from the monitor and look at

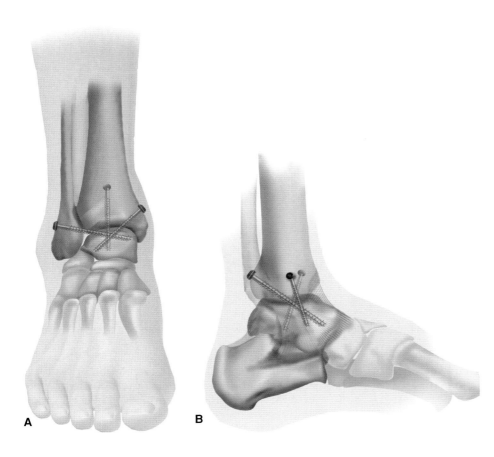

Figure 11–8.   **A:** AP and **B:** lateral view of the traditional "home run screw" technique, 1 screw from the posterior tibia into the talar neck, 1 screw from the fibula into the talus, and 1 screw from the medial tibia into the talus.

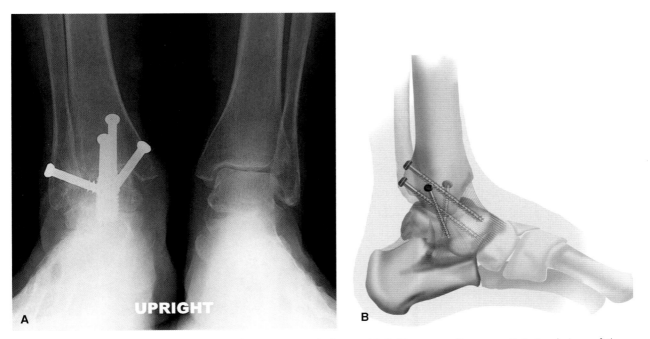

Figure 11–9.   **A:** AP of the ankle showing the 4 screw technique with 2 "home run" screws. **B:** Lateral view of the 4 screw technique with 2 "home run" screws.

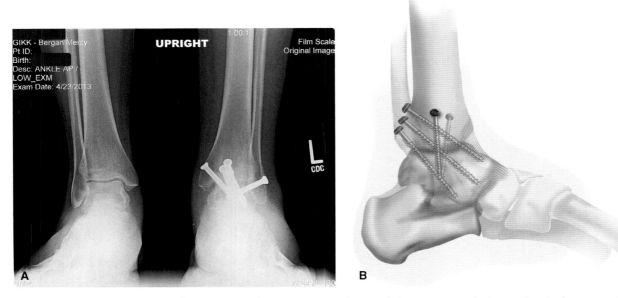

Figure 11–10. **A:** AP example of a 5 screw technique. **B:** Lateral view of the 5 screw technique using 3 "home run" screws.

the ankle. You know the anatomy. Put your finger or thumb on the malleoli and use a curette to clean out the gutters (Fig. 11–15A,B).

2. If you are having trouble evacuating the debris from the joint use a large cannula to drain the joint (Fig. 11–16).

3. Use a 4-mm arthroscope and large joint resectors to give you better visualization and better evacuation of debris (Fig. 11–17).

4. Adapt the composition and orientation of your fixation. Use the combination of screws that works best for your patient's anatomy. In general, more fixation is better than less.

5. Use the padded Mayo stand technique to insert your "home run" screw. Foot of bed flexed, bump removed from ipsilateral buttock to allow for external rotation. One good positioning has the primary surgeon sit while assistant holds ankle in

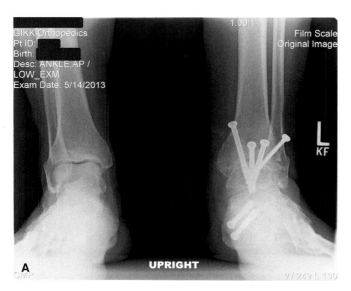

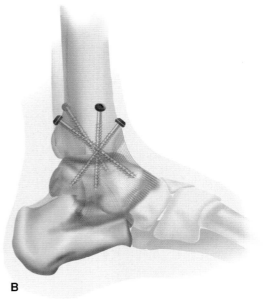

Figure 11–11. **A:** AP x-ray depicting variation of the technique with 1 "home run" screw, 1 anterior-medial screw, 1 anterior-lateral screw, and a fully threaded screw across the fibular-talar joint. **B:** Lateral x-ray depicting this technique variation.

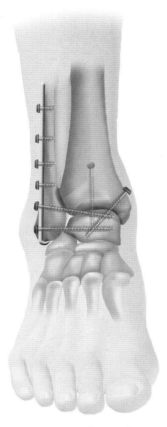

Figure 11–12. Depiction of an arthroscopic ankle fusion with previous open reduction and internal fixation with a fibular plate. Note the fibular plate is left in. Two of the small fragment screws have been removed and have been replaced with longer, partially threaded screws.

proper position. The fluoroscope comes in from the ipsilateral side (Fig. 11–18).

COMPLICATIONS

As noted above in our initial series with the use of skeletal distraction techniques, our complication rate was greater than 50%, almost exclusively due to the problems associated with pin tracts. This included pin tract infections and stress fractures. After we discontinued the use of skeletal distraction, complications associated with AAA have been minimal. Nonunion using arthroscopic method occurs 5% to 8% depending on which study is reviewed. However, in our experience, even if there is incomplete union, despite adequate fixation, many of these patients do quite well with a painless nonunion.

If painful nonunion does occur, either a revision arthroscopic ankle fusion is performed or an open fusion is performed. We now use supplemental fixation in some of these patients. Bone marrow may be aspirated and inserted into the nonfusion site; as may morselized bone

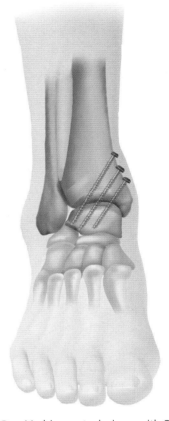

Figure 11–13. Yoshimura technique with 3 medial screws.

graft. Supplemental percutaneous screws are inserted, if required.

Nerve injuries can occur in any arthroscopic procedure. The most common injuries are paresthesias of neuropraxic origin associated with the sensory nerves in and around their arthroscopic portals. These injuries are usually self-limited but can be symptomatically treated with physiotherapy and associated modalities.

REHABILITATION PROTOCOL

Patients may or may not be admitted overnight. Although arthroscopically aided arthrodesis is usually much less painful than the traditional open procedures a supplemental regional anesthetic block is performed in most patients. If not performed preoperatively, it may be done in the recovery room. Two weeks postoperatively or before the patient is placed in a short-leg well-padded non–weight-bearing fiberglass cast.

At 1 month from surgery, the patient's cast is removed, all sutures are removed, and x-rays are obtained. If all is well, a short-leg well-padded fiberglass cast is reapplied. Progressive weight bearing may be started as early as 5 weeks postoperatively, although some wait a few weeks longer. Weight bearing is started with 25% body weight for the first couple

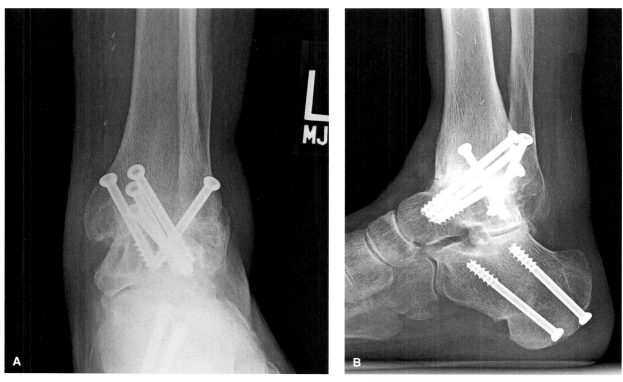

Figure 11–14. **A:** AP view of an arthroscopic ankle fusion with 5 arthroscopic ankle fusion screws with additional lateral displacement calcaneal osteotomy for cavus deformity. **B:** Lateral x-ray depicting the arthroscopic ankle fusion with lateral displacement calcaneal osteotomy.

of days, then 50% body weight for a couple of days, with gradual weaning away from crutches completely.

Cannon, Brown, and Cooke in 2004 published a study comparing early to late weight bearing that concluded patients who were allowed to weight bear immediately did just as well as those patients who began weight bearing at 8 weeks.[45]

Two months following surgery the cast is removed, and x-rays are obtained. If all is well, the patient is placed in a removable walking boot and is allowed to weight

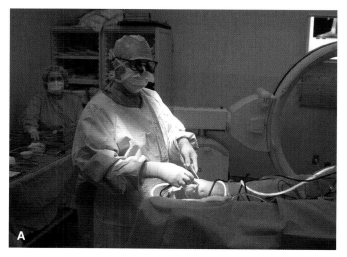
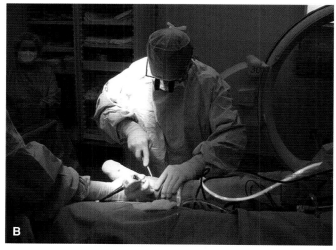

Figure 11–15. **A:** Example of surgeon viewing the monitor during the arthroscopic ankle fusion. **B:** Example of surgeon taking his head away from the monitor looking directly at the ankle to help with completing the procedure especially in the medial and lateral gutters. Always remember you know your anatomy and looking directly at the ankle structures can help with completing the joint preparation.

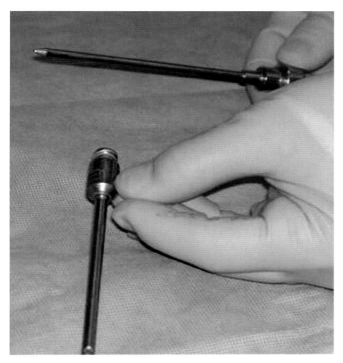

Figure 11–16. Example of a large Dyonics cannula used to help remove some of the larger fragments during the arthroscopic preparation.

bear as tolerated. The patient is allowed to remove the boot for range-of-motion exercises but is required to have the boot on for weight bearing

At 3 months x-rays are obtained. If there is satisfactory evidence of bony consolidation, we recommend the patient be fitted with an extra depth shoe with a soft insole and a rocker bottom sole. The patient is then

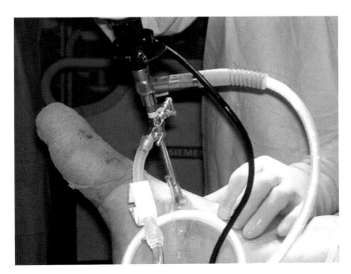

Figure 11–17. Picture depicting the use of the large arthroscope rather than the small arthroscope for this procedure. This helps not only with visualization but also with irrigation and evacuation of large fragments.

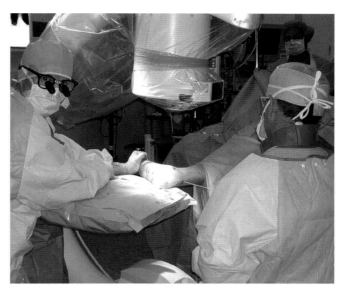

Figure 11–18. Example of the surgeon and assistant inserting the home run screw. Note that the bump has been removed from the patient's buttock allowing the leg to be externally rotated. The foot is placed on the padded Mayo stand and lateral x-ray visualization can then be performed relatively easily. This position helps greatly with the insertion of the "home run" screw.

weaned out of the removable walking boot and uses an ASO ankle brace. While the patient is in the pneumatic boot, some type of antiswelling measure, (e.g., a compression stocking) is used and continued even when they transition into a shoe.

Physical therapy is normally not necessary, since there is no joint to mobilize, but at 4½ months from surgery, if patients are struggling with gait abnormalities, we may consult physical therapy.

OUTCOME

The vast majority of patients in our experience are happy with this procedure. Ankle fusion does not make them normal, but it takes away their pain. It is relatively straightforward, and with the fusion rates being higher, this has become a very acceptable and successful procedure.

REFERENCES

1. Crosby LA, Yee PC, Formanek TS, et al. Complications following arthroscopic ankle arthrodesis. *Foot Ankle Int.* 1996;17:340–342.
2. Bonnin M, Carret JP. Arthrodesis of the ankle under arthroscopy: Apropos of 10 cases reviewed after a year. *Rev Chir Orthop Reparatrice Appar Mot.* 1995;81:128–135.
3. Bresler F, Mole D, Schmidt D. A tibiotalar arthrodesis under arthroscopy. *Rev Chir Orthop Reparatrice Appar Mot.* 1994;80:744–748.

4. Corso SJ, Zimmer TJ. Technique and clinical evaluation of arthroscopic ankle arthrodesis. *Arthroscopy.* 1995;11:585–590.

5. Crosby LA, Formanek TS, Fitzgibbons TC. Arthroscopic ankle fusion utilizing demineralized bone matrix and bone marrow grafting. In: Proceedings of the American Academy of Orthopaedic Surgeons 59th Annual Meeting. Washington, DC. Park Ridge, IL, American Academy of Orthopaedic Surgeons 309, 1992.

6. Dent CM, Patil M, Fairclough JA. Arthroscopic ankle arthrodesis. *J Bone Joint Surg Br.* 1993;75:830–832.

7. de Waal Malefijt MC, van Kampen A. Arthroscopic ankle arthrodesis: A new technique. *Ned Tijdschr Geneeskd.* 1992;136:2585–2588.

8. Fleis DJ. Letter: Arthroscopically assisted arthrodesis for osteoarthritic ankles. *J Bone Joint Surg Am.* 1994;76A:1112.

9. Glick JM, Morgan CD, Myerson MS, et al. Ankle arthrodesis using arthroscopic method: Long term follow-up of 34 cases. *Arthroscopy.* 1996;12:428–434.

10. Morgan CD. Arthroscopic tibiotalar arthrodesis. In: McGinty JB, Caspari RB, Jackson RW, Poehling GG, eds. *Operative arthroscopy.* New York, NY: Lippincott Williams & Wilkins; 1991:695–701.

11. Myerson MS, Allon SM. Arthroscopic ankle arthrodesis. *Contemp Orthop.* 1989;19:21–27.

12. Ogilvie-Harris DJ, Lieberman I, Fitsialos D. Arthroscopically assisted arthrodesis for osteoarthritic ankles. *J Bone Joint Surg Am.* 1993;75:1167–1174.

13. Schneider D. Arthroscopic ankle fusion. *Arth Video J.* 1983;3:35–47.

14. Turan I, Wredmark T, Fellander-Tsai L. Arthroscopic ankle arthrodesis in rheumatoid arthritis. *Clin Orthop Relat Res.* 1995;320:110–114.

15. Abicht BP, Roukis TS. Incidence of nonunion after isolated arthroscopic ankle arthrodesis. *Arthroscopy.* 2013;29(5):949–954.

16. Cameron SE, Ullrich P. Arthroscopic arthrodesis of the ankle joint. *Arthroscopy.* 2000;16(1):21–26.

17. Collman DR, Kaas MH, Schuberth JM. Arthroscopic ankle arthrodesis: Factors influencing union in 39 consecutive patients. *Foot Ankle Int.* 2006;27(12):1079–1085.

18. Dannawi Z, Nawabi DH, Patel A, et al. Arthroscopic ankle arthrodesis: Are results reproducible irrespective of preoperative deformity? *Foot Ankle Surg.* 2011;17(4):294–299.

19. Ferkel RD, Hewitt M. Long-term results of arthroscopic ankle arthrodesis. *Foot Ankle Int.* 2005;26(4):275–280.

20. Fitzgibbons TC. Arthroscopic ankle débridement and fusion: Indications, techniques, and results. *Instr Course Lect.* 1999;48:243–248.

21. Glick JM, Mann JA. Ankle arthrodesis using an arthroscopic method. *Foot Ankle Clin.* 1996;1(1):163–174.

22. Gougoulias NE, Agathangelidis FG, Parsons SW. Arthroscopic ankle arthrodesis. *Foot Ankle Int.* 2007;28(6):695–706.

23. Kats J, van Kampen A, de Waal-Malefijt MC. Improvement in technique for arthroscopic ankle fusion: Results in 15 patients. *Knee Surg Sports Traumatol Arthrosc.* 2002;11(1):46–49.

24. Jerosch J, Steinbeck J, Schroder M, et al. Arthroscopically assisted arthrodesis of the ankle joint. *Arch Orthop Trauma Surg.* 1996;115(3–4):182–189.

25. Jerosch J. Arthroscopic assisted arthrodesis (AAA) of the ankle – a standardized surgical technique. *FussSprungg.* 2003;1:66–75.

26. Nihal A, Gellman RE, Embil JM, et al. Ankle arthrodesis. *Foot Ankle Surg.* 2008;14:1–10.

27. Raikin SM. Arthrodesis of the ankle: Arthroscopic, mini-open, and open techniques. *Foot Ankle Clin.* 2003;8(2):347–59.

28. Rippstein P, Kumar B, Muller M. Ankle arthrodesis using the arthroscopic technique. *Oper Orthop Traumatol.* 2005;17(4–5):442–456.

29. Saragas NP. Results of arthroscopic arthrodesis of the ankle. *Foot Ankle Surg.* 2004;10:141–143.

30. Stone JW. Arthroscopic ankle arthrodesis. *Foot Ankle Clin.* 2006;11(2):361–368.

31. Tasto JP, Frey C, Laimans P, et al. Arthroscopic ankle arthrodesis. *Instr Course Lect.* 2000;49:259–280.

32. Cottino U, Collo G, Morino L, et al. Arthroscopic ankle arthrodesis: A review. *Curr Rev Musculoskelet Med.* 2012;5:151–155.

33. Wang DY. Arthroscopic ankle arthrodesis: A preliminary report. *Zhonghua Yi Xue Za Zhi (Taipei).* 1998;61(12):694–699.

34. Zvijac JE, Lemak L, Schurhoff MR, et al. Analysis of arthroscopically assisted ankle arthrodesis. *Arthroscopy.* 2002;18(1):70–75.

35. Winson IG, Robinson DE, Allen PE. Arthroscopic ankle arthrodesis. *J Bone Joint Surg Br.* 2005;87(3):343–347.

36. Myerson MS, Quill G. Ankle arthrodesis. A comparison of an arthroscopic and an open method of treatment. *Clin Orthop Relat Res.* 1991;268:84–95.

37. Nielsen KK, Linde F, Jensen NC. The outcome of arthroscopic and open surgery ankle arthrodesis: A comparative retrospective study of 107 patients. *Foot Ankle Surg.* 2008;14(3):153–157.

38. O'Brien TS, Hart TS, Shereff MJ, et al. Open versus arthroscopic ankle arthrodesis: A comparative study. *Foot Ankle Int.* 1999;20(6):368–374.

39. Panikkar KV, Taylor A, Kamath S, et al. A comparison of open and arthroscopic ankle fusion. *Foot Ankle Surg.* 2003;9:169–172.

40. Peterson KS, Lee MS, Buddecke DE. Arthroscopic versus open ankle arthrodesis: A retrospective cost analysis. *J Foot Ankle Surg.* 2010;49:242–247.

41. Townshend D, Di Silvestro M, Kraus F, et al. Arthroscopic versus open ankle arthrodesis: A multicenter comparative case series. *J Bone Joint Surg Am.* 2013;95:98–102.

42. Holt ES, Hansen ST, Mayo KA, et al. Ankle arthrodesis using internal screw fixation. *Clin Orthop Relat Res.* 1991;268:21–28.

43. Odutola AA, Sheridan BD, Kelly AJ. Headless compressive screw fixation prevents symptomatic metalwork in arthroscopic ankle arthrodesis. *Foot Ankle Surg.* 2012;18:111–113.

44. Yoshimura I, Kanazawa K, Takeyama A, et al. The effect of screw position and number on the time to union of arthroscopic ankle arthrodesis. *Arthroscopy.* 2012;28(12):1882–1888.

45. Cannon LB, Brown J, Cooke PH. Early weight bearing is safe following arthroscopic ankle arthrodesis *Foot Ankle Surg.* 2004;10:135–139.

CHAPTER 12

Arthroscopic Triple Arthrodesis

Tun Hing Lui   Lung Fung Tse

INDICATIONS

Triple arthrodesis is a commonly used procedure in treating varied foot and ankle problems, including hindfoot joint arthrosis and deformity. Traditionally, it is an open procedure that involves extensive exposure of subtalar, talonavicular, and calcaneocuboid joints. Performing triple arthrodesis in an open fashion may increase the potential for complications. The talonavicular joint is the most common site of nonunion. It is probably related to the difficulty of reaching the plantar and the lateral aspect of the joint and the tendency toward excessive bone resection in order to reach the deep part of the joint.

Arthroscopic triple arthrodesis[1] has been described. The advantages of this approach include better intra-articular visualization, more complete cartilage debridement, preservation of subchondral bone, decreased soft tissue dissection, and better cosmetic results. The ability to completely prepare fusion surfaces with minimal bone removal and preservation of the surrounding soft tissue contributes to the minimization of nonunion risk of the talonavicular joint.[2]

PATIENT POSITIONING

Under general or regional anesthesia, the patient is placed in the supine position. We use a thigh tourniquet to maintain bloodless field. No traction is required.

SURGICAL APPROACHES

Arthroscopic triple arthrodesis comprises arthroscopic subtalar arthrodesis and arthroscopic transverse tarsal arthrodesis.

The subtalar joint comprises anterior, middle, and posterior articulations. The middle and posterior facets are separated by the sinus tarsi and tarsal tunnel. The posterior subtalar joint has a separate joint capsule and does not communicate with other joints. The talocalcaneonavicular articulation includes the posterior articular facet of the navicular bone, the plantar calcaneonavicular (spring) ligament, as well as the anterior and middle calcaneal facets articulating with the talus.

The subtalar portals include the anterolateral, middle, posterolateral, posteromedial, medial tarsal canal, medial midtarsal and dorsomedial portals (Figs. 12–1 and 12–2).

The anterolateral portal is located at the angle of Gissane. The middle portal is just anterior and plantar to the lateral malleolar tip. The posteromedial and posterolateral portals are at the medial and lateral side of the Achilles tendon respectively. They are close to the tendon insertion and just above the superoposterior calcaneal tubercle. The medial tarsal canal portal is at the medial opening of the tarsal canal and just posterior to the sustentaculum tali. The medial midtarsal portal is just proximal and dorsal to the navicular insertion of the posterior tibial tendon.[3] The dorsolateral midtarsal portal is located at the junction between the calcaneocuboid and talonavicular joints.

Arthroscopic arthrodesis of the posterior subtalar joint can be performed by either the lateral approach (anteromedial and middle portals) or the posterior approach (posteromedial and posterolateral portals). The lateral approach is the preferred approach in case of arthroscopic triple arthrodesis because the patient should be put in supine position for the midtarsal arthrodesis. To avoid painful neuroma formation, we create portals by skin incision, followed by blunt dissection of underlying subcutaneous tissue with a hemostat. A 2.7-mm 30-degree arthroscope is used for this procedure. The arthroscope is inserted in the capsular gutter and the junctions between the articular cartilage and the subchondral bone can be identified. The articular cartilage is denuded from the subchondral bone with a small periosteal elevator or an arthroscopic osteotome. The deep part of the cartilage can be removed with an arthroscopic curette. It is important to preserve the subchondral bone as much as possible. Subchondral bone is then microfractured with an arthroscopic awl.

The fusion area can be extended into the anterior subtalar joint. The anterior subtalar joint is approached through the anterolateral and dorsolateral portals. The anterolateral portal is the visualization portal and the 2.7-mm arthroscope is introduced through the superficial and intermediate roots of the inferior extensor retinaculum to the anterior subtalar joint. The dorsolateral portal is the working portal and the lateral capsuloligamentous structures of the anterior subtalar joint are removed by an arthroscopic shaver. The anterior subtalar joint is then exposed and the articular cartilage can be denuded. The subchondral bone is microfractured to prepare the surfaces for triple arthrodesis.[1,4]

Four transverse tarsal portals are used for the arthroscopic arthrodesis of the talonavicular and calcaneocuboid joints. The dorsolateral and the medial portals

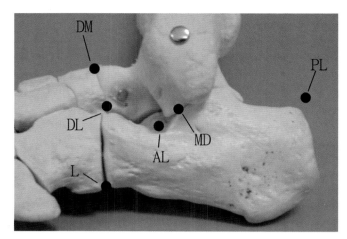

Figure 12–1. Sawbone model showing the lateral side of the subtalar and midtarsal joints and the associated portals. PL, posterolateral portal; MD, middle portal; AL, anterolateral portal; L, lateral portal; DL, dorsolateral portal; DM, dorsomedial portal.

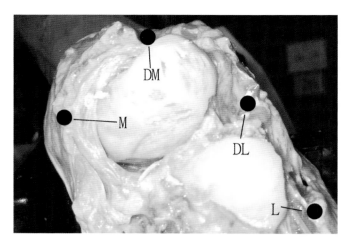

Figure 12–3. Cadaveric model of the midtarsal joint with the talar head and the cuboid exposed. The midtarsal portals were marked. M, medial portal; DM, dorsomedial portal; DL, dorsolateral portal; L, lateral portal.

have been described above. The dorsomedial portal is at the midpoint between the medial and dorsolateral portals. The lateral portal is at plantar lateral corner of calcaneocuboid joint (Fig. 12–3). The calcaneocuboid joint is approached through the lateral and dorsolateral portals. The talonavicular joint is approached through the dorsolateral, dorsomedial, and medial portals. Most of the time, the portals can be located by the surface anatomic landmarks. In the presence of dorsal osteophytes of the talonavicular joint or the presence of severe deformity the dorsomedial portal may be difficult to localize. Fluoroscopy can be used if localization is difficult. The dorsal capsule of the talonavicular joint can be stripped with a small periosteal elevator and fibrous

tissue of the dorsal capsular gutter can be debrided with an arthroscopic shaver to identify the joint line. If after this the joint line is still ill defined, overhanging dorsal osteophytes can be removed by an arthroscopic burr. The portals are interchangeable as the visualization and instrumentation portals. The arthroscope is introduced into the capsular gutter to identify the joint line and the junction between the articular cartilage and subchondral bone. The cartilage is then denuded from the subchondral bone (Fig. 12–4).

Because of the three-dimensional anatomy of the transverse tarsal joint, the talonavicular joint is anatomically dorsal to the calcaneocuboid joint. The dorsolateral portal allows one to reach the plantar lateral aspect of talonavicular and then completes debridement of cartilage of the deep part of the talonavicular joint without the need for excessive bone resection. The dorsolateral portal is the single most important portal of this procedure because the medial aspect of the calcaneocuboid joint, the lateral and plantar aspects of the talonavicular joint, and the potential space between the talonavicular and calcaneocuboid joints can be approached through this portal.[4–6] It is important to recognize that the anterior subtalar joint and the talonavicular joint share the same capsule and form the talocalcaneonavicular joint anatomically. The lateral part of the joint including the spring ligament can be approached through the anterolateral subtalar and dorsolateral transverse tarsal portals.

DEFORMITY CORRECTION

Triple arthrodesis is indicated in the case of severe, rigid deformity especially when arthritic change of the hindfoot occurs. It is important that the arthroscopic triple fusion have potential for deformity correction before it can be considered as a viable alternative to the open

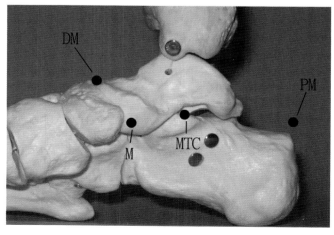

Figure 12–2. Sawbone model showing the medial side of the subtalar and midtarsal joints and the associated portals. PM, posteromedial portal; MTC, medial tarsal canal portal; M, medial portal; DM, dorsomedial portal.

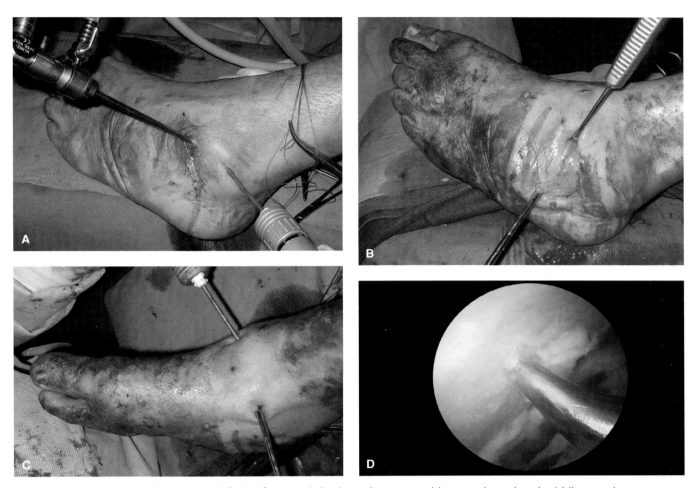

Figure 12–4.   A case of neglected left clubfoot. **A:** Subtalar arthroscopy with anterolateral and middle portals. **B:** Calcaneocuboid arthroscopy with lateral and dorsolateral portals. The cartilage was denuded with an arthroscopic osteotome through the dorsolateral portal. **C:** Talonavicular arthroscopy with dorsolateral and medial portals. **D:** Arthroscopic view showing microfracture of the subchondral bone with an arthroscopic awl after removal of articular cartilage.

approach. "Closing wedge procedure" and arthroscopic capsuloligamentous release through the portals can increase the power of deformity correction of the arthroscopic triple fusion. After the fusion surfaces are prepared as described above "closing wedge procedure" and arthroscopic release of the corresponding joint can be performed as indicated. Arthroscopic lateral subtalar capsuloligamentous release can be performed in case of valgus heel deformity. "Closing wedge procedure" of the subtalar joint is indicated in case of varus heel deformity. Similarly, dorsal "closing wedge procedure" of transverse joint is indicated for correction of cavus foot deformity and plantar "closing wedge procedure" for correction of flat foot deformity. Combined capsular release and "closing wedge procedure" is usually needed for correction of abduction, supination, or pronation deformity of the forefoot.

A 2-mm Isham straight flute burr is used for the "closing wedge procedure." In case of correction of varus heel deformity, a lateral wedge of bone is burred out through

the anterolateral or middle subtalar portal while applying a valgus force to the heel. In case of correction of supination–pronation deformity of the forefoot, a 2-mm K-wire is inserted into the navicular to serve as a joystick and the midfoot is derotated. If it fails to derotate the midfoot, the capsuloligamentous structures can be released by a small periosteal elevator through the talonavicular portals. The Isham straight flute burr is inserted into the talonavicular portals to remove the impinging bone (Fig. 12–5).

The subtalar joint and midtarsal joints are reduced and subtalar joint is transfixed with 7.3-mm cannulated screw and talonavicular and calcaneocuboid joints are transfixed with 4.0-mm cannulated screw using percutaneous screw technique.

Deformity correction with the arthroscopic procedure should follow the same principles of the open procedure. Soft tissue procedure especially the balancing of the tendons should also be performed either as an open or minimally invasive approach.[7] Then, we can titrate the correction of the hindfoot deformity with the "closing

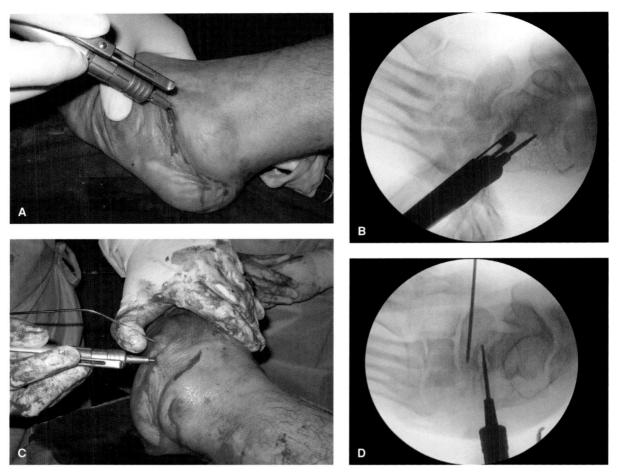

Figure 12–5. **A, B:** "Closing wedge procedure" of the subtalar joint. **C:** "Closing wedge procedure" of the calcaneocuboid joint with a K-wire in the cuboid in order to derotate the midfoot. **D:** "Closing wedge procedure" of the talonavicular joint with a K-wire in the navicular. The Isham burr was inserted through the dorsomedial portal.

wedge procedure" described above. The capsuloligamentous structure can be released through the portals of the corresponding joint. The resection of impinging bone can also be performed through the portals and the resulting morselized bone left in the joint to aid fusion. We believe that with the addition of "closing wedge procedure," the indication of arthroscopic assisted triple fusion can be extended into the correction of severe hindfoot deformity including moderate to severe clubfoot deformity. The most important limiting factor is the stretching of the posterior tibial neurovascular bundle and potential subsequent impairment of perfusion of the skin of medial heel after correction of the varus hindfoot deformity. This was the reason that we perform open posterior tibial tendon transfer rather than the percutaneous procedure, as we can release the tarsal tunnel at the same time. We also had to release the tourniquet after the correction to examine the skin perfusion of medial heel and the distal circulation.[7] Lateral capsular and ligamentous release of the subtalar joint can be performed through the middle and anterolateral portals.[8]

Arthroscopic debridement of the talonavicular joint is possible. Because of the risk of damage to the lateral terminal branch (LTB) of the deep peroneal nerve (DPN), an alternative to the dorsolateral portal should be considered. The anatomy and function of the LTB have not been well studied, and the consequence of damage is unknown. Anatomic studies suggest that in addition to innervating the extensor digitorum brevis muscle, the lateral branch innervates the talonavicular capsule, the lateral tarsometatarsal joints, and the sinus tarsi.[9–11]

Despite innervating these structures, functional deficits or arthropathy are not likely if the LTB was damaged. There have been no reports of functional deficits after the extensor digitorum brevis has been harvested as a flap to cover wounds of the foot and ankle[12] or used as an interposition material after coalition resection.[13] Animal studies involving complete denervation of stable joints and clinical studies on partial joint denervation do not support the risk of arthropathy.[14,15] The more likely impairment after injury to the lateral branch of the DPN would be neuropathic pain. Compression of the LTB resulting in neuropathic pain has recently been described. Kennedy et al.[9] described a series of patients with recalcitrant dorsolateral foot pain after ankle sprain who had symptoms of neurogenic pain radiating to the fourth and fifth metatarsals after compression of the LTB. There is a possibility that such symptoms could arise after damage to the LTB during arthroscopic debridement of the talonavicular joint.

In patients with foot deformity as a result of neuromuscular problems, such as postpolio syndrome, a soft tissue procedure (e.g., tendon release or transfer) is an important component of surgical correction, in addition to triple arthrodesis. In such patients, as well as those with severe hindfoot deformity, in whom much bony reconstruction is required, open triple arthrodesis is preferable.[16]

BONE GRAFTING

The junction between the four bones and the three joint spaces can be grafted through corresponding portals. "Four-corner arthrodesis" at the junction of the four hindfoot bones will aid stabilization of the position and fusion of the subtalar, talonavicular, and calcaneocuboid joints.

The junction of the four bones is packed with autologous cancellous bone graft, which is harvested from the ipsilateral iliac wing using a small bone trephine. Bone graft can also be packed into the three joint spaces through corresponding portals. The dorsomedial, dorsolateral, and lateral portals can be used to prepare the junction of the calcaneum, talus, navicular, and cuboid for fusion. Usually, the dorsomedial and lateral portals are the visualization portals and the dorsolateral portal is the working portal. The cortical bone of the bones bounding the junction is prepared for fusion using an arthroscopic burr.

In patients without foot deformity, bone grafting of the subtalar, talonavicular, and calcaneocuboid joints is not needed. In patients with correction of hindfoot deformity, bone grafting may be needed to fill in the gap of the joints and achieve solid fusion.

FIXATION

The subtalar joint and transverse tarsal joints are then reduced into the desired positions and transfixed with cannulated screws. The subtalar joint is transfixed with a 7.3-mm cannulated screw. The talonavicular and calcaneocuboid joints are transfixed with 4.0-mm cannulated screws using a percutaneous screw technique.

In patients with foot deformity caused by neuromuscular problems, such as in postpolio syndrome, a soft tissue procedure, for example, tendon release or transfer, is an important component of surgical correction, in additional to triple arthrodesis. However, in patients with hindfoot deformity due to intra-articular pathology, for example, rheumatoid arthritis, capsular contracture can be released through the portals obviating additional incisions.[1]

COMPLICATIONS

The structures at risk at the lateral portal include the peroneal tendons and sural nerve.

Long extensor tendons and the intermediate dorsal cutaneous branch of the superficial peroneal nerve are close to the dorsolateral portal. The motor branch to the extensor digitorum brevis muscle can also be at risk.[17]

The extensor hallucis longus tendon and deep peroneal nerve are at risk with work through the dorsomedial portal. There are potential risks of damage to the cutaneous nerves especially at the dorsomedial portal. Although the working areas of the dorsolateral and medial portals covered most of both surfaces, they cannot be visualization portals for each other because they are located at the ends of the equator of the hemispheric talonavicular joint; arthroscopic visual fields of each other will be obscured by the talar head. Even though it has the highest risk of neurovascular injury, the dorsomedial portal has an important role in being the visualization portal of the other two and its working area covered the dorsal side of both surfaces. Careful blunt soft tissue dissection down to the joint capsule before insertion of the instrument is crucial to avoid injury to the neurovascular structures, especially for the dorsomedial portal. Most of the talar and navicular surfaces can be prepared for fusion without the need of excessive bone removal during arthroscopic triple arthrodesis. Careful surgical technique is most important to avoid injury to the neurovascular structures, especially for the dorsomedial portal.[2]

REHABILITATION PROTOCOL

Postoperatively, the foot is protected with a short leg cast and the patient should be nonweight bearing on the operative foot for 8 weeks. They then proceed to protected weight bearing, walking with rocker boot for another 4 weeks.[18]

OUTCOME

Most of the talar and navicular surfaces can be prepared for fusion without the need of excessive bone removal during arthroscopic triple arthrodesis. Reported rates of nonunion after triple arthrodesis range from 6% to 33%, with the majority of pseudarthroses involving the talonavicular joint.[17] In a single surgeon's series, all the operated feet fused solidly. The average time for solid fusion was 21 weeks (16 to 22 weeks). The overall American Orthopaedic Foot & Ankle Society (AOFAS) ankle–hindfoot score was 81.5.[18]

REFERENCES

1. Lui TH. New technique of arthroscopic triple arthrodesis. *Arthroscopy.* 2006;22:464.e1–e5.
2. Lui TH, Chan LK. Safety and efficacy of talonavicular arthroscopy in arthroscopic triple arthrodesis. A cadaveric study. *Knee Surg Sports Traumatol Arthrosc.* 2010;18: w607–611.
3. Lui TH. Medial subtalar arthroscopy. *Foot Ankle Int.* 2012;33:1018–1023.
4. Lui TH. Clinical tips: Anterior subtalar (talocalcaneonavicular) arthroscopy. *Foot Ankle Int.* 2008;29:94–96.
5. Lui TH. Arthroscopic resection of the calcaneonavicular coalition or the "Too Long" anterior process of the calcaneus. *Arthroscopy.* 2006;22:903.e1–e4.
6. Lui TH, Chan KB, Chan LK. Portal safety and efficacy of anterior subtalar arthroscopy: A cadaveric study. *Knee Surg Sports Traumatol Arthrosc.* 2010;18:233–237.
7. Lui TH. Case report: Correction of neglected club foot deformity by arthroscopic assisted triple arthrodesis. *Arch Orthop Trauma Surg.* 2010;130:1007–1011.
8. Lui TH. Arthroscopic subtalar release of post-traumatic subtalar stiffness. *Arthroscopy.* 2006;22:1364.e1–e4.
9. Kennedy JG, Brunner JB, Bohne WH, et al. Clinical importance of the lateral branch of the deep peroneal nerve. *Clin Orthop Relat Res.* 2007;459:222–228.
10. Ucerler H, Ikiz AA, Uygur M. A cadaver study on preserving peroneal nerves during ankle arthroscopy. *Foot Ankle Int.* 2007;28(11):1172–1178.
11. Hammond AW, Phisitkul P, Femino J, et al. Arthroscopic debridement of the talonavicular joint using dorsomedial and dorsolateral portals: A cadaveric study of safety and access. *Arthroscopy.* 2011;27:228–234.
12. Chattar-Cora D, Pederson WC. Experience with the extensor digitorum brevis muscle flap for foot and ankle reconstruction. *Ann Plast Surg.* 2006;57(3):289–294.
13. Okada M, Saito H. Resection interposition arthroplasty of calcaneonavicular coalition using a lateral supramalleolar adipofascial flap: Case report. *J Pediatr Orthop B.* 2013;22(3):252–254.
14. Wu Z, Toh K, Nagata K, et al. Effect of the resection of the sciatic nerve on the Th1/Th2 balance in the synovia of the ankle joint of adjuvant arthritic rats. *Histochem Cell Biol.* 2004;121(2):141–147.
15. Machner A, Pap G, Schwarzberg H, et al. [Deterioration of sensory joint innervation as an enabling factor for development of arthrosis. An animal experiment study of the rat model]. *Z Rheumatol.* 1999;58(3):148–154.
16. Lui TH. Arthroscopy and endoscopy of the foot and ankle: Indications for new techniques. *Arthroscopy.* 2007; 23:889–902.
17. Hammond AW, Phisitkul P, Femino J, et al. Arthroscopic debridement of the talonavicular joint using dorsomedial and dorsolateral portals: A cadaveric study of safety and access. *Arthroscopy.* 2011;27:228–234.
18. Lui TH. Arthroscopic triple arthrodesis in patients with Müller Weiss disease. *Foot and Ankle Surgery.* 2009;15: 119–122.

CHAPTER 13

Axial Screw Technique for Charcot Midfoot Neuropathic Dislocation

V. James Sammarco

INDICATIONS

Charcot neuroarthropathic foot deformity is inherently difficult to treat. For the neuroarthropathic patient, dislocation through the midfoot can progress to a rigid, irreducible deformity, or alternately, the foot may develop gross instability at the level of the dislocation which is unbraceable and difficult to manage. Either sequela may lead to chronic ulceration, infection, osteomyelitis, and eventual amputation. Historically, management of the Charcot foot has included extended periods of casting and nonweight bearing until the foot "consolidates," then treating residual deformity with a functional brace. In the past, surgery was limited to excision of bony prominences in the area of ulceration. More recently, attention has shifted toward surgical restoration of a plantigrade foot by reduction of the dislocation and arthrodesis of the midfoot joints at the level of dislocation. We described the technique of surgical reconstruction with long axial intramedullary screws which span the level of dislocation.[1,2] The screws can be applied percutaneously either proximally or distally. Applying fixation in this manner can facilitate reduction of the deformity and diminishes the required surgical exposure compared to plate, or more standard crossed screw techniques.

The initial treatment of neuropathic foot dislocations in most cases is nonoperative. However, some cases warrant initial treatment using operative means. Published classification systems may aid in deciding which patients warrant initial surgical therapy. Neuropathic midfoot dislocation has been classified by Sammarco and Conti and by Schon et al. based on the anatomic pattern of the involved joints and osseous structures.[3,4] Schon et al. classified the degree of deformity with either type alpha or beta designation. A beta stage indicates more severe deformity and is assigned if one or more of the following criteria are met: (1) a dislocation is present, (2) the lateral first metatarsal angle is ≥30 degrees, (3) the lateral calcaneal-fifth metatarsal angle is ≥0 degrees, or (4) the AP talar-first metatarsal angle is ≥35 degrees. In cases where the patient continues to have ulceration despite appropriate brace management, surgery is indicated. We believe that patients who either present with, or develop Schon-type beta deformity are best served by deformity correction with arthrodesis (Fig. 13–1). Some patients who have progressive deformity may warrant surgical intervention earlier, particularly if the foot is grossly unstable through the midfoot on physical examination. Patients with acute dislocation often represent an indication for reduction and arthrodesis. Assal and Stern[5] presented a similar technique for the treatment of intractable ulceration in patients with midfoot dislocation.

Preoperative medical optimization cannot be overemphasized. Poorly controlled medical comorbidities will impede healing at the surgical site and can lead to wound breakdown and infection which in turn can lead to amputation. Vascular assessment is critical, as dysvascular limbs will not heal and are prone to rapid deterioration. It is important to resolve infection prior to surgery and this may require staged procedures including a formal incisional debridement, usually combined with a provisional reduction and use of an external fixator. It is our opinion that open ulceration with gross infection or underlying osteomyelitis is a contraindication to implanting permanent hardware, and that every effort should be made to resolve ulceration prior to surgery.

As this technique involves passing large screws through the articular surfaces of normal joints, it is only appropriate in patients with an insensate foot, as is typically found in diabetic or other forms of neuropathy.

PATIENT POSITIONING

The patient is placed supine on the operating room table on a large bean bag with the toes pointing toward the ceiling. This allows access to both the medial and lateral columns of the foot. A pneumatic tourniquet is applied to the proximal thigh. Once prepped and draped, a stack of sterile towels is placed beneath the leg at the level of the midcalf to facilitate circumferential access to the foot. Intraoperative fluoroscopy is required throughout the procedure.

SURGICAL APPROACHES

The foot should be viewed as having three columns, and incisions are planned at the level of dislocation. Smaller incisions can be used in cases where the Charcot process is relatively acute and confined to one region of the foot, without significant bone dissolution or fragmentation.

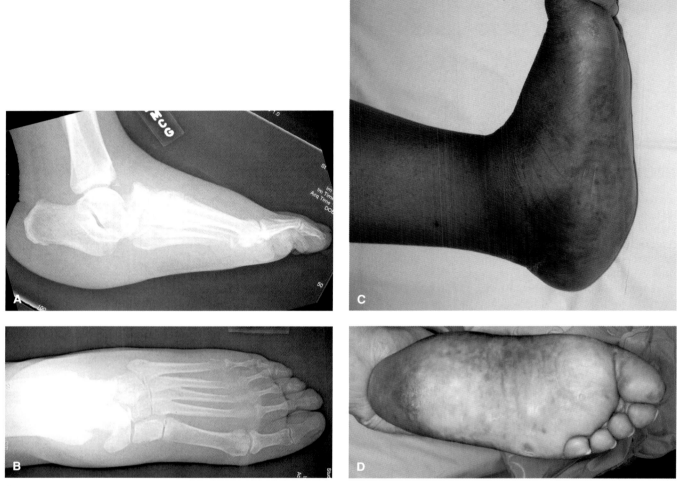

Figure 13–1. **A, B:** Radiographs of a 47-year-old woman with insulin-dependent diabetes mellitus who presented with a spontaneous midfoot dislocation at Chopart joint. The patient developed deformity approximately 3 months prior to presentation. Note "bayoneting" of the forefoot on the hindfoot and marked equinus positioning of the talus. **C, D:** Clinical photographs demonstrating the rocker bottom deformity and an area of preulceration plantar to the cuboid.

More chronic neuropathic patterns will require a full extensile incision with significant bone resection.

The medial approach is used for dislocation at the talonavicular, naviculocuneiform, and first tarsometatarsal joints (Fig. 13–2A). A longitudinal incision is made along the medial border of the foot. The abductor hallucis muscle is elevated with the underlying periosteal sleeve and care is taken to identify the tibialis anterior tendon insertion. In cases where the dislocation is long-standing, the tibialis anterior tendon may need to be detached to allow reduction. In these cases, the tendon is repaired directly to bone with nonabsorbable suture at closure.

The lateral (fourth and fifth) tarsometatarsal joints and calcaneocuboid joints require a dorsolateral incision at the level of deformity (Fig. 13–2B) Often the cuboid is dislocated plantarly, but reduction can usually be achieved through the single lateral incision. A full thickness exposure directly to bone can be utilized in this area, although care needs to be taken not to transect the peroneal tendons.

In cases where the dislocation is at the level of the tarsometatarsal joint, often a middle column exposure is needed. We have not found this necessary for more proximal level Charcot deformity where bone resection can be accomplished through the medial and lateral incisions. If the second and third metatarsals are bayoneted on the dorsum of the cuneiforms, a dorsal incision will be necessary at that level for adequate bone resection to allow reduction. A dorsal incision is made lateral to the second metatarsal base. Care must be taken at this level to identify and protect the medial dorsal cutaneous nerve in the subcutaneous tissues and the dorsalis pedis artery and deep peroneal nerve which must be elevated from the periosteum and meticulously protected to avoid vascular embarrassment of the forefoot.

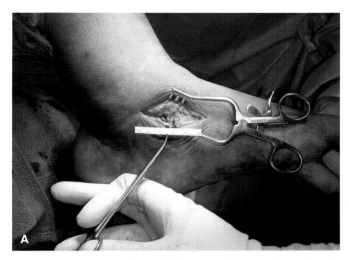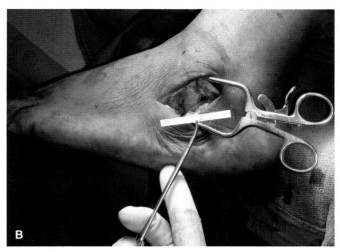

Figure 13–2.   A: The medial approach is used for reduction and arthrodesis of the medial column. The exposure is typically less extensile than that required for plating of the fusion. **B:** A full-thickness dorsolateral exposure allows for reduction of the lateral tarsometatarsal and calcaneocuboid joints. Often the middle column can be reduced through the medial and lateral incision, although sometimes an additional dorsocentral incision will be necessary.

PREPARATION FOR ARTHRODESIS AND REDUCTION OF DEFORMITY

In planning reduction of the deformity, it is helpful to think of the foot as two segments rather than as multiple joint and bones. Consider the hindfoot as one segment and the forefoot as another. Often the bone at the level of the deformity is comminuted, avascular, and fibrotic. The goal of surgery is to align the hindfoot segment with the forefoot and to create a plantigrade surface for

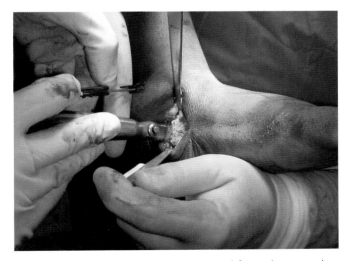

Figure 13–3.   Bone must be removed from the central area of dislocation to allow a tension-free reduction. This can be done with a saw as shown here, or with osteotomes and a rongeur. Over-resection of bone should be avoided. The goal is to create apposition of cancellous bone at the desired fusion level which is relatively tension free.

weight bearing. Bone from the central area of Charcot dissolution is removed to allow a tension-free reduction. The axial screws bridge this area allowing for fixation in the more solid bone proximally and distally (Fig. 13–3). In some cases, structural bone graft is necessary to fill large voids.

Equinus deformity must be addressed before beginning reduction (Fig. 13–4). This may be accomplished by recession of the gastrocnemius and soleus muscle aponeuroses, or by percutaneous tendo-Achilles lengthening. Often both are needed. If adequate tension cannot be generated in the myotendinous unit by dorsiflexion of the foot due to the dislocation, a large Steinmann pin can be inserted in the calcaneus from posteriorly and used as a lever to pull traction on the Achilles tendon during the lengthening procedure.

Once the Achilles is lengthened and the deformity exposed, resection of bone and articular cartilage is preformed with a small oscillating saw. Adequate bone resection must be accomplished in order to allow a tension-free reduction. If the forefoot is bayoneted dorsally, the dorsal soft tissues will be contracted and the foot must be shortened to allow realignment. This is performed through small, incremental bone resections at the arthrodesis site, usually resecting more bone plantarly and medially to recreate the longitudinal arch and to correct forefoot abduction. Care must be taken not to resect too much bone medially or laterally, but to resect enough that the forefoot can be realigned with the hindfoot, while creating even apposition of cancellous bone at the level of the fusion.

Reduction and provisional fixation is achieved by the temporary placement of guidewires in the intramedullary canals of the metatarsals, then by using these guidewires to secure the fusion site and hold the foot reduced. Once adequate reduction is achieved, cannulated screws can

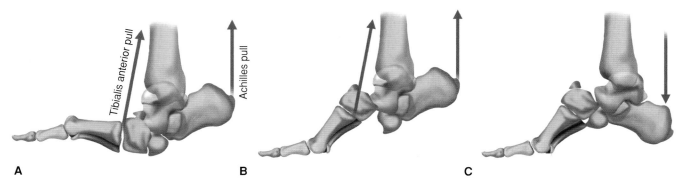

Figure 13–4. **A:** Typical Charcot midfoot deformity due to neuroarthropathy. Note development of rocker bottom and the deforming forces of the Achilles tendon and tibialis anterior tendon. **B:** If left untreated, midfoot instability combined with continued overpull of the tibialis anterior and Achilles tendon can lead to complete dislocation of the forefoot onto the hindfoot. **C:** The first step in reconstruction of the deformity usually involves lengthening of the Achilles tendon, gastrocnemius muscle, or both.

be applied over the guidewires to compress and secure the fusion.

Passing the guidewires into the metatarsal shafts can be difficult, and extra time may be necessary for this part of the procedure. A small image intensifier that can be directly manipulated by the surgeon greatly facilitates this process. Retrograde passage of the wires through the metatarsophalangeal joints is used in most cases, but requires patience and intensive fluoroscopy. The first metatarsal is usually entered first. This can be accomplished by dorsiflexing the hallux and passing a large gauge (typically 3.7 mm) guidewire under fluoroscopic control into the first metatarsal shaft. It is important that the wire is parallel to the shaft both on antero-posterior and lateral radiographs, and that it enters the fusion site centrally. The wire is advanced to the level of dislocation, and then the lesser metatarsals are cannulated. A similar technique can be used for the lesser metatarsals, with smaller (typically 2 mm) guidewires. The first through fourth metatarsals should be cannulated in this way for intercuneiform and tarsometatarsal dislocations. With the guidewires advanced to the level of dislocation, the deformity is reduced and the wires are passed across the level of dislocation into the hindfoot

to restore alignment. Multiplanar fluoroscopy is used at this point to verify reduction and alignment of the forefoot with the hindfoot. The medial wire is most important and this should be parallel with the first meta-tarsal and talar neck on both AP and lateral fluoroscopic images (Fig. 13–5).

Alternate methods of passing the guidewires include passing the wires into the metatarsal shafts from the fusion site (antegrade), which may be more straightforward in the cases of true tarsometatarsal dislocation. Wires can also be passed out the ankle posteriorly through the talus and cal-caneus, then passed antegrade into the metatarsal shafts. This technique can be used in cases of Chopart level dis-location, where arthrodesis of the tarsometatarsal joints is not desired.

Once alignment has been achieved, attention can be focused on applying the final fixation devices.

FIXATION

Reduction of the deformity is the main challenge with this technique. Once reduction has been achieved and held provisionally with guidewires, application of the

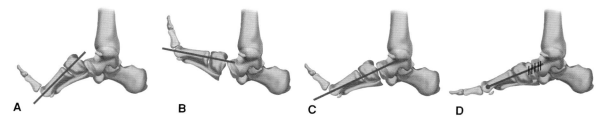

Figure 13–5. Reduction and fixation technique. **A:** After resection of adequate bone for the midfoot and preparation for arthrodesis at the level of deformity, a guidewire is introduced through the first metatarsophalangeal joint. The joint must be dorsiflexed to obtain the correct starting point. **B:** The guidewire is passed to the level of deformity and used to facilitate reduction. **C:** With the deformity held in place, the wire is driven from the forefoot into the talar body, parallel with the talar neck. **D:** A cannulated screw can then be passed over the guidewire and tightened to compress the arthrodesis.

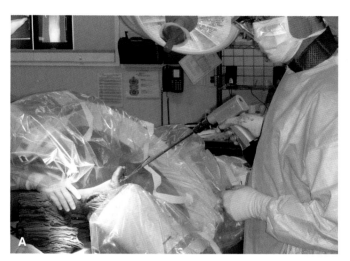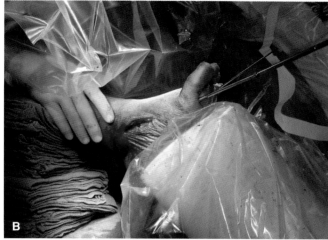

Figure 13–6. **A:** Predrilling the metatarsal shafts is necessary to avoid fracture. **B:** Screws are applied under fluoroscopic control over the guidewires.

final fixation is relatively straightforward. Implant choice is important. The largest diameter screw that will be tolerated by the metatarsal shaft should be used. We have used 6.5-mm, 7.3-mm, and 8.0-mm screws in the medial column, and 4.0-mm, 4.5-mm, 5.0-mm, and (infrequently) 6.5-mm screws in the lesser metatarsals. Our initial study used standard screws with reduced diameter heads to facilitate intramedullary placement. More recently, we have been using headless screws. While the headless screws cause less articular damage when they are passed through joints, they seem to have less fatigue resistance and are more prone to fracture. It is beyond the scope of this text to discuss specific implants, and the reader is encouraged to question manufacturers as to the bending strength and fatigue resistance of the screws considered for use.

Complications including nonunion and implant failure are common with this procedure; therefore, some consideration also needs to be given to implant extraction. We recommend using either polished stainless steel or titanium which has been coated or anodized to avoid bone ingrowth into the metal. We always use cannulated devices for this procedure. Extraction of broken cannulated screws, while challenging, can usually be done percutaneously under fluoroscopic control. This facilitates exchange of hardware without further osseous disruption.

Screws may be applied either proximal to distal or distal to proximal. More proximal level dislocations such as the talonavicular and calcaneocuboid joints may be secured with screws that pass in posteriorly from the talar body and calcaneus respectively. Our initial experience with screws passed from the posterior talar body into the medial column showed that this was technically quite difficult, and we have moved to fixing the medial column retrograde though the first metatarsal head. The middle column is typically secured through the metatarsophalangeal joints. The fourth metatarsal can

be secured either antegrade from the calcaneus (which allows a larger diameter screw to be used), or retrograde through the MTPJ (Fig. 13–6).

Without appropriate preparation of the screw path the metatarsal shaft may shatter. Simply inserting "self-drilling, self-tapping" screws over the guidewires is not adequate. The screw path should be sequentially drilled over the guidewires with increasing diameter cannulated drills. This should be performed under fluoroscopic control, using the fluoroscopic images to determine when the metatarsal cannot be reamed further. This is usually close to the diameter of the desired screw. We also hand tap the entire screw path, and do so under fluoroscopy. If great resistance is felt while tapping in the metatarsal shaft, either further reaming is necessary, or a smaller diameter screw must be used.

Once the screw path is prepared, a cannulated depth gauge is used to determine the proper length of the screws. Ideally, the screw engages the metaphyseal–diaphyseal junction and compresses the arthrodesis. The screws should be applied and then used to compress the fusion, tightening each sequentially under fluoroscopic control. Final radiographs verify alignment and extra-articular positioning of the screw head and tip (Fig. 13–7).

POSTOPERATIVE CARE

A sterile, well-padded postoperative splint is applied with the ankle held in neutral alignment. This is removed within a few days and changed to a total contact cast. Casting is continued for 2 to 3 months until soft tissue swelling has subsided, at which point a diabetic pneumatic boot walker is applied. Weight bearing is started on radiographic consolidation, which is typically 4 to 5 months postoperatively. The patient may be transitioned from the boot walker to an extra depth shoe with a custom

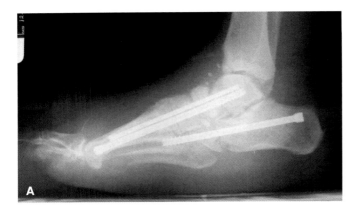

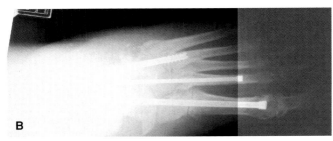

Figure 13–7. A, B: Postoperative radiographs demonstrating reduction of the deformity. Screws were inserted in a retrograde fashion through the first and second metatarsal shafts into the talar neck and body, and in an anterograde fashion from the calcaneus through the calcaneocuboid joint, into the fourth metatarsal base.

molded diabetic inlay usually 6 to 9 months following the surgery.

COMPLICATIONS

As with any surgery, early complications with this technique may occur. The risks of poor wound healing and infection can be minimized by adequate medical optimization including good glucose control, if possible. Edema control is also important and frequent cast changes may be needed as swelling subsides after surgery. The necessity of adequate arterial perfusion cannot be overemphasized. If this type of surgery is performed without adequate perfusion, there is a high likelihood of poor wound healing, infection, loss of blood supply, and even amputation in the postoperative period.

Delayed union is common and it may take a year or more for complete osseous consolidation to occur. Some patients heal only with a fibrous union and some recurrence of the deformity can be expected with time. Frequent follow-up and serial radiography over the course

of 2 years is necessary, particularly in the early period once the patient starts weight bearing. If hardware failure is noted, we have had success by removing the broken screws and exchanging them for new screws percutaneously, without reexposing or grafting the fusion area.

Failure of the fusion accompanied by reactivation of the Charcot process and significant recurrence of deformity can occur, although infrequently. Depending on the overall health of the patient and remaining bone stock, the alternatives include management with a Charcot Restraint Orthosis Walker (CROW), or formal revision of the arthrodesis with bone grafting and replacement of hardware. In cases where osteomyelitis, nonunion, and hardware failure occur simultaneously, amputation should be considered.

OUTCOME

In 2009, two series of midfoot fusion utilizing intramedullary screws were published. Sammarco et al. presented a series where 22 patients underwent midfoot fusion using the technique described above.[2] Durable correction of deformity was achieved in most patients, although complications including nonunion and hardware failure were common in patients where the talonavicular joint was included in the fusion. All patients had successful limb salvage and were able to ambulate without above ankle bracing at a minimum 2-year follow-up. Assal and Stern[5] also reported successful limb salvage where an intramedullary axial screw was used to realign the medial column of the foot in midfoot fusion of neuropathic patients. Plates and crossed screws were used for the lateral and middle columns. Successful limb salvage was achieved in 14 of 15 patients.

REFERENCES

1. Sammarco VJ. Superconstructs in the treatment of charcot foot deformity: Plantar plating, locked plating, and axial screw fixation. *Foot Ankle Clin.* 2009;14:393–407.
2. Sammarco VJ, Sammarco GJ, Walker EW Jr, et al; GUIAO RP. Midtarsal arthrodesis in the treatment of Charcot midfoot arthropathy. *J Bone Joint Surg Am.* 2009;91:80–91.
3. Sammarco GJ, Conti SF. Surgical treatment of neuroarthropathic foot deformity. *Foot Ankle Int.* 1998;19:102–109.
4. Schon LC, Easley ME, Cohen I, et al. The acquired midtarsus deformity classification system–interobserver reliability and intraobserver reproducibility. *Foot Ankle Int.* 2002;23:30–36.
5. Assal M, Stern R. Realignment and extended fusion with use of a medial column screw for midfoot deformities secondary to diabetic neuropathy. *J Bone Joint Surg Am.* 2009;91:812–820.

CHAPTER 14

Ankle Arthroscopy—Basics

Marcus P. Coe
Alastair S.E. Younger
Kevin Wing

INDICATIONS

Ankle arthroscopy has evolved over the course of the last 30 years to provide a minimally invasive means of visualizing and addressing intra-articular pathology in the tibiotalar joint. The use of solely diagnostic ankle arthroscopy has been replaced by advancements in imaging, including MRI and thin-slice CT scans. Currently, ankle arthroscopy is used to surgically address a large range of both bony and soft tissue pathology in the tibiotalar joint. This chapter will focus on the basics of ankle arthroscopy, including setup, positioning, portal placement, portal views, general complications, and rehabilitation. Subsequent chapters will address arthroscopic management of osteochondral lesions of the talus, more complete evaluation and management of syndesmotic injuries, and hindfoot arthroscopy.

Ankle arthroscopy can be used to assist with the treatment of any intra-articular pathology in the tibiotalar joint. Current indications to treat bony pathology include treatment of osteochondral lesions of the talus; assistance in reduction of intra-articular fractures of the ankle and tibial plafond; late treatment of displaced or malreduced fractures; debridement of anterior impingement from bony spurs; excision of the os trigonum or posterior bony spurs; assistance in tibiotalar fusion; and removal of loose bodies. Current indications to address soft tissue pathology are as follows: synovectomy, treatment of the deltoid ligament, the anterior talofibular ligament, and the distal syndesmosis (all of which have intra-articular components).

PATIENT POSITIONING AND EQUIPMENT

Patients may be positioned in either the supine or the prone position. In general, the supine position is preferred when the majority of the pathology to be addressed is in the anterior portion of the ankle and the prone position is preferred when the majority of the pathology to be addressed is in the posterior portion of the ankle. The setup for supine positioning allows excellent access to the anterior portals and adequate access to the posterior portals. We find that the supine position allows more extensive viewing of the joint compared with the prone position. As the extent of ankle pathology cannot always be fully predicted preoperatively anterior ankle arthroscopy is more versatile. Prone positioning should be used for isolated posterior ankle pathology (especially posterior medial pathology); the anterior ankle portals cannot be easily accessed in the prone position.

Supine Positioning

Patients may be anesthetized with general anesthesia, popliteal blocks, regional ankle blocks, or a combination of these. With a popliteal block, dense general sedation is needed if a thigh tourniquet is to be inflated, as the block does not provide sufficient proximal pain control. Our preference is to bolster the hip and place a high thigh tourniquet, which can be inflated at the beginning of the case or if intra-articular bleeding is encountered later in the case (Fig. 14–1). The foot should be even with the edge of

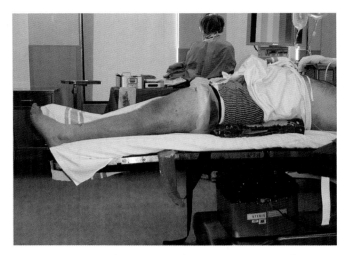

Figure 14–1. Photograph of supine positioning for ankle arthroscopy with a hip bump and a high thigh tourniquet.

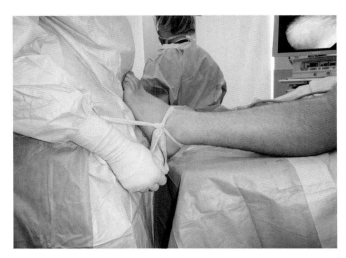

Figure 14–2. Intraoperative photograph of elasticized bandage tied around the foot that is used for dynamic distraction. Note the position of the bandage just below the malleoli.

the bed distally. Leg holders that brace the thigh and hold the hip and knee in flexion are also a viable option for positioning. A calf tourniquet can be used in lieu of a thigh tourniquet, but this compresses the leg muscles, shortening tendons traversing the ankle joint and preventing joint distraction. This represents a significant impediment to ankle arthroscopy under regional anesthesia. A tourniquet can often be avoided as long as a high-flow cannula is used and synovial debridement is kept to a minimum.

Distraction can help open the ankle joint for viewing and allow safe passage of instruments without damaging the articular cartilage. Static invasive distractors may be placed with threaded pins through the calcaneus and the tibia, or with a less invasive sling around the heel and midfoot that is tensioned at the end of the operative table. Our preference is to use dynamic distraction with an elasticized bandage tied around the foot, just below the malleoli, and then around the operative surgeon's waist (Fig. 14–2). This allows for relaxation and distraction when needed, as well as the ability to dorsiflex and plantarflex the ankle with pressure on the sole of the foot from the operative surgeon's abdomen (Fig. 14–3). It carries the added benefit of avoiding prolonged, persistent traction, which may result in skin necrosis or possibly nerve injury. Ergonomically, the surgeon has good control over the position of the foot and comfortable hand position when working through the anteromedial and anterolateral portals (Fig. 14–4). Supine dynamic distraction also allows the surgeon to abduct the ankle over the edge of the table and access the posterior portals by dropping the surgeon's hands posteriorly below the mid-coronal line of the ankle (Fig. 14–5).

Prone Positioning

The prone position is usually more uncomfortable for the awake patient, and also makes access to the airway

harder for the anesthesiologist. This combination of factors favors general anesthesia in the prone patient. Gel rolls or rolled blankets are placed longitudinally along the chest wall to elevate it from the table. Alternately, a prone positioning table such as a Wilson frame table can be used (Fig. 14–6). The sterile field should extend to the knee, but not above it. A thigh tourniquet is typically used. Surgeon hand positioning is similar to supine positioning (Fig. 14–7). Distraction may or may not be used with posterior ankle arthroscopy.

Equipment

A 2.9-mm 30-degree wide-angle arthroscope with a high-flow cannula is the most versatile scope for ankle arthroscopy. It allows a good balance between flow (which keeps

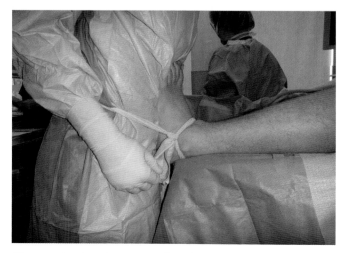

Figure 14–3. Intraoperative photograph of dorsiflexion of the ankle with pressure against the surgeon's abdomen.

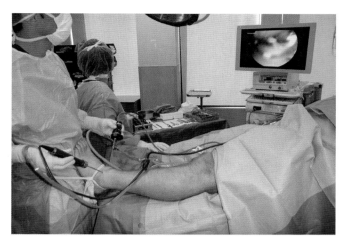

Figure 14–4. Intraoperative photograph of positioning for supine arthroscopy.

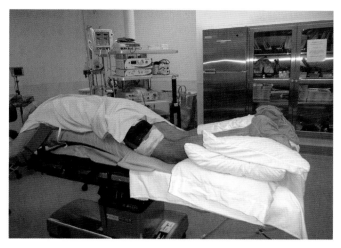

Figure 14–6. Photograph of prone positioning on the Wilson frame table.

the viewing field clear), small diameter (which allows drive-through over the talar dome into the anterior or posterior portion of the ankle), and field of view (which allows visualization of pathology). It is useful to have on hand and be familiar with the use of a 4.0-mm 30-degree scope as well, as this allows high flow and a larger field of view when advanced imaging indicates that drive-through into other compartments will not be necessary. For tight joints, a 2.4-mm 30-degree scope can be used if the 2.9-mm scope cannot be inserted.

An automatic pump may be used to maintain a constant pressure within the ankle joint to aid in distraction and tamponade of bleeding vessels during soft tissue debridement or microfracture of open cancellous bone. Gravity flow with or without a hand pump is also a serviceable option.

Powered shavers are essential for joint visualization as they allow soft tissue debridement as well as variable outflow. For the ankle a 3.5-mm shaver will suffice, and a 4-mm burr will fit in if needed for debridement of anterior

osteophytes, posterior osteophytes, or to prepare articular surfaces for arthroscopically assisted ankle fusions.

A selection of curved and straight curettes (00 or 000) will assist in debridement of OCD lesions. Ring curettes may also be useful for debridement. Straight and curved osteotomes in the 2 to 5 mm range will allow removal

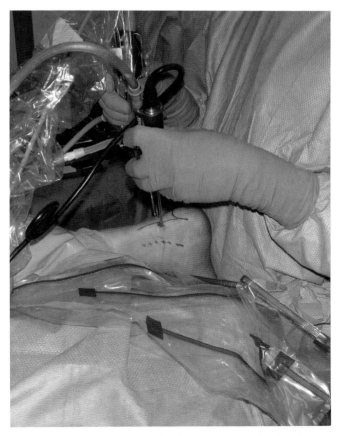

Figure 14–7. Photograph of surgeon positioning for prone arthroscopy.

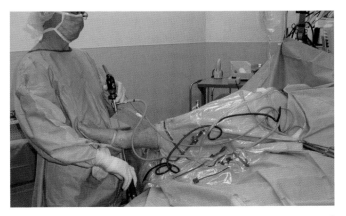

Figure 14–5. Intraoperative photograph of abduction of the leg away from the table to allow access to the posterior portals.

of anterior osteophytes in lieu of a burr. A pituitary rongeur or intra-articular grasper will assist in the removal of bone fragments. Knee instruments are valuable to keep available, including probes and microfracture awls. Drills may be necessary for retrograde drilling of OCD lesions.

PORTAL PLACEMENT

Safe portal placement requires a sound understanding of the anatomy surrounding the ankle and the traversing structures at risk. The ankle affords the advantage of relatively subcutaneous endangered structures, making their identification by palpation and visualization easier than in other joints. Figures 14–8 and 14–9 shows the anatomical relationship of portals to the surrounding soft tissue structures.

Standard anterior portals include the workhorse anteromedial and anterolateral portals, which are located at the "soft spots" of the ankle as shown in Figure 14–10. Posteriorly, the posterolateral portal is the most often used, though a posteromedial portal is a viable option,

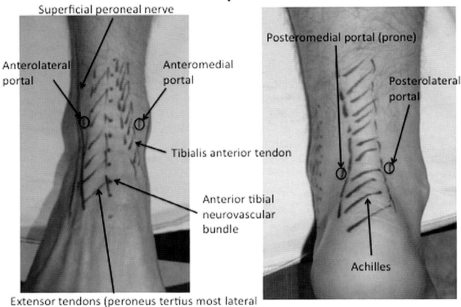

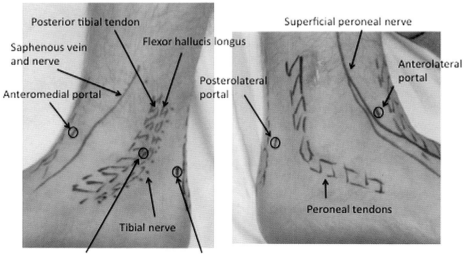

Figure 14–8. Pertinent ankle surface anatomy surrounding **(A)** anterior, posterior medial, and **(B)** medial and lateral arthroscopic portals.

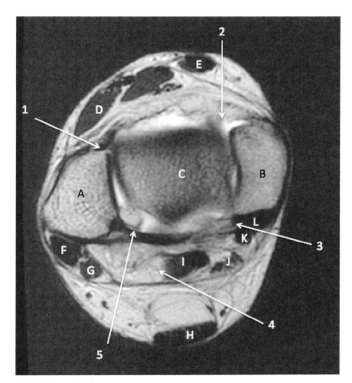

Figure 14–9. Cross-sectional anatomy at the ankle joint of different intervals for portal placement: *(1)* anterolateral portal; *(2)* anteromedial portal; *(3)* posteromedial portal (supine); *(4)* posteromedial portal (prone); *(5)* posterolateral portal; *(A)* lateral malleolus; *(B)* medial malleolus; *(C)* talus; *(D)* peroneus tertius and extensor digitorum longus; *(E)* tibialis anterior; *(F)* peroneus brevis; *(G)* peroneus longus; *(H)* Achilles tendon; *(I)* flexor hallucis longus; *(J)* tibial nerve and posterior tibial artery; *(K)* flexor digitorum longus; *(L)* posterior tibialis tendon.

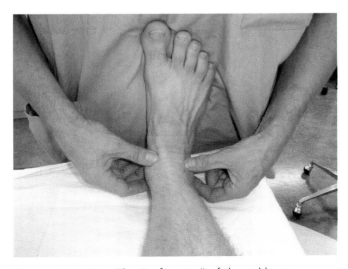

Figure 14–10. The "soft spots" of the ankle are palpated at the joint line just medial to the tibialis anterior tendon (on the left side of the photograph) and just lateral to the peroneus tertius tendon (on the right side of the photograph). Gentle dorsiflexion and plantarflexion help identify the joint line.

especially for addressing posteromedial pathology. The posteromedial portal is made through a different interval depending on whether it is approached in the supine or the prone position. The trans-Achilles portal, the anterocentral portal, and transosseous portals through the medial malleolus are rarely used, though they might have limited use in specific circumstances. Accessory portals can be made over the tip of the medial and lateral malleolus (just inferior to the standard anteromedial and anterolateral portals) to assist in instrumentation and visualization of the gutters.

In general, ankle portals are made using a "nick-and-spread" technique to avoid injury to underlying nerves. Unlike the knee and shoulder, skin nerves are close to the anterior lateral portal and are easily damaged. The superficial branch of the peroneal nerve is particularly at risk.[1]

After correct portal marking, a 15 or 11 blade is used to make a vertical incision through the skin, then a small snap is used to spread down to the level of the joint capsule, which is penetrated with the blunt snap or subsequent trocar. The ankle joint can be injected with arthroscopic fluid prior to portal placement in order to distend the joint and protect the articular surfaces from blindly inserted instruments.

The anteromedial portal is placed between the anterior tibial tendon and the saphenous vein, where a soft spot is palpable at the joint line. The saphenous vein is at risk with this portal. The anteromedial portal is typically the first portal established in a standard arthroscopic examination of the ankle joint. Subsequent portals are established under direct visualization using an 18-gauge needle to establish a location prior to trocar placement.

The anterolateral portal is placed between the peroneus tertius (on the lateral boarder of the extensor digitorum longus) and the superficial peroneal nerve, which is vulnerable to injury. The superficial peroneal nerve can be seen through the skin by inverting the hindfoot and plantarflexing the ankle. It appears as a linear, branching structure sweeping from superior-posterior to anterior-inferior just in front of the lateral malleolus at the level of the joint line. A blunt instrument can be rolled over the nerve perpendicular to its course to identify it. The anterolateral portal is typically the workhorse portal for instrument placement, though swapping of the viewing and working portal medially and laterally is common based on the location of pathology.

The anterocentral portal can provide a view of the central talar dome and distal tibia, but its proximity to the anterior tibial artery and the deep peroneal nerve place these structures at significant risk. Given the overlying extensor tendons, the at-risk structures are not as easily identifiable as they are with the anteromedial and anterolateral portals, and therefore at greater risk.

The posterolateral portal is the most commonly used posterior portal. It lies lateral to the Achilles tendon and just medial to the small saphenous vein and the sural nerve, both of which are at risk with portal placement. It

TABLE 14–1. The 21-Point Comprehensive Ankle Examination

Anterior Ankle	Central Ankle	Posterior Ankle
Deltoid ligament	Medial tibia and talus	Posteromedial gutter
Point 1 Deep Deltoid Ligament	Point 9	Point 15 Deltoid Ligament Posteromedial Gutter
Medial gutter	Central tibia and talus	Posteromedial talus
Point 2 Medial Gutter	Point 10	Point 16
Medial talus	Lateral tibiofibular or talofibular articulation	Posterocentral talus
Point 3 Medial Talar Dome	Point 11	Notch of Harty Point 17
Central talus and overhang	Posterior inferior tibiofibular ligament	Posterolateral talus
Point 4	Point 12 Posterior Inferior Tibiofibular Ligament	Point 18

(*continued*)

Anterior Ankle	Central Ankle	Posterior Ankle
Trifurcation of the talus, tibia, and fibula	Transverse ligament	Posterior talofibular articulation

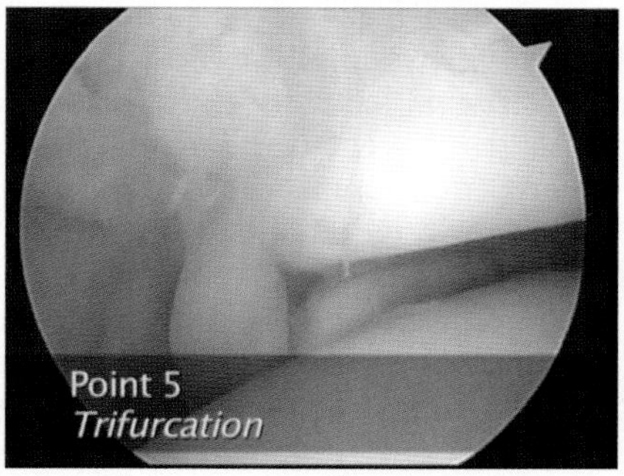

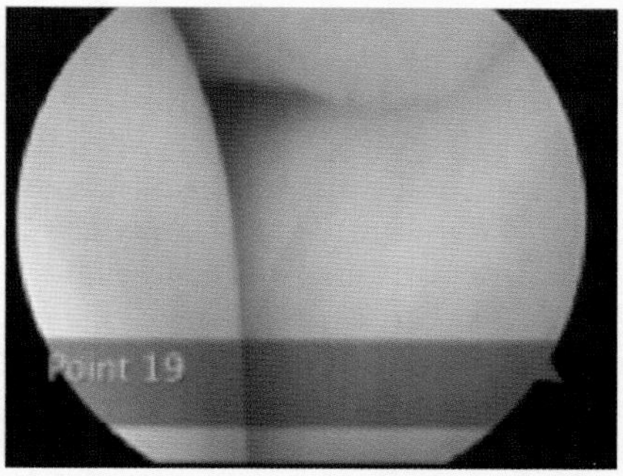

Point 5
Trifurcation

Point 13
Transverse Tibiofibular Ligament

Point 19

Lateral talus and anterior inferior tibiofibular ligament | Reflection of the flexor hallucis longus | Posterolateral gutter and posterior talofibular ligament

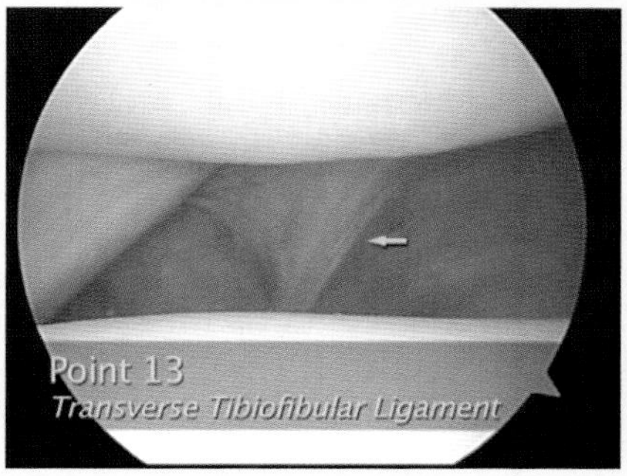

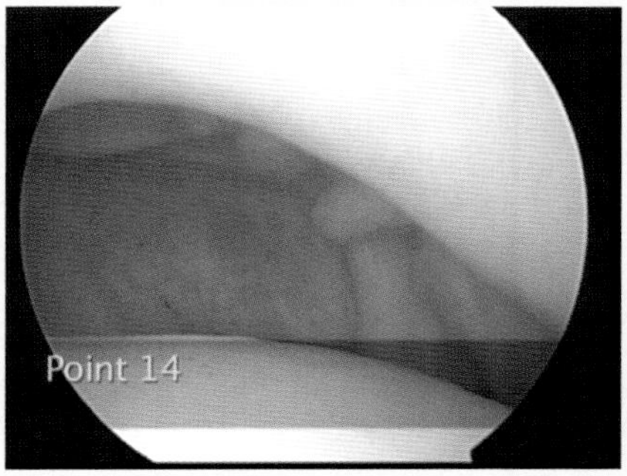

Point 6
Anterior Inferior Tibiofibular Ligament

Point 14

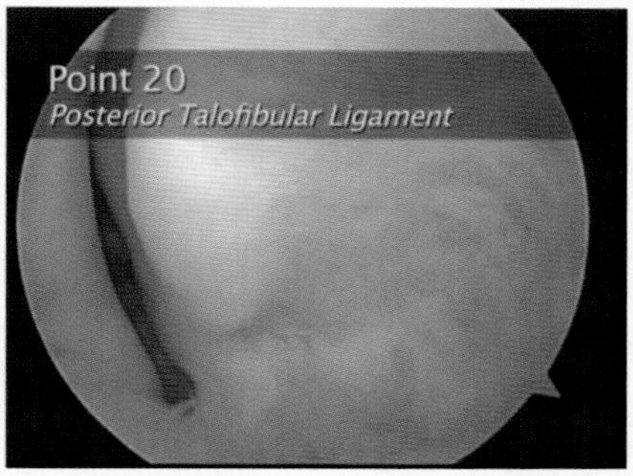

Point 20
Posterior Talofibular Ligament

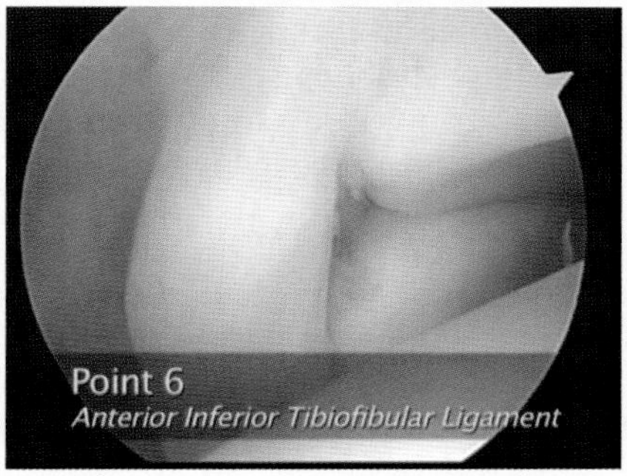

Lateral gutter and anterior talofibular ligament

Posterior gutter

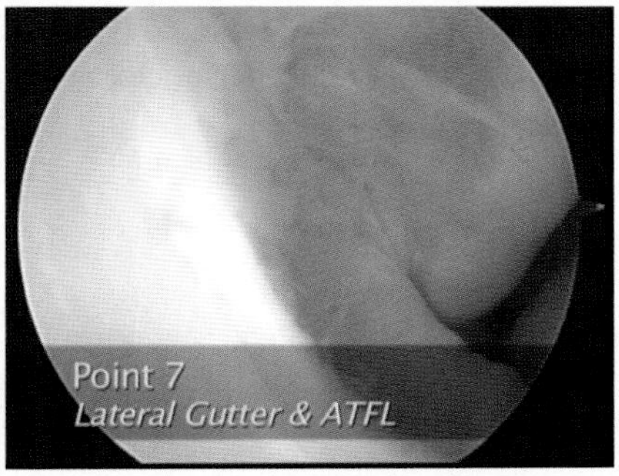

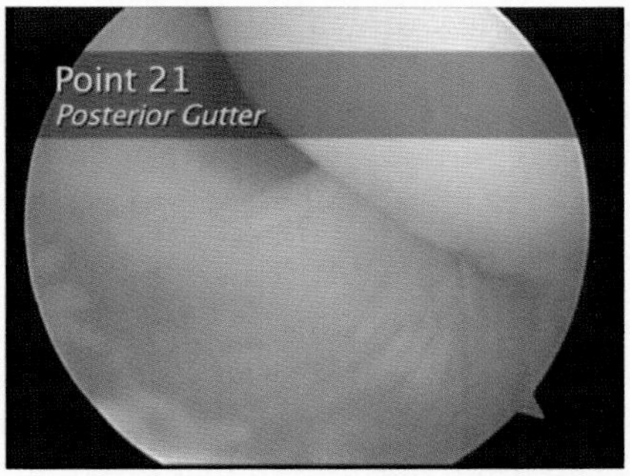

Point 7
Lateral Gutter & ATFL

Point 21
Posterior Gutter

Anterior gutter

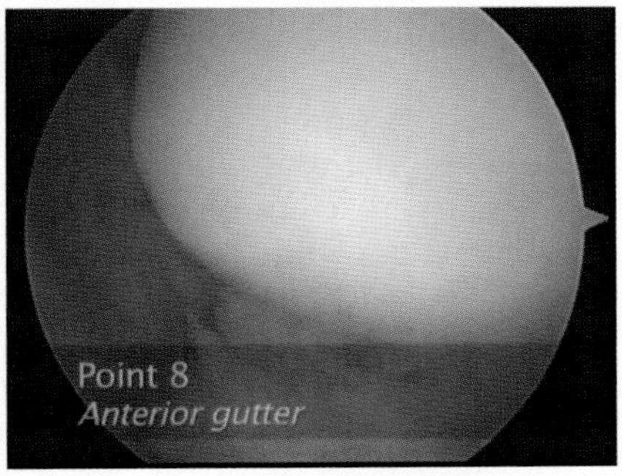

Point 8
Anterior gutter

Photographs with permission from Albritton MJ, Ferkel RD. 21 Point Arthroscopic Examination of the Ankle (Video) AAOS, Rosemont, Illinois; Cheng JC, Ferkel RD. The role of arthroscopy in ankle and subtalar degenerative joint disease. *Clin Orthop Relat Res.* 1998;(349):65–72.

is placed in the same position whether used in the supine or the prone position.

The posteromedial portal is made through two different intervals depending on the positioning of the patient. In the supine position, the leg is abducted over the edge of the bed and the portal is made just behind the medial malleolus in the interval between the posterior tibial tendon and the flexor digitorum longus, which protects the tibial nerve and vessels lying just posterior. In cadaver dissection we have found this portal to go behind the flexor digitorum longus one-third of the time, placing the tibial nerve and vessels at risk. As a result the portal must be used with extreme care. To prevent damage to the tibial nerve the skin incision should be shallow, and sharp obturators should be avoided if the arthroscope is being placed in this portal. If the portal is being used for instrumentation, all power instruments must be viewed with the arthroscope within the joint before being turned on.

When using a posterior medial portal in the prone position, it is typically placed just medial to the Achilles tendon at the level of the ankle joint. The deep plane is always lateral to the flexor hallucis longus tendon at the posterior boarder of the medial flexor tendon/neurovascular bundle to avoid damage to these structures. It is typically used in conjunction with the posterolateral portal. As described by van Dijk, typically the arthroscope is inserted in the posterolateral portal, aiming toward the first web space and resting in the soft tissue at the posterior lateral aspect of the ankle.[2] Instruments are inserted through the posteromedial portal perpendicular to the arthroscope and they are slid down the scope until they come into view. Triangulation by palpation with the instrument tips is necessary prior to turning on the shaver in oscillating mode. Care must therefore be taken to ensure that the shaver starts laterally and progresses medially.

The posteromedial portal may be chosen over the posterior lateral portal because it allows easy access to the posterior side of the ankle in the prone position and is extremely valuable for debriding posterior medial osteochondral defects. In an unpublished internal review of 109 cases using this portal, there were three reported cases of transient numbness in the tibial nerve distribution, all of which resolved with time.

STANDARD ARTHROSCOPIC EVALUATION AND VIEWS

Traditionally, a 21-point examination, described by Ferkel, has been used to describe the stepwise approach to examining the ankle (Table 14–1).[3] This examination traditionally starts with the arthroscope in the anteromedial portal and progresses posteriorly. Illustrations of arthroscopic views from the 21-point examination are shown in Table 14–1. The complete 21-point examination is useful for meticulous examination of the ankle (ensuring that no pathology is missed) and standardization of arthroscopic views. We find that dedicated arthroscopic photos of each view are usually unnecessary, and oftentimes individual points on the examination blend into a dynamic view of specific regions of the ankle.

The most preferable portal for viewing is dependent on the location of pathology, the tightness of the ankle joint, and the position of the patient. The tightness of the ankle, which can be increased by arthritis, contractures, scarring, and tourniquets, affects the amount of the ankle that can be viewed from any individual portal. Figure 14–11 shows the area of the talus that is visible through each of the major viewing areas: anterolateral, anteromedial, and posterior (including both the posteromedial and posterolateral portals). The area that is visible from each portal is decreased in a tight ankle significantly, as shown in the illustrations.

We prefer to modify the approach, order, and focus of the arthroscopic examination dependent on the pathology being treated. For arthroscopic ankle fusion, all joint surfaces must be examined and debrided in a systematic way to allow cartilage removal. In ankle instability the joint is usually loose and mobile, making safe viewing of the joint much easier, especially from the lateral side. The medial and lateral talar dome should be carefully inspected and probed for osteochondral injuries that oftentimes accompany instability. In anterior impingement (bony and soft tissue) an anterior debridement should be done first to allow access to the rest of the joint. The ankle should be dorsiflexed during anterior debridement to avoid injury to the deep branch of the peroneal nerve and the anterior tibial artery, as they sit just anterior to the capsule at the level of the joint. In ankle arthroscopies after fracture, the joint is often stiff and hard to visualize. A smaller scope is often needed and even with care and experience the joint surface may not be fully visualized.

COMPLICATIONS

Early reviews and surveys indicated a very low complication rate from ankle arthroscopy.[4,5] It is likely that these low complication rates (below 2%) were prone to recall and/or reporting bias and not accurate. There have been a handful of relatively large, relatively high-quality series of ankle arthroscopies for a multitude of indications that show an overall complication rate between 7% and 9%.[1,6–8] Other references in the literature broaden the complication rate to between 3% and 13%.[9,10]

In the largest series to date, the most common complication was neurologic injury, specifically to the superficial peroneal nerve, which is in close proximity to the anterolateral portal.[1] Anatomic cadaver studies have demonstrated that the primary neurovascular structures at risk—the superficial peroneal nerve with the anterolateral portal, the saphenous vein and nerve with the anteromedial portal, the sural nerve with the posterolateral portal, and the tibial nerve and vessels with the posteromedial portal—are within 1 cm of their respective portal.[11–13] This emphasizes the importance of two

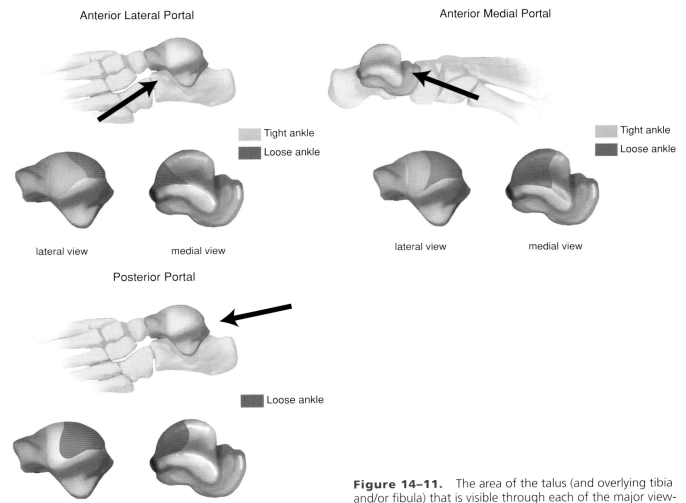

Anterior Lateral Portal

Tight ankle
Loose ankle

lateral view   medial view

Posterior Portal

Loose ankle

lateral view   medial view

Anterior Medial Portal

Tight ankle
Loose ankle

lateral view   medial view

Figure 14–11. The area of the talus (and overlying tibia and/or fibula) that is visible through each of the major viewing areas: anterolateral, anteromedial, and posterior.

things when placing portals: proper knowledge and identification of landmarks and surface anatomy, and careful nick-and-spread portal placement technique.

Other surgical complications related to distractor placement, overzealous or prolonged distraction, damage to tendons and ligaments, chondral damage from instruments, broken or retained instruments, infection, and reflex sympathetic dystrophy are possible as well.[6]

REHABILITATION PROTOCOL

Rehabilitation protocols vary based on whether or not soft tissue or bony repairs require time to heal. In general, arthroscopy allows a faster recovery than open arthrotomies, which require a period of limited range of motion while joint-spanning incisions heal. Smaller portal incisions are typically less painful and more cosmetic than open arthrotomy incisions as well. Portals are typically closed with single sutures to avoid arthrocutaneous fistulas.

OUTCOME

Outcomes are specific to the procedure performed and the tool used to measure outcome. Undoubtedly the ankle arthroscopist's comfort with viewing and addressing pathology has improved over the decades since its widespread adoption—it is impossible to definitively say whether this has resulted in better outcomes. Part of this uncertainty stems from the lack of a single, accurate, validated, universally adopted tool for measuring outcome. Ankle arthroscopy is typically performed on a relatively active population, and tools such as the AOFAS score are likely not sensitive enough to record functional improvements that may be of value to the patient. By the same token, measures of global function such as the EQ-5D and the SF-36 are broader still in their scope. Other tools, such as patient satisfaction and their answer to the question "would you have this procedure again" are prone to significant bias.

Ankle arthroscopy has allowed the creation of new procedures, but it has also allowed established procedures to be performed in less invasive ways. As an example, there is evidence that arthroscopic ankle fusion gives significantly improved results without increases in complications when compared to open ankle fusion.[14] This, ultimately, should be the ankle arthroscopist's goal: to offer new and improved techniques while reducing complications and rehabilitation time and optimizing results.

REFERENCES

1. Ferkel RD, Heath DD, Guhl JF. Neurological complications of ankle arthroscopy. *Arthroscopy.* 1996;12(2):200–208.
2. Dijk CN. Hindfoot endoscopy for posterior ankle pain. *Instr Course Lect.* 2006;55:545–554.
3. Cheng JC, Ferkel RD. The role of arthroscopy in ankle and subtalar degenerative joint disease. *Clin Orthop Relat Res.* 1998;(349):65–72.
4. Small NC. Complications in arthroscopic surgery performed by experienced arthroscopists. *Arthroscopy.* 1988; 4(3):215–221.
5. Small NC. Complications in arthroscopy: the knee and other joints. Committee on Complications of the Arthroscopy Association of North America. *Arthroscopy.* 1986;2(4):253–258.
6. Ferkel RD, Small HN, Gittins JE. Complications in foot and ankle arthroscopy. *Clin Orthop Relat Res.* 2001;(391):89–104.
7. Young BH, Flanigan RM, DiGiovanni BF. Complications of ankle arthroscopy utilizing a contemporary noninvasive distraction technique. *J Bone Joint Surg.* 2011;93(10):963–968.
8. Nickisch F, Barg A, Saltzman CL, et al. Postoperative complications of posterior ankle and hindfoot arthroscopy. *J Bone Joint Surg.* 2012;94(5):439–446.
9. Niek van Dijk C, van Bergen CJ. Advancements in ankle arthroscopy. *J Am Acad Orthop Surg.* 2008;16(11):635–646.
10. Unger F, Lajtai G, Ramadani F, et al. [Arthroscopy of the upper ankle joint. A retrospective analysis of complications]. *Unfallchirurg.* 2000;103(10):858–863.
11. Takao M, Uchio Y, Shu N, et al. Anatomic bases of ankle arthroscopy: Study of superficial and deep peroneal nerves around anterolateral and anterocentral approach. *Surg Radiol Anat.* 1998;20(5):317–320.
12. Feiwell LA, Frey C. Anatomic study of arthroscopic debridement of the ankle. *Foot Ankle Int.* 1994;15(11):614–621.
13. Göksel D, Halil Ibrahim B, Mehmet A, et al. Paper # 211: Relationship of posterior ankle arthroscopy portals with neurovascular structures at different ankle position on fresh cadaver. *Arthroscopy.* 2011;27(10):e211–e212.
14. Younger A, Townshend DN, Di Silvestro M, et al. Prospective comparison of open and arthroscopic ankle arthrodesis using validated outcome score with two-year minimum follow-up (SS-55). *Arthroscopy J Arthroscopic Relat Surg.* 2011;27(5, Supplement):e59.

CHAPTER 15

Arthroscopic Treatment of Osteochondral Lesions of the Talus: Microfracture

Eric Giza   Edward Shin   Stephanie E. Wong

INDICATIONS

Osteochondral lesions of the talus (OLTs) are rare, representing approximately 4% of all such lesions in the body.[1] These lesions also have been termed osteochondritis dissecans, transchondral fracture, talar dome fracture, and osteochondral defect. OLTs consist of a focal cartilage deficit with associated reactive bone edema. Lesions may extend to subchondral bone, causing bone loss. Following traumatic injury to articular cartilage, the capacity for intrinsic repair is limited by chondrocyte encasement in a matrix, limited vascularity, and chondrocyte apoptosis. Full-thickness injuries that extend to subchondral bone allow recruitment of marrow elements, but injuries greater than 2 to 4 mm show a poor potential to heal with normal appearing cartilage.[2]

The talar dome is trapezoidal in shape, and its anterior surface averages 2.5 mm wider than the posterior surface. The medial and lateral articular facets of the talus articulate with the medial and lateral malleoli. The articular surface of these facets is contiguous with the superior articular surface of the talar dome. Approximately 60% of the dome of the talus is covered by the trochlear articular cartilage, which is incapable of supporting intrinsic repair. The cartilage is largely avascular and incapable of healing through the typical inflammatory phase.

The talus has no muscular or tendinous attachments, further limiting the healing potential of cartilage defects. Most of the blood supply of the talus enters through the neck via the sinus tarsi. The dorsalis pedis artery supplies the head and neck of the talus. The artery of the sinus tarsi is formed from branches of the peroneal and dorsalis pedis arteries. The artery of the tarsal canal arises from branches of the posterior tibial artery. The sinus tarsi artery and the tarsal canal artery join to form an anastomotic sling inferior to the talus, from which branches enter the talar neck.

The articular cartilage of the talus is inconsistent in thickness, with the posteromedial corner having a greater depth of cartilage than the anterolateral. This is manifest in geographic mechanical properties and may influence the rate and type of articular injury.[3-5] Various mechanisms have been suggested by authors to describe the location of OLTs although there is no clear consensus. Raikin et al. examined 428 ankles by MRI and developed a nine-cell grid to describe the location of injuries in the talar dome (Fig. 15–1). They found that both medial (53%) and lateral (26%) defects were most common at the equator or mid talar dome.[6]

Patients with OLT typically present with chronic ankle pain along with variable amounts of swelling, catching, stiffness, and instability. Ligamentous instability may be a predisposing factor and should be assessed. Palpation may reveal tenderness behind the medial malleolus when the ankle is dorsiflexed, indicating a posteromedial lesion. Anterolateral lesions may be tender when the anterolateral ankle joint is palpated with the joint in maximal plantar flexion. An effusion in a chronically painful joint usually indicates intra-articular pathology, which could include an OLT.

A history of trauma is documented in more than 85% of patients.[7-11] In most cases, the mechanism of injury is an inversion injury to the lateral ligamentous complex. Although the etiology of nontraumatic OLTs is unknown, a primary ischemic event may be responsible. Nontraumatic OLTs can also be familial, multiple lesions can occur in the same patient, and identical medial talar lesions have occurred in identical twins.[12]

Patients with an acute ankle injury with hemarthrosis or substantial tenderness should first undergo weight-bearing plain radiography in anteroposterior, lateral, and mortise views (Fig. 15–2). Radiographs in varying degrees of plantar flexion and dorsiflexion may help in diagnosing posteromedial and anterolateral lesions, respectively.[13] Plain radiographs of the contralateral ankle should be obtained, as there is a 10% to 25% incidence of a contralateral lesion.[14]

Symptomatic patients with negative findings on plain radiographs should undergo an initial period of immobilization, followed by physical therapy. Patients whose plain images indicate OLTs and patients who remain symptomatic after 6 weeks should undergo additional evaluation with MRI.

Magnetic resonance imaging (MRI) can identify occult injuries of the subchondral bone and cartilage that may not be detected with routine radiographs.[15,16] Classic MRI findings include areas of low signal intensity on T1-weighted images, which suggests sclerosis of the bed of the lesion and that it is chronic (Fig. 15–3).[17,18] T2-weighted images reveal a rim that represents instability of the osteochondral fragment.[17-19] Posttreatment

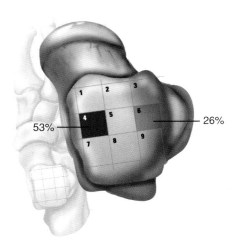

Figure 15–1. Talar dome with grid of areas most frequently involved with osteochondral lesions of the talus. (Modified with permission from Foot and Ankle International, AOFAS.)

MRI should reveal a reduction or disappearance of the low signal intensity on T1-weighted images and the rim on T2-weighted images.

Conservative treatment for symptomatic OLTs may be attempted with smaller lesions in the absence of

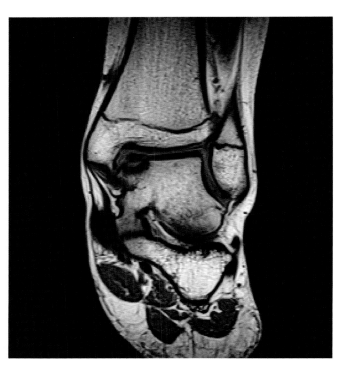

Figure 15–3. T1-weighted coronal ankle MRI of the same patient in Figure 15–2. MRI demonstrates a medial talus OLT with detached, but nondisplaced fragment.

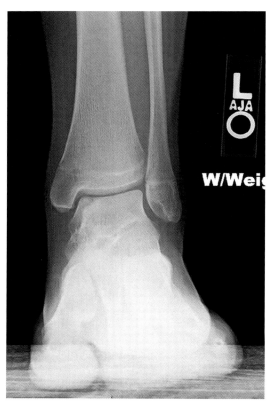

Figure 15–2. Anteroposterior ankle radiograph of a skeletally mature 13-year-old who had pain and swelling with activity following an ankle sprain.

mechanical symptoms. A period of immobilization with weight-bearing restriction and progressive range of motion has been advocated. Studies have shown that a trial of conservative therapy does not adversely affect surgery performed after conservative therapy has failed.[1,20] Arthroscopy is indicated for unstable lesions and those that have failed conservative treatment with stable lesions. The initial surgical treatment for most OLTs involves curettage and microfracture using arthroscopic technique. Best results are seen in patients with small lesions (<1 cm^2) and stable surrounding cartilage. The lesion is debrided to a stable articular rim with marrow stimulation techniques used to create the healing cartilage. This technique is described in detail later in this chapter.

Surgical repair of OLTs is contraindicated when the risks outweigh the perceived benefits. Patients with advanced osteoarthritis and deformity are poor candidates due to compromised healing potential. Risks include active infection in the operative area, the likelihood of patient noncompliance, and patients who are medically unstable. Relative contraindications include degenerative changes of the ankle involving more than an isolated OLT.

The goals of cartilage repair are to restore the articular cartilage surface, match the biochemical and biomechanical properties of normal hyaline cartilage, improve patient symptoms and function, and prevent or slow progression of focal chondral injury. O'Driscoll[21] has posited that articular cartilage injury can be restored, replaced, relieved, or resected (the four r's). Acute restoration is performed on the rare lesion with a bony defined fragment that is technically repairable. Delamination must not be present and the best candidates are young athletes with good healing potential who are able to comply with weight-bearing restrictions. Techniques include open reduction and internal fixation with recessed transchondral screws, retrograde internal fixation, and biodegradable fixation devices. No large scale studies are available to evaluate these techniques.[22] Open reduction, internal fixation (ORIF) is reserved for large acute OLTs and will not be covered here.

Replacing, relieving, or resecting the OLT can be facilitated through open or arthroscopic approaches. Prior to the advent of arthroscopic technology, namely, high-resolution, small-diameter scopes, the open approach was the standard treatment of OLT.[23] Arthrotomies and osteotomies allowed access to the tibiotalar articular surface.

Open treatment for OLT has been well described by Flick and generally requires extensive arthrotomy and dissection.[20] Morbidity with these open approaches is often severe, with reported atrophy and stiffness of the ankle, as well as malleolar malunion or nonunion from transmalleolar osteotomies.[24] Arthroscopy of the ankle has eliminated many of these complications associated with open approaches.

Currently, most primary interventions are performed with the aid of the arthroscope. Arthroscopic treatment of OLT involves one or a combination of the following three principles: removing loose bodies, securing the lesion to the talar dome (ORIF), and/or stimulating development of repair cartilage. In addition to avoiding the morbidity associated with open surgical technique, minimally invasive or arthroscopic treatment of talar dome lesions potentially allows for earlier rehabilitation.

There is significant history of treatment of OLT with either microfracture or autologous osteochondral transplant, with more recent progression to the use of minimally invasive techniques for osteochondral grafting, chondrocyte transplantation, and bulk fresh allograft transplantation. These technologies represent significant developments and ongoing research toward achieving the goals of cartilage repair or restoration in OLT.

This chapter is dedicated to the description of microfracture treatment of OLTs using minimally invasive or arthroscopic technique. The main goals of treatment are to provide relief of pain and mechanical symptoms by stimulating fibrocartilage filling of the defect.

PATIENT POSITIONING

Following induction of general anesthesia, the patient is laid supine on the operating table. A roll is placed under the ipsilateral hip to facilitate optimal rotation of the operative ankle, and a pneumatic tourniquet is applied to the thigh. The operative leg is then placed in a commercially available positioner with the hip and knee flexed approximately 30 degrees (Fig. 15–4). The general room set up with draping is shown in Fig. 15–5.

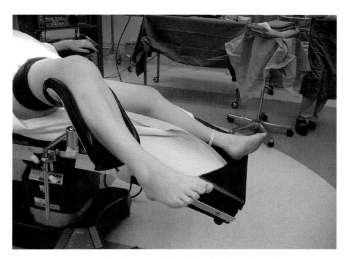

Figure 15–4. Patient positioning before draping.

SURGICAL APPROACHES

The anteromedial portal is established medial to the anterior tibial tendon at the level of the joint (Fig. 15–6). A 30-degree 2.7-mm arthroscope is introduced via an anteromedial portal; however, it is recommended to have a 70-degree 2.7-mm arthroscope and 1.9-mm arthroscope available. Next an anterolateral portal is established under direct visualization just lateral to the peroneus tertius tendon. If possible, the branches of the superficial peroneal nerve should be palpated and marked prior to the procedure in order to decrease the possible complication of neuritis or nerve laceration (Fig. 15–7). If necessary, a posterolateral portal can be used to access posterior lesions.

Access to the joint space is highly dependent on the ligamentous restraint, capsule fibrosis, and bony architecture. A joint distraction system is not always necessary, but

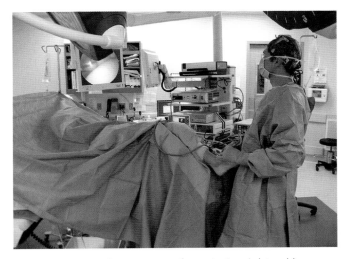

Figure 15–5. Room set up for anterior right ankle arthroscopy. Note that video monitor and arthroscopic equipment is all readily visualized by surgeon in comfortable working position.

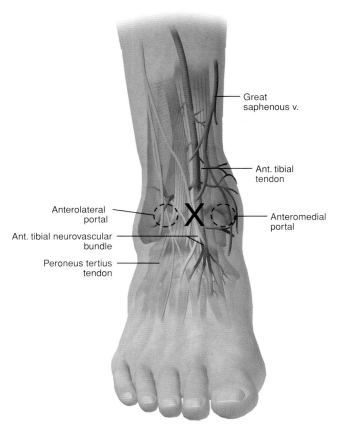

Figure 15–6. Anterior ankle neurovascular structures. Anteromedial and anterolateral portal locations are marked. Anterocentral portal (X) placement should be avoided to minimize risk of neurovascular structure damage.

should be available so that the entire articular surface of the tibia and talus can be inspected thoroughly. Distraction techniques facilitate the placement of the arthroscope and instruments into the tightly configured ankle joint and play an important role in allowing access to

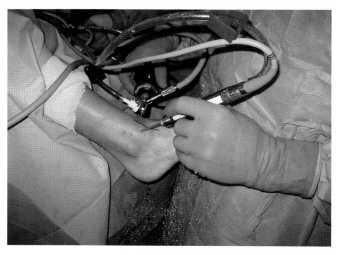

Figure 15–7. Anteromedial and anterolateral portal placement in right ankle arthroscopy.

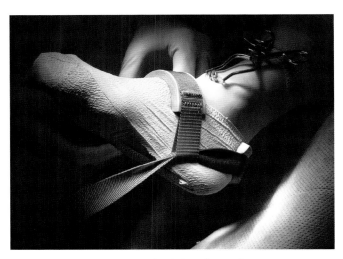

Figure 15–8. Noninvasive joint distraction system.

talar dome lesions. Noninvasive techniques involving straps, harnesses, and outriggers are distraction methods used most commonly and minimize the risk of neurovascular injury and other complications (Fig. 15–8).[25]

Removal of anterior tibial and talar osteophytes should be performed to improve visualization and prevent anterior impingement. Anterior osteophyte removal should be performed without joint distraction to ensure that the anterior neurovascular structures are not tented over the anterior ankle joint.

SURGICAL TECHNIQUES

The microfracture technique for OLTs is based on the success of similar techniques in the knee.[26,27] An overview of the microfracture technique for OLTs is shown in Figure 15–9. Once the lesion is identified, the size and extent of the lesion is carefully probed and any loose or delaminated material is curetted or removed with a shaver (Fig. 15–10). Soft or cystic bone is also removed and the cartilage is debrided to a stable border (Fig. 15–11). The lesion is carefully measured and using arthroscopic awls, microfractures are made approximately 3 to 4 mm apart in the subchondral bone (if intact) while maintaining integrity of the bone plate (Fig. 15–12). The microfracture technique promotes new tissue formation by releasing substances such as mesenchymal stem cells, growth factors, and healing proteins.[26] Ultimately, cartilage-like cells (fibrocartilage) form and fill the original defect. Figure 15–13 shows the microfracture technique completed. A tourniquet is used during the procedure and should be released to confirm a bleeding bed of bone in the area of the microfracture (Fig. 15–14). The technique can be performed entirely through standard arthroscopic portals for lesions at the equator of the dome and anterior.

Retrograde talar drilling can be used to stimulate medullary bleeding in cystic lesions with intact cartilage and subchondral bone.[28] The use of an anterior cruciate

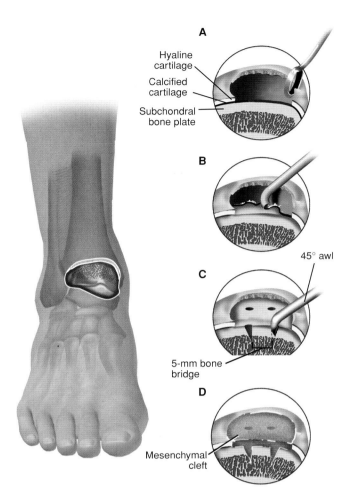

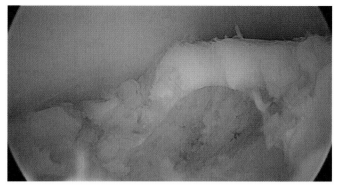

Figure 15–11.   The unstable lesion in Figure 15–10 debrided to a stable border of healthy tissue.

Figure 15–9.   Microfracture technique (first figure) superimposed upon a cross-sectional view of the talar dome (second figure). (**A**) Ring curette is used to achieve stable peripheral border of cartilage. (**B**) Standard curette is used to expose the subchondral bone. (**C**) Microfracture awl is used to perforate the subchondral bone and allow marrow elements to reach the area of the OLT. (**D**) Marrow clot fills articular defect on talus.

ligament (ACL)-type guide and fluoroscopy can be helpful for this technique. A 4 to 6 mm ACL reamer is advanced through the sinus tarsi and lateral neck area with the use of a guidewire. Care is taken not to disrupt the intact cartilage overlying the cyst. Once the lesion has been ablated allograft bone can be placed in the drill hole, at the surgeon's discretion.

Any concomitant ligament stabilization should follow the arthroscopy procedure to avoid trauma to the repaired ligaments. Sample biopsy cartilage, including that from the lesion itself, can be harvested if subsequent chondrocyte implantation is foreseeable.

COMPLICATIONS

Complications of talus microfracture surgery include injury to neurovascular structures in the anterior ankle (such as superficial peroneal neuritis) and need for repeat surgery. In addition, there is risk of standard surgical complications such as wound healing problems, infection, and deep vein thrombosis.

Revision microfracture surgery is indicated for patients with persistent pain who have imaging suggestive of incomplete healing and whom are not candidates for more invasive procedures. Repeat microfracture for continued pain after a primary procedure in some cases

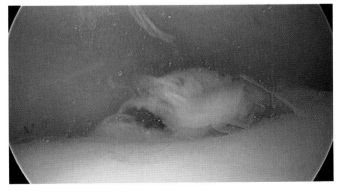

Figure 15–10.   Arthroscopic photograph of the same patient in Figure 15–2 showing an unstable OLT.

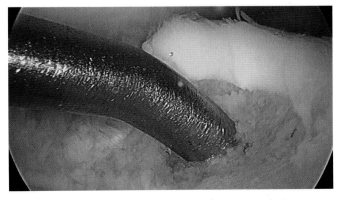

Figure 15–12.   Arthroscopic microfracture awl placement.

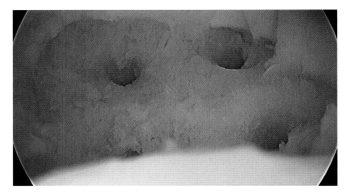

Figure 15–13. Microfracture hole placement in talar bone. These are approximately 3 mm apart from one another.

has been shown to be effective at a mean of 5.9 years. Repeat microfracture or drilling appears to be a reasonable, low complication procedure for patients who have failed primary attempts at healing if the lesion is one that clinically has a high expectation of healing.[29]

REHABILITATION PROTOCOL

Postoperative protocol is individualized for the approach and the techniques used to reestablish the articular surface. Patients who undergo arthroscopic debridement with microfracture do not bear weight for 4 weeks. Non–weight-bearing motion is started at 2 weeks to promote molding of the joint surface in the area of the former OLT and synovial lubrication. Boot walker ambulation is begun at 4 weeks with transfer into a shoe with protective brace occurring at 6 to 8 weeks. Physical therapy, including manual joint mobilizations, is very helpful and is begun at 2 months postoperatively. An ankle effusion is an indication that the joint requires additional time and less mechanical stress and should be used to guide physical therapy and return to sports/activities. Return to activity following arthroscopy and microfracture was shown to average 15.1 ± 4 weeks in stage 2 to 4 OLT lesions of the talus.[30]

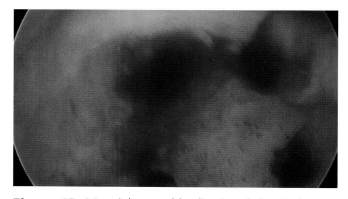

Figure 15–14. Adequate bleeding in subchondral bone after microfracture and tourniquet release.

OUTCOME

Ferkel et al.[31] reported on 59 patients treated with arthroscopic microfracture, with an average follow-up of 40 months. They found good to excellent results in 84% of patients; outcomes were found to be worse in those with pre-existing arthritis. Comparing outcomes of open treatment with those of arthroscopic treatment, the results produced with arthroscopic treatment are equally as good or better.[10,31–33] Most lateral lesions are located on the anterior talar dome and are easily accessible for microfracture surgery through the standard anterolateral arthroscopy approach.[34] However, certain large OLTs may require an open approach. For example, most medial lesions are located on the posterior talar dome and a medial malleolus osteotomy is generally required for access to this lesion.[34]

Several techniques are described to stimulate healing and include drilling (both transmalleolar and through an arthrotomy), retrograde talar drilling, curettage and microfracture. Although rare, cystic lesions with intact cartilage and subchondral bone can be retrograde drilled to stimulate medullary bleeding through subchondral bone.[28] More advanced lesions with full-thickness loss of surface cartilage necessitate antegrade drilling with 1.2-mm Kirschner wires or curettage and microfracture with awls. Transmalleolar drilling allows access to posteromedial lesions that are troublesome to visualize from standard arthroscopic portals.[35] A comparison of transmalleolar drilling and retrograde drilling of undetached fragments by Kono showed no significant difference between the two techniques at 2 years with similar outcomes for clinical improvement of American Orthopaedic Foot & Ankle Society (AOFAS) score and MRI findings.[36]

Clinical improvement in pain is seen in 85% of people in a number of studies with long-term follow-up.[8,37,38] Schuman studied a combined group of 38 patients with 22 patients receiving microfracture with arthroscopic technique as a primary procedure and 16 patients following a failed index procedure with a mean follow-up of 4.8 years. The revision group showed 75% good or excellent results and the primary group had 86% good or excellent results. The longest follow-up has been an average 71 months (24 to 152 months) with 72% excellent/good results, 20% fair and 8% poor. The average outcome AOFAS score was 84 but there was no preoperative baseline for comparison. The arthroscopic grade correlated with outcome and was best in patients with intact cartilage who received a drilling intervention to stimulate healing.

Overall, arthroscopic technique remains our preferred method for treating the majority of talar dome lesions with curettage and microfracture or drilling. Open procedures are reserved for lesions that are inaccessible by arthroscopic means (i.e., posteromedial lesions) or for ankles in which arthroscopic technique may be contraindicated (i.e., excessive scar tissue).

Although the goals of cartilage repair include matching the normal properties of hyaline cartilage, defects treated with drilling and microfracture usually heal with fibrocartilage. Fibrocartilage is predominately type I cartilage, which lacks the organized structure of normal hyaline cartilage, and thus, has inferior wear characteristics. Failed procedures after 4 months of healing and physical therapy should be scrutinized for concomitant pathology such as subtle instability or impingement of both bone and soft tissue. To ensure optimal outcome, alignment and stability should be restored along with the cartilage treatment, which has been described at the time of microfracture or in a staged lesion. Recalcitrant lesions in active patients are candidates for grafting procedures. At this time, there are no long-term studies of treated defects that demonstrate the time to secondary procedures for ankle arthritis, such as ankle fusion or arthroplasty.

Kissing Lesions

Ferkel et al.[39] reviewed 880 consecutive ankle arthroscopies and identified 23 patients (2.6%) with osteochondral lesions of the distal tibia. They reported on 17 patients with distal tibial OLT treated with microfracture. Six (35%) had osteochondral lesions of the tibia and talus; 11 had isolated lesions of the distal tibia. Treatment included excision, curettage, and abrasion arthroplasty in all patients. Five patients had transmalleolar drilling of the lesion, two had microfracture, and two had iliac bone grafting. Preoperatively, the median AOFAS Ankle–Hindfoot score was 52, and postoperatively, it was 87. The authors recommended arthroscopic treatment by means of debridement, curettage, abrasion arthroplasty, and, in some patients, transmalleolar drilling, microfracture, or iliac crest bone grafting. They found excellent and good results in 14 of 17 patients at 44 (24 to 99) months.

REFERENCES

1. Alexander AH, Lichtman DM. Surgical treatment of transchondral talar-dome fractures (osteochondritis dissecans). Long-term follow-up. *J Bone Joint Surg Am.* 1980;62(4): 646–652.
2. Whittaker JP, Smith G, Makwana N, et al. Early results of autologous chondrocyte implantation in the talus. *J Bone Joint Surg Br.* 2005;87(2):179–183.
3. Sugimoto K, Takakura Y, Tohno Y, et al. Cartilage thickness of the talar dome. *Arthroscopy.* 2005;21(4):401–404.
4. Wan L, de Asla RJ, Rubash HE, et al. Quantification of ankle articular cartilage topography and thickness using a high resolution stereophotography system. *J Orthop Res.* 2008;26(8):1081-1089.
5. Millington S, Grabner M, Wozelka R, et al. A stereophotographic study of ankle joint contact area. *J Orthop Res.* 2007; 25(11): 1465–1473.
6. Elias I, Zoga AC, Morrison WB, et al. Osteochondral lesions of the talus: Localization and morphologic data from 424 patients using a novel anatomical grid scheme. *Foot Ankle Int.* 2007;28(2):154–161.
7. Anderson IF, Crichton KJ, Grattan-Smith T, et al. Osteochondral fractures of the dome of the talus. *J Bone Joint Surg Am.* 1989;71(8):1143–1152.

8. Baker CL Jr., Morales RW. Arthroscopic treatment of transchondral talar dome fractures: A long-term follow-up study. *Arthroscopy.* 1999;15(2):197–202.
9. Parisien JS. Arthroscopic treatment of osteochondral lesions of the talus. *Am J Sports Med.* 1986;14(3):211–217.
10. Pettine KA, Morrey BF. Osteochondral fractures of the talus. A long-term follow-up. *J Bone Joint Surg Br.* 1987; 69(1):89–92.
11. Van Buecken K, Barrack RL, Alexander AH, et al. Arthroscopic treatment of transchondral talar dome fractures. *Am J Sports Med.* 1989;17(3):350–355; discussion 355–356.
12. Woods K, Harris I. Osteochondritis dissecans of the talus in identical twins. *J Bone Joint Surg Br.* 1995;77(2):331.
13. Stroud CC, Marks RM. Imaging of osteochondral lesions of the talus. *Foot Ankle Clin.* 2000;5(1):119–133.
14. Stone JW. Osteochondral lesions of the talar dome. *J Am Acad Orthop Surg.* 1996;4(2):63–73.
15. Elias I, Jung JW, Raikin SM, et al. Osteochondral lesions of the talus: Change in MRI findings over time in talar lesions without operative intervention and implications for staging systems. *Foot Ankle Int.* 2006;27(3):157–166.
16. Loredo R, Sanders TG. Imaging of osteochondral injuries. *Clin Sports Med.* 2001;20(2):249–278.
17. Higashiyama I, Kumai T, Takakura Y, et al. Follow-up study of MRI for osteochondral lesion of the talus. *Foot Ankle Int.* 2000;21(2):127–133.
18. Mesgarzadeh M, Sapega AA, Bonakdarpour A. Osteochondritis dissecans: Analysis of mechanical stability with radiography, scintigraphy, and MR. *Radiology.* 1987;165(3):775–780.
19. De Smet AA, Fisher DR, Burnstein MI, et al. Value of MR imaging in staging osteochondral lesions of the talus (osteochondritis dissecans): Results in 14 patients. *AJR Am J Roentgenol.* 1990;154(3):555–558.
20. Flick AB, Gould N. Osteochondritis dissecans of the talus (transchondral fractures of the talus): Review of the literature and new surgical approach for medial dome lesions. *Foot Ankle.* 1985;5(4):165–185.
21. O'Driscoll SW. The healing and regeneration of articular cartilage. *J Bone Joint Surg Am.* 1998;80(12):1795–1812.
22. Kumai T, Takakura Y, Kitada C, et al. Fixation of osteochondral lesions of the talus using cortical bone pegs. *J Bone Joint Surg Br.* 2002;84(3):369–374.
23. Ghul JF. Operative arthroscopy. *Am J Sports Med.* 1979;7: 328–335.
24. Stetson WB, Ferkel RD. Ankle arthroscopy: II. Indications and results. *J Am Acad Orthop Surg.* 1996;4(1):24–34.
25. Frey CC. Foot and ankle arthroscopy and endoscopy. In: Myerson MS, ed. *Foot and ankle disorders.* Philadelphia, PA: WB Saunders, 2000.
26. Steadman JR, Rodkey WG, Rodrigo JJ. Microfracture: Surgical technique and rehabilitation to treat chondral defects. *Clin Orthop Relat Res.* 2001;(391 Suppl):S362–S369.
27. Sledge SL. Microfracture techniques in the treatment of osteochondral injuries. *Clin Sports Med.* 2001;20(2):365–377.
28. Taranow WS, Bisignani GA, Towers JD, et al. Retrograde drilling of osteochondral lesions of the medial talar dome. *Foot Ankle Int.* 1999;20(8):474–480.
29. Savva N, Jabur M, Davies M, et al. Osteochondral lesions of the talus: Results of repeat arthroscopic debridement. *Foot Ankle Int.* 2007;28(6):669–673.

30. Saxena A, Eakin C. Articular talar injuries in athletes: Results of microfracture and autogenous bone graft. *Am J Sports Med.* 2007;35(10):1680–1687.

31. Ferkel RD, Sgaglione NA, Del Pizzo W. Arthroscopic treatment of osteochondral lesions of the talus: Technique and results. *Orthop Trans.* 1990;14:172–173.

32. Pritsch M, Horoshovski H, Farine I. Arthroscopic treatment of osteochondral lesions of the talus. *J Bone Joint Surg Am.* 1986;68(6):862–865.

33. Loomer R, Fisher C, Lloyd-Smith R, et al. Osteochondral lesions of the talus. *Am J Sports Med.* 1993;21(1):13–19.

34. Navid DO, Myerson MS. Approach alternatives for treatment of osteochondral lesions of the talus. *Foot Ankle Clin.* 2002;7(3):635–649.

35. Kumai T, Takakura Y, Higashiyama I, et al. Arthroscopic drilling for the treatment of osteochondral lesions of the talus. *J Bone Joint Surg Am.* 1999;81(9):1229–1235.

36. Kono M, Takao M, Naito K, et al. Retrograde drilling for osteochondral lesions of the talar dome. *Am J Sports Med.* 2006;34(9):1450–1456.

37. Becher C, Thermann H. Results of microfracture in the treatment of articular cartilage defects of the talus. *Foot Ankle Int.* 2005;26(8):583–589.

38. Schuman L, Struijs PA, van Dijk CN. Arthroscopic treatment for osteochondral defects of the talus. Results at follow-up at 2 to 11 years. *J Bone Joint Surg Br.* 2002;84(3):364–368.

39. Ferkel RD, Zanotti RM, Komenda GA, et al. Arthroscopic treatment of chronic osteochondral lesions of the talus: Long-term results. *Am J Sports Med.* 2008;36(9):1750–1762.

CHAPTER 16

Osteochondral Lesion of the Talus (OLT) Treated by Matrix-Based Techniques (Matrix-Induced Chondrocyte Implantation [MACI] and Autologous Matrix-Induced Chondrogenesis [AMIC])

Markus Walther

INDICATION

Matrix-induced chondrocytes implantation (MACI) and autologous matrix-induced chondrogenesis (AMIC) are surgical treatment options for symptomatic cartilage defects. MACI is a two-step procedure in which in vitro cultured chondrocytes are cultured and seeded onto an acid collagen scaffold which is transplanted to the defect and fixed in place with fibrin glue. AMIC is a one-step procedure combining microfracture of the vascular subchondral bone with the application of a bilayer collagen matrix. Microfracturing causes release of blood and bone marrow that form a super clot containing the requisite building blocks for cartilage repair: multipotent mesenchymal progenitor cells, cytokines, and growth factors. The collagen matrix secures the clot and improves its overall stability. Furthermore, it provides an environment where cells can adhere, proliferate, and produce repair tissue in a protected setting.[1]

Compared to other cartilage reconstruction techniques, MACI and AMIC provide a stable cartilage rim which can be maintained at the site of the lesion. Large defects can be readily addressed with this technique. The use of the matrix makes it much easier to manage shoulder lesions of the talus (Fig. 16–1). Finally a matrix can be glued to the bone surface with fibrin glue. Gluing the matrix to the bone helps to avoid osteotomies in nearly all cases.[2]

MACI and AMIC are best suited for patients between 18 and 50 years of age. They are indicated for management of symptomatic osteochondral lesions failing debridement, drilling, or microfracture.[3–5]

Primary MACI or AMIC can be considered in focal cartilage defects of the talus (ICRS Grade III and IV) >1.5 cm^2 or in osteochondral lesions of the talus (OLT) associated with expansive subchondral cysts (Scranton Stage V lesion).[4,6]

However, there are some disadvantages of MACI for the talus. These include high cost and the need for a two-stage procedure to allow time for chondrocyte culture. Harvesting cells for culturing is considered to be a part of a drug-producing process. Therefore special permission has to be requested by the local healthcare administration. Standard operating procedures (SOPs) for harvesting and transportation of the cartilage cells are mandatory for the accreditation process.

AMIC is an off the shelf product to be used in a one-step procedure. Both, AMIC and MACI are not approved by the Food and Drug Administration (FDA) for the use in foot and ankle surgery (as of July 2012). Therefore informed consent and extended patient education are imperative.

Contraindications for MACI or AMIC include generalized degenerative changes in the joint, cartilage defects in the corresponding opposite joint surface, inflammatory joint disease, crystal arthropathy, and neuroarthropathy. Instability and axis malalignment do not represent contraindications if these can be addressed along with cartilage reconstruction.

For larger OLTs or OLTs failing prior surgical management, both techniques provide patients and their treating surgeons a potentially successful treatment avenue that did not exist prior to MACI or AMIC.

Patient Positioning to Harvest Chondrocytes (Only Indicated for MACI)

The patient position to harvest chondrocytes is that used for a standard arthroscopy of the ankle. Harvest of chondrocytes can be performed with conventional knee or ankle arthroscopy. Suitable locations for harvesting expendable articular cartilage from the knee include peripheral superomedial or superolateral femoral condyle or the intercondylar notch. Alternatively, Giannini et al.[7] have demonstrated that the detached OLT fragment at the time of index arthroscopic debridement/drilling or microfracture may be an acceptable source of chondrocytes for MACI, however these results have not been confirmed by Candrian et al.[8] Another possible harvest area is the anterior part of the talus.[6]

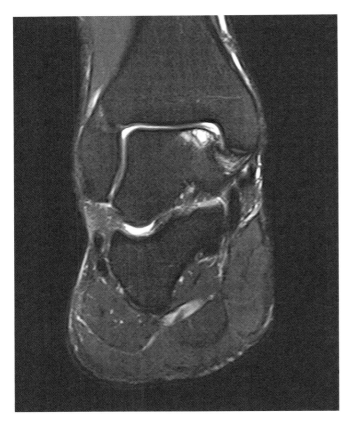

Figure 16–1. MRI (T2-weighed, coronary view) of an osteochondral defect at the medial talar shoulder.

By using a curette, two to three full-thickness articular grafts are harvested, grafts that include the superficial layer of the subchondral bone. The grafts are transferred to a sterile container with nutrient medium and transported to the laboratory. Using a patented procedure, the articular cartilage matrix is enzymatically disrupted to isolate the chondrocytes. Culturing of chondrocytes requires approximately 2 to 6 weeks; the length is dependent on the method used by the company that the performs the culture.

Patient Positioning for Transplantation of MACI or AMIC

The procedure can be performed using several types of anesthesia. Homeostasis is maintained using a thigh tourniquet inflated 100 mm Hg above the systolic blood pressure. A radiation protection mat is placed from the middle of lower thigh proximally over the patient. An image intensifier is used only if an osteotomy is utilized.

Dependent on the location of the defect, the patient is positioned supine with a slightly internal or external rotated lower extremity. Lateral recumbent position is used in case of dorsomedial approach, and on the contralateral side in case of dorsolateral approach. The affected leg is positioned free to be able to flex the knee; otherwise, adequate dorsal extension of the ankle joint is not possible.

If iliac crest graft is to be obtained, the pelvis needs to be prepped and draped as well and the ipsilateral pelvis supported with a bump. Alternatively, bone graft may be harvested from the calcaneus, distal tibia, or proximal tibia, all of which are locations prepped into the surgical field for ankle surgery.[9] A vacuum mattress can be helpful to adjust the patient's position during the procedure.

SURGICAL APPROACHES

Depending on the location of the cartilage defect, a ventromedial, ventrocentral, or ventrolateral approach is used. The ventromedial approach is carried out between the medial malleolus and the anterior tibial tendon (Fig. 16–2). The ventrocentral access is between the anterior tibial and the extensor hallucis longus tendon (Fig. 16–3). The neurovascular bundle is retracted laterally with a blunt Hohmann retractor. With that, the entire ankle joint can be visualized well. This approach is particularly useful for treating defects on the medial and lateral talus shoulder as well as for centrally located defects.

The ventrolateral approach (Ollier approach) is carried out lateral to the peroneus tertius tendon ventral to the lateral malleolus (Fig. 16–4). Lesions of the lateral

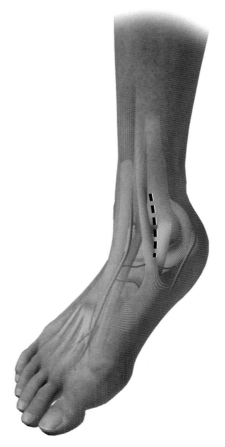

Figure 16–2. Ventromedial approach between the medial malleolus and the anterior tibial tendon.

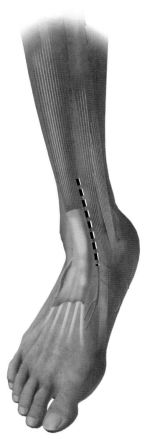

Figure 16–3.   Ventrocentral approach between the anterior tibial and the extensor hallucis longus tendon.

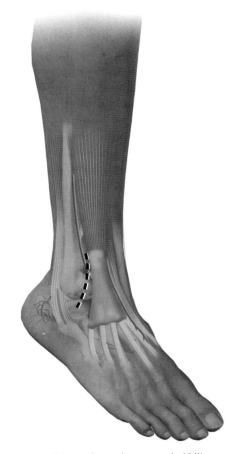

Figure 16–4.   Ventrolateral approach (Ollier approach) lateral to the peroneus tertius tendon and ventral to the lateral malleolus.

talus shoulder can be addressed well with this approach. The capsule closure can be combined with stabilization of the external ligaments.

Dorsal approaches are seldom necessary, since with adequate distraction of the joint with K-wire distractor, deeper-lying defects can also be accessed. The dorsolateral approach runs dorsal to the lateral malleolus, and enables medial or lateral retraction of the peroneal tendons (Fig. 16–5).

For a dorsomedial approach between the medial malleolus and the posterior tibial tendon (Fig. 16–6), the patient is positioned on the affected side. The contralateral leg is well padded, and the affected leg is positioned in a freely moveable fashion. Using a short vacuum beanbag positioner considerably facilitates the procedure. Here too, adequate flexion of the knee is necessary.

Surgical Technique to Implant the Matrix

The further surgical steps are illustrated using the example of a case of an OLT with subchondral cyst of the medial talar shoulder using a medial approach (Fig. 16–1).

The skin incision is marked medial between the medial malleolus and the anterior tibial tendon (Fig. 16–2). After dissection to the level of the joint capsule, the joint is opened by a longitudinal incision. A 2.0-mm K-wire is drilled into the distal tibia, a second one parallel to it, in the talus. Placing the wires using the K-wire distractor as drill guide facilitates precise positioning of the wires. The joint is then distracted in maximum plantar flexion (Fig. 16–7).

Unstable cartilage is debrided. A stable cartilage edge must be established adjacent to a healthy osteochondral border. Oval-shaped preparation of the defect facilitates insertion of the collagen matrix. All necrotic bone is removed and cysts curetted. The underlying sclerotic zone is perforated using multiple small drill holes (1.2-mm K-wire) with adequate cooling or with microfracture (Fig. 16–8).

The osseous defect is reconstructed to the level of the subchondral bone lamella using autologous cancellous bone. Particular attention must be paid to ensure that the bone graft does not extend higher than the level of the subchondral bone lamella, which can lead to delamination of the collagen matrix. Cancellous

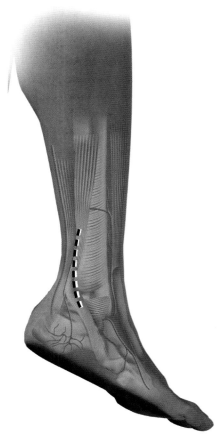

Figure 16–5. Dorsolateral approach dorsal to the lateral malleolus.

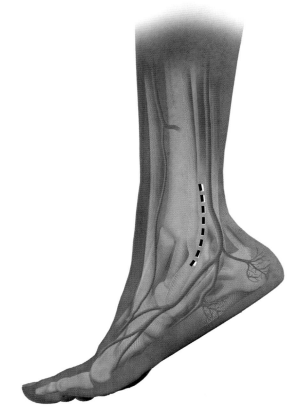

Figure 16–6. Dorsomedial approach between the medial malleolus and the posterior tibial tendon.

bone harvested from the ipsilateral calcaneus is adequate in most cases. It is also possible to harvest cancellous bone from the tibial plafond or iliac crest (Fig. 16–9).

Next the matrix is prepared for placement over the bone-grafted area. The defect size is measured using aluminum foil, which is pressed into the defect with forceps so that the borders of the cartilage are clearly depicted. The foil is then cut to size and its exact fit within the talar lesion is checked once again. The collagen matrix (MACI taken from the transport medium or AMIC hydrated in a physiologic saline solution) is then cut to shape with the help of the template. The matrix has a rough side which should face the bone; the smooth side faces the joint (Fig. 16–10).

The cancellous bone graft is covered with commercially available fibrin glue, and the matrix is glued onto it. Additional suturing is not required. Care should be taken that the matrix does not overlap the edge of the adjacent cartilage which increases the risk of delamination when the joint is moved (Fig. 16–11). If the surrounding cartilage is very thick or if there is just one defect zone 1 to 2 mm deep, two layers of the collagen matrix can be implanted using a sandwich technique. Both matrices

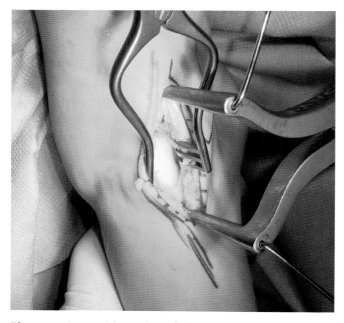

Figure 16–7. Distraction of the ankle to facilitate access to the cartilage lesion. The joint is opened through a longitudinal incision and distracted in maximum plantar flexion. A dorsoventral approach is shown. The foot is at the bottom of the image.

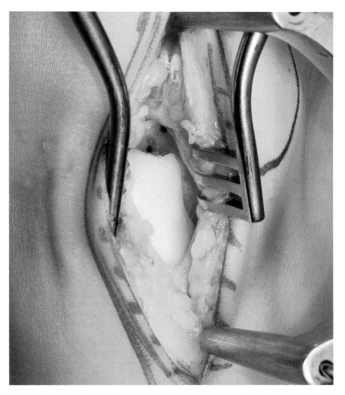

Figure 16–8. Debridement of unstable cartilage, necrotic bone, and cysts. A close-up view of Figure 16–7 is shown. Note the stable osteochondral edge, healthy bone bed, and perforated base to facilitate ingress of marrow elements.

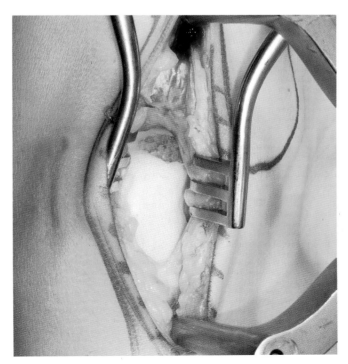

Figure 16–9. Reconstruction of the defect with cancellous bone. Note that the graft material does not extend more superficial than the level of the subchondral bone.

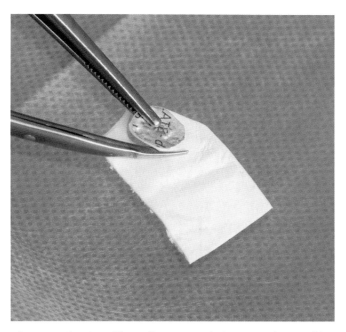

Figure 16–10. The collagen matrix is cut to shape with the help of the template. The smooth side of the matrix is facing up in this image.

are glued with the rough surface facing the bone and the smooth surface facing the joint.

After consolidation of the fibrin glue, the distractor is removed and the joint moved throughout the range of motion several times. If the matrix remains in place,

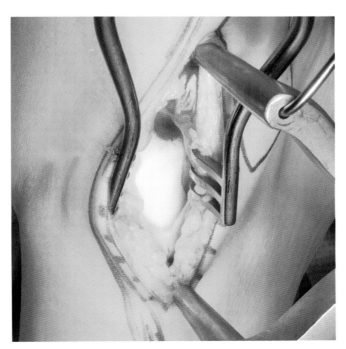

Figure 16–11. Matrix within the talar defect after it has been fixed with fibrin glue.

one can assume the implantation to be stable. If delamination occurs, possible overlap of the matrix with the surrounding cartilage should be looked for and excess matrix shaved off. Bone graft exceeding the level of the subchondral bone can also lead to delamination of the matrix. In this case, the excess graft should be reduced and the matrix reglued in place. Finally, the soft tissues, including the capsule, are closed in layers with resorbable suture material. A drain without suction can be inserted if necessary. After applying an elastic compression bandage, the ankle is immobilized with a dorsal plaster splint for the first 48 hours postoperatively.

COMPLICATIONS

Delamination of the matrix can be caused by a protrusion at the edge of the adjacent cartilage. If the bone graft is too thick, the surface layer should be ablated and the matrix reglued over it.

Deep wound infection is managed by removal of the sutures, wound swab, debridement, and appropriate antibiotic treatment after surgical debridement.

In the case of incomplete healing of bone graft with new cyst formation,[10] it is possible to repeat the procedure. However, after failure of surgery, it is important to reassess the axial malalignment or instability as possible causes.

Pain is regularly encountered during the beginning of full weight bearing and physical therapy after immobilization. The source of pain from an OCL remains ill defined, and cartilage resurfacing is certainly not 100% effective. Even without obvious complication, pain may persist.[11,12]

If the clinical outcome is not satisfactory and follow-up imaging studies are suggestive of graft compromise, ankle arthroscopy is warranted. Fibrous tissue may form at the graft–host articular junction or within the ankle, causing impingement. This can be effectively debrided by arthroscopy to relieve symptoms. Second-look arthroscopy may demonstrate that the cartilage resurfacing procedure was successful, but was inadequate to resurface what proved to be a larger area of diseased talus than originally identified.[11]

General surgical complications like deep venous thrombosis, wound healing problems, or infection can occur.

Rehabilitation Protocol

The ankle is completely immobilized in neutral for 48 hours. After 48 hours a drain if inserted is removed and continuous passive motion is started limited to a range of 20 degrees plantarflexion to 20 degrees dorsiflexion. A splint is applied for 2 weeks until wound healing is complete. From week 1 to 6, partial weight bearing of 10 kg is recommended. From week 7 to 12 the patient can stepwise increase weight bearing (20 kg every 2 weeks).

From week 13 onwards, the patient is permitted to incur stress from activities of daily living, cycling, and swimming. Sports involving impact loading or rapid change of direction should be avoided for at least 12 months. Whether return to professional sports is possible after cartilage reconstruction has not yet been conclusively established.

OUTCOME

To date, only results of level IV studies reporting on the results of talar cartilage repair at the talus are available (Table 16–1). The reported AOFAS scores achieved by the matrix-based techniques are between 85 and 90 points.[6,11,13,14] The only prospective study with a randomized trial comparing microfracture, OATS, and autologous chondrocyte implantation with a periosteal flap by Gobbi et al.[15] was withdrawn 2 years later due to technical limitations.[16]

A larger number of studies are available on cartilage reconstruction of the knee. Gooding et al.[17] compared two ACI techniques for treatment of osteochondral defects in the knee: One in which a periosteal flap and the other in which a type I/III collagen scaffold is used for covering the defect. They found a significant number in the periosteum group with hypertrophic grafts requiring secondary shaving. These findings clearly suggest the superiority of matrix-based techniques.

Several studies have shown that the bilayer collagen matrix with its compact cell-occlusive layer protects the so-called superclot and attracts to its porous cell-adhesive layer the pluripotent mesenchymal progenitor stem cells released by microfracturing. These cells enhance chondrogenic differentiation.[1] The fibrin glue with which the scaffold is fixed over the defect supports migration and proliferation of the mesenchymal cells and stimulates chondrocytes to deposit proteoglycan, abundantly present in healthy cartilage.[18] Microfracturing also releases cytokines, and transforming growth factors-beta from the subchondral bone.[19]

Giza et al.[13] reported a retrospective case study which included 10 patients treated with MACI. The mean age was 40.2 (25 to 59) with a follow-up of 24 months. They found an improvement in the AOFAS score from a mean 61 (42 to 76) to a mean 73.3 (42 to 90) points. In our cohort (12 patients, mean age 38.5 [21 to 58]), we found an improvement in the AOFAS score from a mean of 54.3 (43 to 72) to a mean of 78.2 (62 to 96) at the 24-month follow-up.

We followed up 15 patients 30 to 36 months after AMIC treatment of the talus. What was the mean time postprocedure of evaluation. The AOFAS scores improved significantly from 48 to 88 points.[10] There was no significant difference in the leg circumference or in the range of motion between the treated and the untreated ankle, which can be interpreted to be an indicator of normal leg function (Fig. 16–12). It is unclear whether seeding

TABLE 16–1. Results of the Different Techniques of Cartilage Reconstruction.[6,10,11,13,14,20,21]

	Product	n	Age	Follow-Up (months)	AOFAS Pre	AOFAS Post	Good Results (%)	Sat. Results (%)	Level of Evidence
Baums, *JBJS* 2006	Codon	12	29.7 (18–42)	63 (48–84)	43.5	88.4	92	8	IV
Giannini, *Am J Sports Med* 2008	Hyalograft	46	31.4 (20–47)	36	57.2	89.5	82	18	IV
Thermann, *Orthopaede* 2008	Hyalograft	9	29 (16–41)	43 (31–58)	n.a.	n.a.	77	23	IV
Schneider, *FAI* 2009	MACI	20	36 (19–61)	21.1 (9–42)	60	87	90	10	IV
Giannini, *Clin Orthop Relat Res* 2009	Hyaluronic acid membrane	24	28.5 ± 9.5	24	66.2 ± 10.5	92.8 ± 5.3	96	4	IV
Giza, *FAI* 2010	MACI	10	40.2 (21–58)	24	61.2 (42–76)	73.3 (42–90)	90	10	IV
Walther, unpublished data	MACI	12	38.5 (18–63)	24	54 (43–72)	78 (62–95)	88	12	IV
Walther, *Fuss und Sprung-gelenk* 2012	AMIC Chondro-Gide	15	40.1 (18–63)	32 (30–36)	48 (38–60)	88 (75–100)	93	7	IV

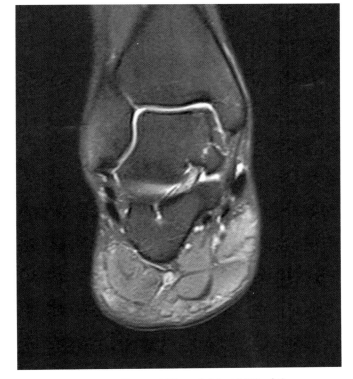

Figure 16–12. Coronal T2-weighted MRI of the same patient shown in Fig. 16–1 1 year after MACI procedure. Note complete coverage of the former defect at the medial talar shoulder.

the cell-free matrix with autologous stem cells prior to implantation into the defect might lead to improved results.[20]

REFERENCES

1. Dickhut A, Dexheimer V, Martin KT, et al. Chondrogenesis of human mesenchymal stem cells by local transforming growth factor-beta delivery in a biphasic resorbable carrier. *Tissue Eng Part A*. 2010;16:453–464.
2. Young KW, Deland JT, Lee KT, et al. Medial approaches to osteochondral lesion of the talus without medial malleolar osteotomy. *Knee Surg Sports Traumatol Arthrosc*. 2010;18:634–637.
3. Al-Shaikh RA, Chou LB, Mann JA, et al. Autologous osteochondral grafting for talar cartilage defects. *Foot Ankle Int*. 2002;23:381–389.
4. Brittberg M, Peterson L, Sjogren-Jansson E, et al. Articular cartilage engineering with autologous chondrocyte transplantation. A review of recent developments. *J Bone Joint Surg Am*. 2003;85-A Suppl 3:109–115.
5. Mandelbaum BR, Gerhardt MB, Peterson L. Autologous chondrocyte implantation of the talus. *Arthroscopy*. 2003; 19 Suppl 1:129–137.
6. Baums MH, Heidrich G, Schultz W, et al Autologous chondrocyte transplantation for treating cartilage defects of the talus. *J Bone Joint Surg Am*. 2006;88:303–308.
7. Giannini S, Buda R, Grigolo B, et al. The detached osteochondral fragment as a source of cells for autologous chondrocyte implantation (ACI) in the ankle joint. *Osteoarthritis Cartilage*. 2005;13:601–607.

8. Candrian C, Miot S, Wolf F, et al. Are ankle chondrocytes from damaged fragments a suitable cell source for cartilage repair? *Osteoarthritis Cartilage.* 2010;18(8):1067–1076.

9. Raikin SM, Brislin K. Local bone graft harvested from the distal tibia or calcaneus for surgery of the foot and ankle. *Foot Ankle Int.* 2005;26:449–453.

10. Walther M, Becher C, Volkering C, et al. Treatment of chondral and osteochondral defects of the talus by autologous matrix induced chondrogenesis. *Fuß und Sprunggelenk.* 2012;10:121–129.

11. Schneider TE, Karaikudi S. Matrix-induced autologous chondrocyte implantation (MACI) grafting for osteochondral lesions of the talus. *Foot Ankle Int.* 2009;30:810–814.

12. Zheng MH, Willers C, Kirilak L, et al. Matrix-induced autologous chondrocyte implantation (MACI): biological and histological assessment. *Tissue Eng.* 2007;13:737–746.

13. Giza E, Sullivan M, Ocel D, et al. Matrix-induced autologous chondrocyte implantation of talus articular defects. *Foot Ankle Int.* 2010;31:747–753.

14. Giannini S, Buda R, Vannini F, et al. Arthroscopic autologous chondrocyte implantation in osteochondral lesions of the talus: surgical technique and results. *Am J Sports Med.* 2008;36:873–880.

15. Gobbi A, Francisco RA, Lubowitz JH, et al. Osteochondral lesions of the talus: randomized controlled trial comparing chondroplasty, microfracture, and osteochondral autograft transplantation. *Arthroscopy.* 2006;22:1085–1092.

16. Gobbi A. Error in level of evidence. *Arthroscopy.* 2008; 24:247.

17. Gooding CR, Bartlett W, Bentley G, et al. A prospective, randomised study comparing two techniques of autologous chondrocyte implantation for osteochondral defects in the knee: Periosteum covered versus type I/III collagen covered. *Knee.* 2006;13:203–210.

18. Kirilak Y, Pavlos NJ, Willers CR, et al. Fibrin sealant promotes migration and proliferation of human articular chondrocytes: possible involvement of thrombin and protease-activated receptors. *Int J Mol Med.* 2006;17:551–558.

19. Finnson KW, Parker WL, Chi Y, et al. Endoglin differentially regulates TGF-beta-induced Smad2/3 and Smad1/5 signalling and its expression correlates with extracellular matrix production and cellular differentiation state in human chondrocytes. *Osteoarthritis Cartilage.* 2010;18: 1518–1527.

20. Giannini S, Buda R, Vannini F, et al. One-step bone marrow-derived cell transplantation in talar osteochondral lesions. *Clin Orthop Relat Res.* 2009;467:3307–3320.

21. Thermann H, Driessen A, Becher C. Autologous chondrocyte transplantation in the treatment of articular cartilage lesions of the talus. *Orthopade.* 2008;37:232–239.

CHAPTER 17

Arthroscopic Treatment of Osteochondral Lesions of the Talus: Juvenile Articular Cartilage Allograft

Eric Giza   Edward Shin   Stephanie E. Wong

INDICATIONS

The surgical management of refractory talar osteochondral lesions of the talus (OLTs) has generally produced good results. Initial management of these lesions most often involves arthroscopy and microfracture/curettage.[1,2] The resulting regenerative tissue is fibrocartilage (Fig. 17–1). Symptomatic improvement is experienced in approximately 85% of cases in studies with long-term follow-up.[1–3] Larger lesions (>1 cm^2) and lesions with cystic change often require secondary procedures such as osteochondral allograft/autograft transfer system (OATS) or autologous chondrocyte implantation (ACI).[4–7] Traditionally, these procedures require the use of an open technique, often with the added morbidity associated with osteotomies for adequate exposure.

The recent introduction of fresh juvenile allograft chondrocytes for the treatment of osteochondral lesions has created a potential tool for the treatment of OLTs refractory to microfracture. This method, which also obviates the need for tibial or fibular osteotomies, reproduces hyaline cartilage architecture (see Fig. 17–1) without the morbidity and technical difficulties attendant to other currently available restorative techniques. Juvenile articular allograft currently is available as a pre-packaged, off-the-shelf finely diced preparation from donors aged less than 13 years with a high chondrocyte viability (Fig. 17–2). Current recommendations suggest the use of one package for coverage of up to a 2.5-cm^2 defect.

DeNovo NT offers an efficient, one-step allogeneic alternative to ACI for treatment of osteochondral lesions of the talus. Benefits include readily available young and healthy chondrocytes, no donor-site morbidity, and lack of time delay for chondrocyte culturing as is necessary for ACI or matrix-induced autologous chondrocyte implantation (MACI).[8] In addition, the use of DeNovo NT does not exclude the possibility of using other cartilage restoration techniques if needed in the future. A disadvantage of this technology is that harvested cartilage must be used within 2 weeks. As a result, it is imperative to plan to have the appropriate amount of graft available for the size of the lesion so that there is no shortage or excess.

The ideal patient for the use of DeNovo NT is a young patient (<50 years) with a symptomatic isolated talar osteochondral lesion that has failed conservative treatment and previous microfracture. Large lesions (>1 cm^2) are less likely to respond to microfracture and are a relative indication. Large cystic bone defects are still an indication for OATS. Kissing lesions, global osteoarthritis, or active infection are contraindications.[9] Standing weight-bearing ankle radiographs, as well as magnetic resonance and computed tomography scans, are valuable in localizing the lesion and assessing depth of bone involvement. Instability or malalignment of the ankle must be corrected at the time of surgery.

PATIENT POSITIONING

Following the induction of anesthesia, the patient is positioned supine on the operating table. A roll is placed under the ipsilateral hip to facilitate optimal rotation of the ankle, and a pneumatic thigh tourniquet is applied. The leg is then placed in a commercially available positioner with the hip and knee flexed approximately 30 degrees (Fig. 17–3). Adequate padding is placed under the positioner to avoid injury to neurovascular structures, specifically the common peroneal nerve and popliteal artery.

SURGICAL APPROACHES

Routine ankle arthroscopy with anteromedial and anterolateral portals is performed without traction and anterior osteophytes are removed as discussed in Chapter 15 (Figs. 15–4 through 15–7 from Chapter 15 on microfracture). Important landmarks, including the tibialis anterior, peroneus tertius, and superficial peroneal nerve are marked while the patient is in the preoperative holding area. If necessary, a noninvasive distraction device is used to enhance access to the joint (Fig. 17–5).

As with microfracture, any loose or delaminated articular cartilage is excised with a curette and a stable chondral border is established (Figs. 17–6 and 17–7). An arthroscopic probe is used to measure the lesion in two dimensions. Any bony cysts underlying the lesion should also be debrided at this time. The placement of autograft or allograft bone into cysts greater than 5 mm in depth is recommended in order to restore the architecture of talus.

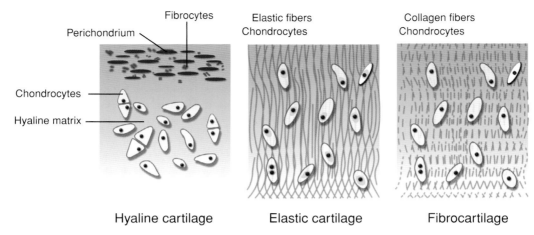

Figure 17–1. Hyaline cartilage produced as a result of juvenile articular cartilage allograft, compared to fibrocartilage produced after microfracture.

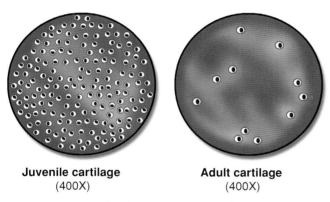

Figure 17–2. Histologic comparison of juvenile cartilage and adult cartilage, showing an increased number of viable chondrocytes in juvenile cartilage.

For lesions in which the calcified cartilage layer is present, gentle curettage is recommended to prepare the surface. Deep perforation of the subchondral bone is avoided.

FIXATION

Once preparation of the defect is complete, the ankle is evacuated of any arthroscopic fluid and the remainder of the procedure is performed "dry." The portal providing the most direct access to the lesion is sufficiently enlarged (usually to 15 to 20 mm) to provide unencumbered access to the lesion (Fig. 17–8). Approximately one package of particulated juvenile allograft cartilage is used for 2.5 cm^2 of defect size. Please refer to the product

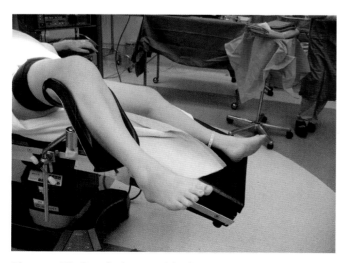

Figure 17–3. Patient positioning.

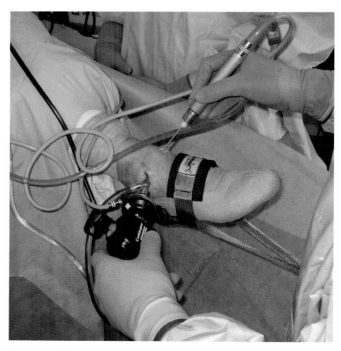

Figure 17–4. Portal placement.

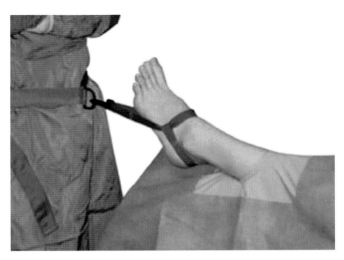

Figure 17–5. Joint distraction system.

instructions to determine the recommended quantity to use. The packaging fluid is removed using a 25-gauge needle and the graft is loaded retrograde into a small-joint arthroscopy cannula (Figs. 17–9 and 17–10). The graft is then set aside until implantation.

Under arthroscopic visualization the lesion is dried of any fluid utilizing fine-tip suction and pledgets, with care taken to ensure that there is no excessive bony bleeding from the surface of the lesion (Fig. 17–11). The tourniquet is inflated during this portion of the case to avoid dilution of the fibrin/DeNovo NT as the fibrin sets. The surface of the lesion is then covered with a thin layer of fibrin glue (Figs. 17–12 and 17–13). While the fibrin glue is still liquid, the graft is expressed from the cannula using the trocar and is gently spread with an elevator to cover the defect (Figs. 17–14 and 17–15). A second layer of fibrin glue is then applied to cover and secure the graft in position (Fig. 17–16). The fibrin glue is allowed to set for 5 minutes and then the ankle is ranged. Arthroscopic visualization of the graft after range of motion is performed to ensure that the graft does not delaminate (Fig. 17–17). The wounds are then closed with nylon suture and the operative ankle is immobilized in a plaster splint.

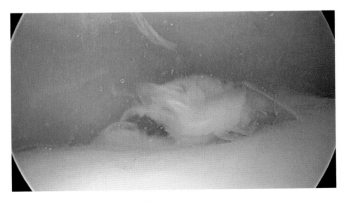

Figure 17–6. Unstable lesion.

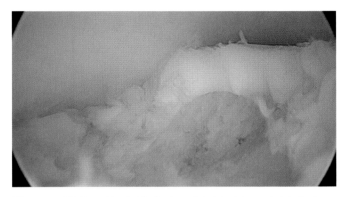

Figure 17–7. Unstable lesion debrided to a stable lesion.

COMPLICATIONS

Complications of arthroscopic transplantation of juvenile chondrocytes include injury to the neurovascular structures of the anterior ankle (e.g., superficial peroneal

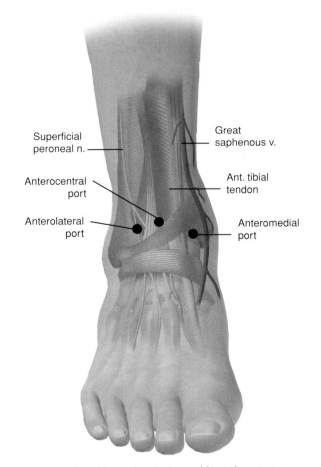

Figure 17–8. Normal anterior ankle arthroscopy anterolateral and anteromedial portals shown (5 mm). These portals can be extended longitudinally to 15 to 20 mm length for placement of juvenile articular cartilage allograft. The anterocentral portal should rarely be used because of risk of damage to the anterior neurovascular bundle.

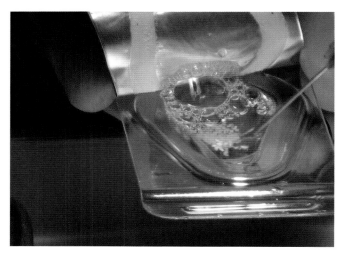

Figure 17–9. Juvenile articular cartilage graft.

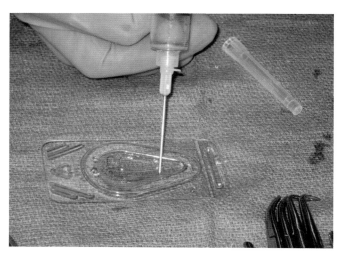

Figure 17–10. Loading graft into syringe.

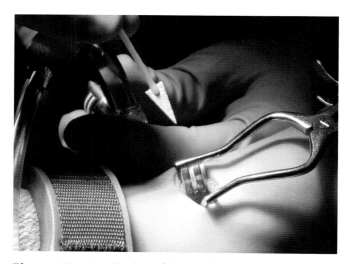

Figure 17–11. Drying of the graft site.

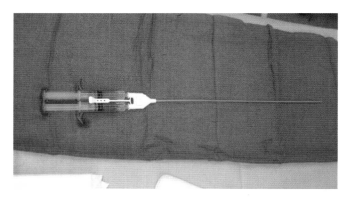

Figure 17–12. Fibrin glue in applicator syringe.

neuralgia) and other standard surgical complications such as wound healing problems, infection, and deep vein thrombosis.

Juvenile articular cartilage allograft is considered a failed intervention if the patient has continued pain at 1 to 2 years postoperatively. Since the use of DeNovo NT does not exclude the possibility of using other cartilage restoration techniques, OATS or ACI can be performed in the event of persistent symptoms.

There is risk of disease transmission and immunogenic reaction as DeNovo NT is an allogeneic tissue graft; however, to date, there have been no reports of such complications.

REHABILITATION PROTOCOL

The patient is kept nonweight bearing for 6 weeks. At 2 weeks postoperatively the splint is exchanged for a cast boot. Gentle active and passive range-of-motion exercises are initiated to prevent anterior scar formation. Strengthening and elastic band resistance exercises may also be initiated, although plantarflexion is limited to 20 degrees to ensure graft containment. A night splint can be used depending on lesion size. At 6 weeks postoperatively, the patient is advanced to weight-bearing as-tolerated in a

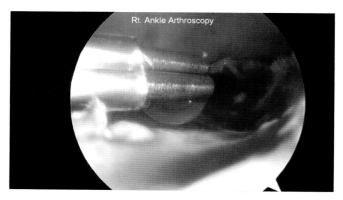

Figure 17–13. Application of the first layer of fibrin glue into the graft site.

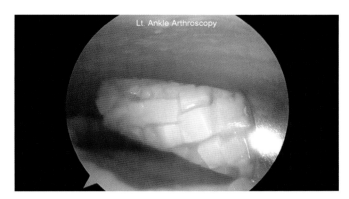

Figure 17–14. Injecting graft into lesion.

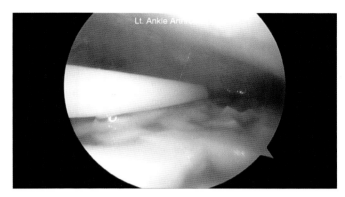

Figure 17–16. Placement of second layer of fibrin glue over the graft.

boot, with increasing ROM exercises, stationary bike, nonimpact cardiotherapy, and pool therapy. From weeks 12 to 24, the patient is encouraged to walk and gradually increase activity. Between postoperative weeks 24 and 52, the patient may return to running and loading activities.

OUTCOMES

The DeNovo NT is an FDA-approved allograft that has been in use since 2007 with over 1,700 grafts placed in the ankle, knee, and shoulder. Farr et al.[10] presented data in 2010 at the International Cartilage Repair Society Meeting on 48 patients with focal chondral defects of the knee treated with particulate juvenile cartilage allograft. At 20 months, the average VAS resting scores improved from 2.1 to 0.8 and maximal pain scores improved from 6.3 to 4.3. An equine study compared histologic results of cartilage defects filled with fibrin alone to cartilage defects filled with DeNovo NT and fibrin.[11] At 12 months, the DeNovo NT specimens had complete filling of the defect.

Cartilage from juvenile donors has been shown to proliferate more robustly in vitro and resist differentiation while in culture, retaining an articular cartilage phenotype more reliably than adult chondrocytes with 10 times more cartilage cell density.[12] In a laboratory study, the chondrogenic activity of freshly isolated human articular chondrocytes from juvenile (<13 years old) and adult (>13 years old) donors were measured by proteoglycan assay, gene expression analysis, and histology.[13] The investigators found that the proteoglycan content in juvenile neocartilage was 100 times greater than neocartilage produced by adult cells. They also found that juvenile cells grew significantly faster in monolayer cultures than adult cells ($p = .002$), and that juvenile chondrocytes did not stimulate lymphocyte proliferation.

Osteochondral allografts have been utilized for reconstructive procedures with few adverse graft-related reactions reported over three decades.[14] In addition, arthroscopic transplantation of juvenile chondrocytes avoids many of the disadvantages of conventional restorative techniques for treatment of talar cartilage lesions. An all-arthroscopic or extended-portal technique is a single-stage procedure that obviates the need for malleolar osteotomy or cartilage biopsy and eliminates donor-site morbidity. At the authors' institution, this procedure has shown favorable short-term results in selected patients and its clinical promise warrants further investigation. Currently, prospective trials of arthroscopic treatment of large OLTs are underway at the authors' institution.

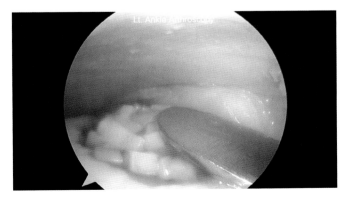

Figure 17–15. Tamping down graft.

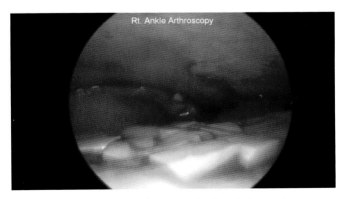

Figure 17–17. Completed graft after being set for approximately 5 minutes.

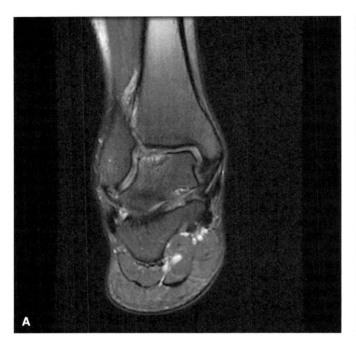
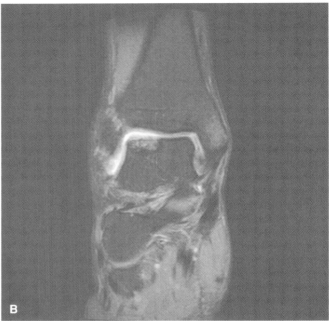

Figure 17–18.   **A:** Case 1: Preoperative T2-weighted coronal ankle MRI showing OLT and bone edema. **B:** Case 1: Six-month postoperative T2-weighted coronal ankle MRI demonstrating a visible cartilage layer with resolving bone edema.

CASE EXAMPLE

Case 1 is a 36-year-old female soccer player. She presented 3 years following an inversion injury with recurrent ankle swelling and pain with daily activities. After conservative treatment with rest, the patient had continued symptoms.

Preoperative MRI demonstrated a large lesion with unstable cartilage delamination and reactive edema in the talus (Fig. 17–18A). MRI 6 months postoperatively demonstrated a visible cartilage layer with resolving bone edema (Fig. 17–18B). At 1 year postoperatively, the patient had no complaints of pain and had returned to full activities.

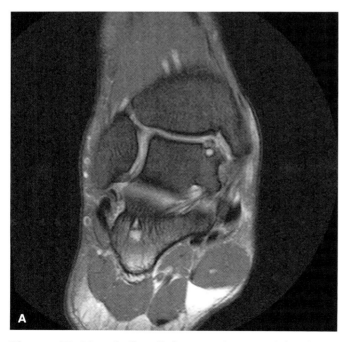
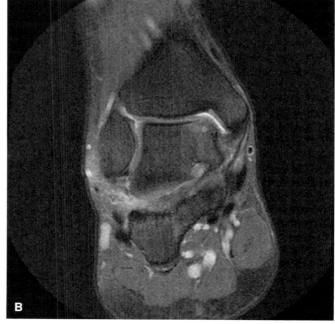

Figure 17–19.   **A:** Case 2: Preoperative T2-weighted coronal ankle MRI showing OLT with cystic change. **B:** Case 2: Six-month postoperative T2-weighted coronal ankle MRI showing a visible cartilage layer with partial resolution of cyst.

The patient for Case 2 is a 33-year-old male who presented with dull ankle pain 2 years following an inversion injury. The patient underwent ankle arthroscopy and debridement at an outside institution 1 year prior. He had continued pain and preoperative MRI demonstrated a cystic talar defect (Fig. 17–19A). The patient had allograft bone placed in the cyst along with a particulated allograft juvenile cartilage transplantation procedure. An MRI at 6 months postoperatively demonstrated a visible cartilage layer with partial resolution of the cyst (Fig. 17–19B). The American Orthopaedic Foot and Ankle Society hindfoot/ankle score improved from 29 preoperatively to 79 points at 6 months postoperatively.

REFERENCES

1. Baker CL Jr., Morales RW. Arthroscopic treatment of transchondral talar dome fractures: A long-term follow-up study. *Arthroscopy*. 1999;15(2):197–202.
2. Schuman L, Struijs PA, van Dijk CN. Arthroscopic treatment for osteochondral defects of the talus. Results at follow-up at 2 to 11 years. *J Bone Joint Surg Br*. 2002;84(3):364–368.
3. Becher C, Thermann H. Results of microfracture in the treatment of articular cartilage defects of the talus. *Foot Ankle Int*. 2005;26(8):583–589.
4. Aurich M, Bedi HS, Smith PJ, et al. Arthroscopic treatment of osteochondral lesions of the ankle with matrix-associated chondrocyte implantation. *Am J Sports Med*. 2011;39(2):311–319.
5. Giannini S, Buda R, Vannini F, et al. Arthroscopic autologous chondrocyte implantation in osteochondral lesions of the talus. *Am J Sports Med*. 2008;36(5):873–880.
6. Hangody L, Hangody L. The mosaicplasty technique for osteochondral lesions of the talus. *Foot Ankle Clin*. 2003;8(2):259–273.
7. Giza E, Sullivan M, Ocel D, et al. Matrix-induced autologous chondrocyte implantation of talus articular defects. *Foot Ankle Int*. 2010;31(9):747–753.
8. Hatic SO, 2nd, Berlet GC. Particulated juvenile articular cartilage graft (DeNovo NT Graft) for treatment of osteochondral lesions of the talus. *Foot Ankle Spec*. 2010;3(6):361–364.
9. Choi WJ, Park KK, Kim BS, et al. Osteochondral lesion of the talus. *Am J Sports Med*. 2009;37(10):1974–1980.
10. Farr J, Kercher J, Salata M, et al. Particulated juvenile cartilage allograft transplantation for repair of high grade chondral lesions. Poster Presentation. International Cartilage Repair Society Meeting, Barcelona, Spain, September 26–28, 2010.
11. Frisbie DD. Future directions in treatment of joint disease in horses. *Vet Clin North Am-Equine Pract*. 2005;21(3):713–724.
12. Feder J, Adkisson HD, Kizer N, et al. In: Sandell L, Grodzinsky A, eds. *Tissue engineering in musculoskeletal clinical practice*. Rosemont, IL: American Academy of Orthopaedic Surgeons, 2004.
13. Adkisson HD, Martin JA, Amendola RL, et al. The potential of human allogeneic juvenile chondrocytes for restoration of articular cartilage. *Am J Sports Med*. 2010;38(7):1324–1333.
14. Gross AE, Shasha N, Aubin P, et al. Long-term followup of the use of fresh osteochondral allografts for posttraumatic knee defects. *Clin Orthop Relat Res*. 2005;(435):79–87.

CHAPTER 18

Arthroscopic Management of Distal Lower Extremity Syndesmosis Injuries

Tun Hing Lui   Lung Fung Tse

INTRODUCTION

The distal tibiofibular syndesmosis consists of the interosseous tibiofibular ligament (IOL), the anterior-inferior tibiofibular ligament (AITFL), the posterior-inferior tibiofibular ligament (PTFL), and the transverse tibiofibular ligament (TL).[1] Approximately 20% of the AITFL is intra-articular. Ankle syndesmotic injury is not uncommon. It is reported to occur in 1% to 11% of soft tissue injuries about the ankle.[2,3] Ebraheim et al.[4] reported that 8% of all ankle fractures have syndesmotic disruptions and that this kind of injury should receive special care owing to the increased risk of associated complications. Burns et al.[5] reported that a complete disruption of the syndesmosis caused a 39% decrease in the tibiotalar contact area and a 42% increase in the tibiotalar contact pressure.[3,6] Purely ligamentous injuries of the syndesmosis, or high ankle sprains, occur when the external rotation force is insufficient to create a fracture.[3,7] Unstable syndesmosis injuries are associated with a high risk of articular surface injury to the talar dome.[8]

Injury to the syndesmosis occurs through rupture or bony avulsion of the syndesmotic ligament complex.[1,9,10] These injuries result most often from an external rotation mechanism.[3,11] In anatomic specimens the proportional contribution to syndesmotic stability of the individual syndesmotic ligaments to syndesmotic stability was found to be 35% for the AITFL, 33% for the TL, 22% for the IOL, and 9% for the PITFL.[12] The AITFL is the weakest of the four syndesmotic ligaments and is the first to yield to forces that create an external rotation of the fibula around its longitudinal axis. As the PITFL is a thick and strong ligament, excessive stress results more often in a posterior malleolus avulsion fracture rather than a ligamentous injury. During external rotation of the foot the fibula is translated posteriorly and rotated externally, which results in increased tension on the AITFL. This may result in isolated rupture of the AITFL.[13] Rupture of the AITFL, in turn, can result in instability of the syndesmosis and ankle mortise.[1,8,9,13,14]

The diagnosis and reduction of syndesmostic injuries, either isolated or in conjunction with an ankle fracture, can be challenging. Previous studies have demonstrated that standard radiographic measurements used to evaluate the integrity of the syndesmosis are inaccurate.[15–17] Many surgically stabilized syndesmotic injuries were malreduced on CT scan but went undetected by plain radiographs. Radiographic measurements did not accurately reflect the status of the distal tibiofibular joint. Furthermore, postreduction radiographic measurements were inaccurate for assessing the quality of the reduction.

Historically, it has been difficult to treat neglected syndesmosis disruption. Reconstructive salvage procedures include syndesmotic fusion and ligamentous reconstruction. Although it has not been correlated to functional outcomes, the known morbidity of postoperative syndesmotic malreduction should lead to heightened vigilance for assessing accurate syndesmosis reduction intraoperatively.[10]

INDICATION

The role of arthroscopy in the management of syndesmotic injury includes

1. Diagnosis of syndesmosis injury
2. Guidance of reduction
3. Ability to assess and treat associated intra-articular pathology

1. Diagnosis of syndesmosis injury

Ankle fractures are among the most common operatively treated lower extremity injuries. Displaced fractures require anatomic reduction to ensure restoration of joint surfaces and normalization of tibiotalar contact forces to minimize the risk of posttraumatic arthritis.[10,18] Although AO Weber type C ankle fractures have traditionally been associated with syndesmotic injuries, injury to the syndesmosis may occur with other fibular fracture patterns.[10,19] Complete disruption of this complex often manifests in diastasis that is visible on plain radiographs; however, more subtle injuries can go undetected. Increasing evidence exists that the traditional radiographic parameters for determining the status of the syndesmosis may be inaccurate.[10,20] None of the specific syndesmotic stress tests was uniformly positive in the presence of a syndesmotic rupture.[6] No definite diagnosis should be made based on the medical history and the physical examination alone.[6]

Arthroscopic evaluation of ankle fractures has the advantage of being minimally invasive while providing excellent visualization of the ankle joint intraoperatively.[21] When, based on medical history and physical examination, syndesmotic injury is suspected, but standard radiographs of the ankle show no indication that syndesmotic injury is present or the diagnosis is still open to debate, additional evaluation of the syndesmosis can be desirable. During arthroscopy of the ankle, injury of the anterior syndesmosis can be confirmed with more certainty.[6,11,15,22–24] The arthroscopic stress test is useful for evaluating the stability of the tibiofibular articulation.[24] By means of ankle arthroscopy, the pattern of syndesmosis disruption can be assessed in three planes (coronal, sagittal, and frontal).[14]

2. Guidance of anatomic reduction

An accurate initial reduction of a disrupted syndesmosis is crucial to the long-term stability and function of the ankle.[25] Failure to reduce and stabilize a disruption of the syndesmosis that occurs in association with some rotational ankle fractures is associated with poor outcomes. A recent study of human cadaver specimens concluded that no optimal radiographic measurement exists to assess syndesmotic integrity, and that repeated radiographs of the ankle are of little value because of the inability to reproduce ankle positioning even under optimal laboratory conditions.[7] In the setting of ankle fractures with syndesmosis disruption, fixing the fibula in as much as 30 degrees of external rotation may go undetected using intraoperative fluoroscopy alone. These findings are clinically relevant since in both supination-external rotation and pronation-external rotation injuries of the ankle, which constitute the majority of ankle fractures, the distal fibula is displaced in external rotation[26] and may therefore be subject to malreduction and fixation in this position. As it may be difficult to obtain an accurate lateral fluoroscopic view and there is no definition of the anatomic location of the syndesmosis on the lateral view, the integrity of the syndesmosis in the sagittal plane is difficult to assess radiographically.[15] Assessment of the three-dimensional position of the distal fibula within the incisura is difficult when relying on two-dimensional imaging. The incidence of incongruity of the distal tibiofibular joint after operative reduction and internal fixation for syndesmotic injury was higher than previously reported the literature.[10] The prevalence of postoperative syndesmotic malreduction has been reported to be between 0% and 16%.[8,16,21,27]

3. Ability to assess and treat associated intra-articular pathology

Arthroscopy is a useful tool for investigating intra-articular disorders of the ankle joint. Rotational fractures of the ankle joint in particular can lead to the development of these intra-articular disorders. Ono et al.[28] evaluated the arthroscopic findings and surgical outcome for fresh malleolar fractures and reported that intra-articular disorders were identified in no less than 50%. With regard to the treatment for such lesions, the efficacy of nonsurgical treatments is uncertain. However, the clinical results of each type of surgical treatment have been reported to be satisfactory. During arthroscopy the presence and extent of chondral pathology can easily be assessed. Chondral lesions can be the direct result of ankle fracture or indirect result of the instability of the ankle mortise, contributed to by injury of the syndesmosis.[6] Syndesmosis disruption portends a particularly high risk of articular surface injury to the talar dome that would otherwise remain unrecognized on conventional radiographs.

The advantages of ankle arthroscopy are that clinicians can correctly diagnose and treat the intra-articular lesion with minimal soft tissue disruption under direct visualization.[2] Arthroscopy may provide prognostic information regarding the functional outcome of these injuries. We believed that there was a high incidence of concomitant intra-articular disorders and therefore performed arthroscopic investigation and treatment for these lesions at the time of fracture surgery to avoid the development of residual ankle disability.[13] Therefore, ankle arthroscopy is particularly well suited for clarifying the accompanying intra-articular disorders in distal fibular fractures.[29]

CONTRAINDICATION

Absolute contraindications include open fractures, neurovascular injury, and severe soft tissue swelling.

Patient Position

Under general or regional anesthesia, the patient is placed in the supine position with folded blankets under the ipsilateral hip/buttock. We use a well-padded tourniquet on the proximal thigh to maintain a bloodless field. No traction is required.

Surgical Approaches

We perform ankle arthroscopy through standard anteromedial and anterolateral portals using a 30-degree 2.7-mm arthroscope. A standard 4-mm arthroscope may be used, however, a 2.7-mm arthroscope provides easy access. Instruments usually include 2.5- or 3.5-mm arthroscopic shaver, thermal ablation device, and small arthroscopic manual instruments (biter and grasper devices). Loose osteocartilaginous debris and soft tissue are removed from the joint.

During anterior ankle arthroscopy with standard anteromedial and anterolateral portals, easy passage of the arthroscope or arthroscopic instrument into the lateral ankle gutter is a hint to the presence of syndesmosis diastasis.[15] The AITFL, synovialized portion of the syndesmosis, the PITFL, and the TL can be seen during arthroscopy. The IOL cannot be seen normally as it is located above the joint line. However, in case of significant syndesmosis diastasis the ruptured IOL can be seen with

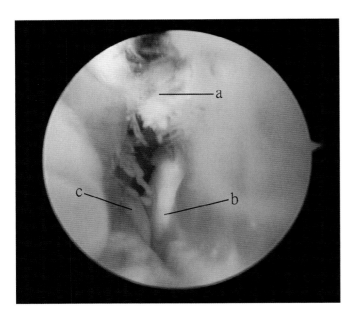

Figure 18–1.   The torn interosseous ligament *(a)* can be seen in case of significant syndesmosis diastasis; *(b)* lateral articular edge of distal tibia; *(c)* medial articular edge of distal fibula.

the arthroscope passed between the distal tibia and fibula (Fig. 18–1).

Open reduction and fixation techniques may not be accurate if there is a posterior malleolar fracture or a posterior syndesmotic ligament rupture. The posterior malleolar fracture can be fixed to provide a stable posterior fulcrum on which to base reduction of the syndesmosis. However, this is only feasible when the PITFL is intact. In contrast, arthroscopic assessment of the syndesmosis allows for assessment of syndesmotic reduction under these conditions. Specifically, comprehensive assessment of anterior edge of the syndesmosis, intra-articular portion, and posterior part of the syndesmosis can be made via the standard two portal arthroscopy. Arthroscopic syndesmotic assessment has another advantage over conventional open syndesmotic reduction in that there is no need for release of the extensor retinacular fibers (which run anterior and parallel to the anterior syndesmotic ligamentous fibers) from the anterior surface of the fibula.

However, it may be difficult to assess the reduction of syndesmosis in conditions like high fibular fracture and complete syndesmotic ligament rupture in case of Maisonneuve fracture and floating fibula. Moreover, the shortened fibula (loss of longitudinal syndesmosis reduction) after malreduction of a comminuted fibular fracture cannot be appreciated via arthroscopy. Fluoroscopy is needed to assess the fibular length.[15,30]

Reduction Technique

We perform open reduction and internal fixation of the distal fibular fracture by 3.5-mm one-third tubular plate

through the standard lateral approach. For medial malleolar fractures, we use two 4.0-mm cannulated screws for fracture fixation. After fixation, we use fluoroscopy to check the reduction and look for any gross coronal or longitudinal syndesmosis disruption. We also perform an anterior drawer test of the ankle. If the drawer test is positive, we dorsiflex the ankle during stabilization of the syndesmosis and insertion of a syndesmotic screw. Otherwise, the ankle was kept in neutral position during insertion of the screw. This can avoid plantar or anterior translation of the talar body with syndesmosis stabilization in case of extensive collateral ligament damage (Fig. 18–2). Next, we perform ankle arthroscopy with direct visualization to evaluate syndesmosis integrity. The syndesmosis is examined for any diastasis in the coronal, sagittal, and rotational planes (Fig. 18–3). Stress is applied to detect any occult diastasis (Fig. 18–4). We apply laterally directed stress to the distal fibula with a bone hook to assess coronal plane stability of the syndesmosis. Anteroposterior force is applied to assess sagittal plane stability. Finally, external rotation stress is applied through the tibiotalar joint to assess rotational plane stability. Coronal and sagittal syndesmosis instability is defined by 2 mm or more displacement of the lateral malleolus in the coronal (lateral displacement) or sagittal (posterior displacement) plane, respectively.[11,15,24] Rotational syndesmosis instability (external rotation of the distal fibula) is defined as displacement of the anterior border of the lateral malleolus at least 2 mm more than displacement of the posterior border of the lateral malleolus relative to the tibia. The definition of occult syndesmotic diastasis is the same as those for disruption in different planes but is evident only in response to applied stress.

After thorough analysis of the integrity of the syndesmosis, the disrupted syndesmosis is reduced under arthroscopic guidance by lining up the anterior leading edge of the fibular syndesmotic articulation with that of the tibia and eliminating gapping or space (Fig. 18–5). The syndesmosis is then fixed. Two screws are inserted in case of Maisonneuve fracture.[31] The syndesmotic screw was removed 6 weeks later when second-look ankle arthroscopy was also performed.[15,30]

The posterior complex, which may be destabilized by either a tear of the posterior-inferior tibiofibular ligament or a posterior malleolar fracture, plays a significant role in the stability of the syndesmosis and ankle mortise.[3,11,18,24] It is unclear to what degree the posterior malleolar fractures contribute to syndesmotic malreductions. However, anatomic reduction and fixation of the posterior malleolar fragment may allow for restoration of a more congruous incisura and result in a better reduction of the tibiofibular joint. In that series reported by Cottom et al.,[9] another possible cause of malreduction may be nonanatomic reduction of the fibula. Although no gross fibular malreductions were seen on radiographs postoperatively, subtle incongruencies may have occurred and led to a mildly asymmetric

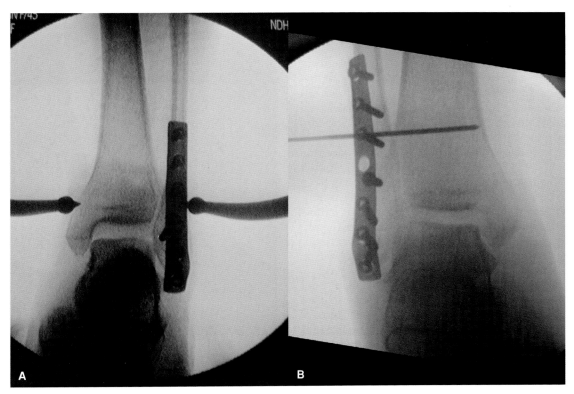

Figure 18–2.   The talar body was plantarly displaced during temporary stabilization of the syndesmosis with the ankle in neutral position as a result of significant damage of the collateral ligaments of the ankle. Intraoperative fluoroscopic anteroposterior view of **(A)** a case with reduction forceps applied and **(B)** of a case after reduction was held provisionally with a guidewire.

tibiofibular reduction, particularly in cases with significant fibular comminution. Finally, infolded ligaments or other soft tissue debris within the incisura may account for malreduced cases.[10]

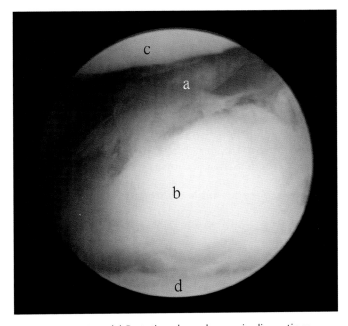

Figure 18–3.   *(a)* Rotational syndesmosis disruption; *(b)* lateral malleolus; *(c)* tibial plafond; *(d)* talar dome.

Open reduction and internal fixation of the posterior malleolar fragment is often performed in conjunction with open reduction of the syndesmosis. In our experience, the posterior malleolar fracture usually does not hinder arthroscopic-assisted syndesmosis reduction. Failed arthroscopic-assisted syndesmosis reduction has occurred in some cases of Maisonneuve fracture with floating fibula. In these cases, the posterior syndesmotic ligament was ruptured rather than a posterior malleolar fracture. The lateral malleolus can be freely rotated along the fibular axis in these cases.

COMPLICATIONS

Acute compartment syndrome is one of the complications that can occur after ankle arthroscopy. While Ferkel et al.[1] reported that excessive extravasation during arthroscopy can cause this complication, other authors have reported that it may be due to the perioperative position of the lower extremity.[2,3] Olson and Glasgow[2] reported that traction of the lower extremity with the ankle in the plantar-flexed position caused increased pressure in the anterior compartment. In addition, Meyer et al. reported that hemilithotomy positions were implicated in the development of perioperative compartment syndrome of the lower extremity. We feel that there are three reasons why acute compartment syndrome may

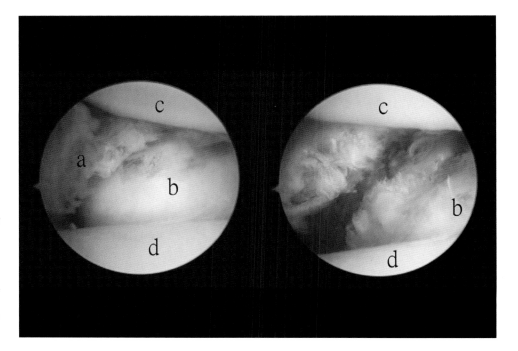

Figure 18–4. Occult sagittal syndesmosis disruption. The left image is shown at rest. Posterior force has been applied to the same ankle in the image to the right demonstrating diastasis between the ligament and the fibula. *(a)* Torn anterior syndesmotic ligament; *(b)* lateral malleolus; *(c)* tibial plafond; *(d)* talar dome.

develop. First, increasing intracompartmental pressure resulting from the extensive disruption of the interosseous membrane. Second, excessive extravasation of irrigation fluids during the arthroscopic procedure, which might have run through the ruptured interosseous membrane or have expanded subcutaneously. The third reason involves the operative position, and specifically keeping the patient in the hemilithotomy position throughout surgery. We believe that the synergistic effects of these reasons may lead to the development of this condition.

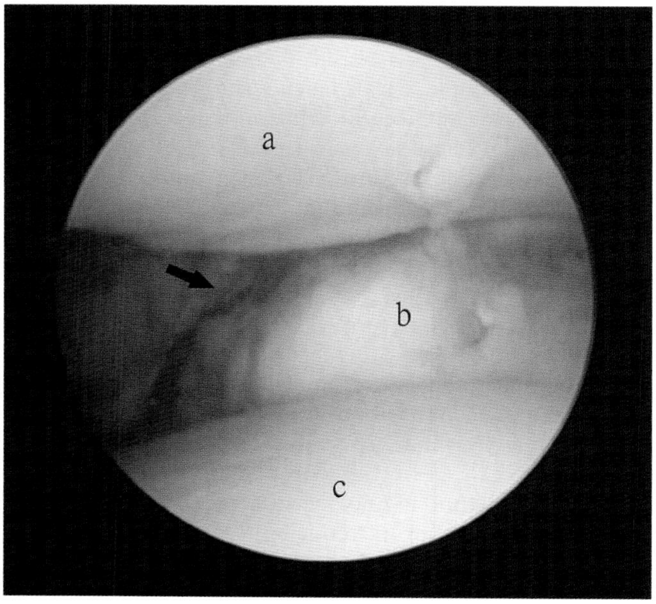

OUTCOME

Ankle fractures with syndesmotic injury treated using fluoroscopic reduction and standard trans-syndesmotic fixation may have malreduction rate of 23%.[32] Ankle arthroscopy allows more direct intraoperative assessment of the accuracy of the syndesmotic reduction.[33] An ankle with an incongruous mortise, chronic diastasis of the syndesmosis, and arthritis can be salvaged with reduction and arthrodesis of the distal tibiofibular articulation. Nevertheless, our research as well as that of others demonstrates that arthrodesis can reduce pain, improve function, correct alignment, and delay the progression of radiographic signs of arthritis.[25,34] These results further demonstrate that reduction and arthrodesis of the distal tibiofibular articulation is a viable alternative to ankle arthrodesis and that it postpones, and may obviate, the need for an ankle arthrodesis or arthroplasty in the future.[25,34]

There is debate as to whether arthroscopy may lead to excessive diagnosis of syndesmotic injury, and potentially overtreatment.[35] AP views are reported to be between 44% and 48% sensitive and mortise views are reported to be between 64% and 65% sensitive of syndesmosis disruption.[23,24] Stress radiographs are often negative.[36] Even allowing for the low sensitivity, the exact radiologic criteria are debatable. The reported measurements vary, making the assessment of the syndesmosis

Figure 18–5. The reduced syndesmosis. Arthroscopic image of the ankle shown in Figure 18–4 after reduction. The torn ends of the anterior syndesmotic ligament were apposed *(arrow)*. *(a)* Tibial plafond; *(b)* lateral malleolus; *(c)* talar dome.

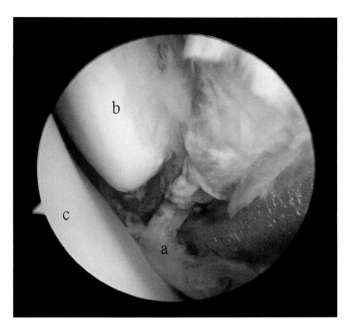

Figure 18–6. The deep deltoid ligament *(a)* avulsed from the medial malleolus *(b)*. *(c)* Medial facet of the talar body.

controversial.[35] As such, it remains controversial as to whether or not the arthroscopic identification of an isolated syndesmotic injury requires treatment.

Ankle fractures have a high incidence of concomitant intra-articular pathology with syndesmosis disruption portending a particularly high risk of articular surface injury to the talar dome. Arthroscopy is a valuable tool in identifying and treating intra-articular damage that would otherwise remain unrecognized; although the prognostic importance of traumatic articular lesions is unclear. Unstable syndesmosis injuries are associated with a significantly high risk of articular surface injury to the talar dome. Although uncommon, an interposed deltoid ligament may also impede reduction of the fibula or talus, requiring a medial arthrotomy. Routine arthroscopic evaluation and debridement of the medial gutter may preclude the need for an open medial approach to address interposed tissue (Fig. 18–6).

SUMMARY

Arthroscopic evaluation of acute ankle fractures has the advantages of minimal surgical trauma and excellent visualization of the joint surfaces for assessing alignment and treating the articular surface damage. The procedure also permits evaluation and debridement of ligament tears and removal of loose debris that may cause third body articular damage. Furthermore, arthroscopic visualization may facilitate reduction and internal fixation in certain fracture patterns.[8,13,14]

Nevertheless, criteria for syndesmotic disruption on arthroscopy have not been completely established. Further,

extended follow-up will be necessary to determine if early arthroscopic intervention will improve clinical outcome.

REFERENCES

1. Bartonicek J. Anatomy of the tibiofibular syndesmosis and its clinical relevance. *Surg Radiol Anat.* 2003;25:379–386.
2. Olson SA, Glasgow RR. Acute compartment syndrome in lower extremity musculoskeletal trauma. *J Am Acad Orthop Surg.* 2005;13(7):436–444.
3. Cottom JM, Hyer CF, Philbin TM, et al. Transosseous fixation of the distal tibiofibular syndesmosis: Comparison of an interosseous suture and endobutton to traditional screw fixation in 50 cases. *J Foot Ankle Surg.* 2009;48(6):620–630.
4. Ebraheim NA, Elgafy H, Padanilam T. Syndesmotic disruption in low fibular fractures associated with deltoid ligament injury. *Clin Orthop Relat Res.* 2003;(409):260–267.
5. Burns WC, Prakash K, Adelaar R, et al. Tibiotalar joint dynamics: Indications for the syndesmotic screw—a cadaver study. *Foot Ankle Int.* 1993;14:153–158.
6. Wagener ML, Beumer A, Swierstra BA. Chronic instability of the anterior tibiofibular syndesmosis of the ankle. Arthroscopic findings and results of anatomical reconstruction. *BMC Musculoskeletal Disorders.* 2011;12:212.
7. Chan KB, Lui TH. Isolated anterior syndesmosis diastasis without fracture. *Arch Orthop Trauma Surg.* 2007;127:321–324.
8. Loren GJ, Ferkel RD. Arthroscopic assessment of occult intra-articular injury in acute ankle fractures. *Arthroscopy.* 2002;18:412–421.
9. Cottom JM, Hyer CF, Philbin TM et al. Treatment of syndesmotic disruptions with the Arthrex Tightrope: A report of 25 cases. *Foot Ankle Int.* 2008;29(8):773–780.
10. Gardner MJ, Demetrakopoulos D, Briggs SM, et al. Malreduction of the tibiofibular syndesmosis in ankle fractures. *Foot Ankle Int.* 2006;27:788–792.
11. Han SH, Lee JW, Kim S, et al. Chronic tibiofibular syndesmosis injury: The diagnostic efficiency of magnetic resonance imaging and comparative analysis of operative treatment. *Foot Ankle Int.* 2007;28:336-342.
12. Hermans JJ, Beumer A, de Jong TAW, et al. Anatomy of the distal tibiofibular syndesmosis in adults: A pictorial essay with a multimodality approach. *J Anat.* 2010;217:633–645.
13. Imade S, Takao M, Miyamoto W, et al. Leg anterior compartment syndrome following ankle arthroscopy after Maisonneuve fracture. *Arthroscopy.* 2009;25(2):215–218.
14. Lui TH. Tri-ligamentous reconstruction of the distal tibiofibular syndesmosis: A minimally invasive approach. *J Foot Ankle Surg.* 2010;49:495–500.
15. Lui TH, Ip KY, Chow HT. Comparison of radiologic and arthroscopic diagnoses of distal tibiofibular syndesmosis disruption in acute ankle fracture. *Arthroscopy.* 2005;21:1370–1374.
16. Beumer A, Hemert WV, Niesing R, et al. Radiographic measurement of the distal tibiofibular syndesmosis has limited use. *Clin Orthop Relat Res.* 2004;423(6):227–234.
17. Nielson JH, Gardner MJ, Peterson MGE, et al. Radiographic measurements do not predict syndesmotic injury

in ankle fractures. An MRI study. *Clin Orthop Relat Res.* 2005;436:216–221.

18. Thordarson DB, Motamed S, Hedman T, et al. The effect of fibular malreduction on contact pressures in an ankle fracture malunion model. *J Bone Joint Surg.* 1997;79A:1809–1815.

19. Kennedy JG, Soffe KE, Dalla Vedova P, et al. Evaluation of the syndesmotic screw in low Weber C ankle fractures. *J Orthop Trauma.* 2000;14:359–366.

20. Nielson JH, Sallis JG, Potter HG, et al. Correlation of interosseous membrane tears to the level of the fibular fracture. *J Orthop Trauma.* 2004;18:68–74.

21. Yoshimura I, Naito M, Kanazawa K, et al. Arthroscopic findings in Maisonneuve fractures. *J Orthop Sci.* 2008;13: 3–6.

22. Oae K, Takao M, Naito K, et al. Injury of the tibiofibular syndesmosis: Value of MR imaging for diagnosis. *Radiology.* 2003;227:155–161.

23. Takao M, Ochi M, Naito K, et al. Arthroscopic diagnosis of tibiofibular syndesmosis disruption. *Arthroscopy.* 2001; 17:836–843.

24. Takao M, Ochi M, Oae K, et al. Diagnosis of a tear of the tibiofibular syndesmosis. The role of arthroscopy of the ankle. *J Bone Joint Surg.* 2003;85B:324–329.

25. Olson KM, Dairyko GH Jr, Toolan BC, Salvage of chronic instability of the syndesmosis with distal tibiofibular arthrodesis. Functional and radiographic results. *J Bone Joint Surg Am.* 2011;93:66–72.

26. Morris MW, Rice P, Schneider TE. Distal tibiofibular syndesmosis reconstruction using a free hamstring autograft. *Foot Ankle Int.* 2009;30(6):506–511.

27. Marmor M, Hansen E, Han HK, et al. Limitations of standard fluoroscopy in detecting rotational malreduction of the syndesmosis in an ankle fracture model. *Foot Ankle Int.* 2011;32(6):616–622.

28. Ono A, Nishikawa S, Nagao A, et al. Arthroscopically assisted treatment of ankle fractures: Arthroscopic findings and surgical outcomes. *Arthroscopy.* 2004;20(6):627–631.

29. Takao M, Uchio Y, Naito K, et al. Diagnosis and treatment of combined intra-articular disorders in acute distal fibular fractures. *J Trauma.* 2004;57:1303–1307.

30. Lui TH, Chan KB, Ngai WK. Premature closure of distal fibular growth plate: A case of longitudinal syndesmosis-instability. *Arch Orthop Trauma Surg.* 2008;128:45–48.

31. Sagi HC, Shah AR, Sanders RW. The functional consequence of syndesmotic joint malreduction at a minimum 2-year follow-up. *J Orthop Trauma.* 2012;26:439–443.

32. Moon SW, Kim JW. Usefulness of intraoperative three-dimensional imaging in fracture surgery: A prospective study. *J Orthop Sci.* 2014;19:125–131.

33. Miller AN, Carroll EA, Parker RJ, et al. Direct visualization for syndesmotic stabilization of ankle fractures. *Foot Ankle Int.* 2009;30:419–426.

34. Yasui Y, Takao M, Miyamoto W, et al. Anatomical reconstruction of the anterior inferior tibiofibular ligament for chronic disruption of the distal tibiofibular syndesmosis. *Knee Surg Sports Traumatol Arthrosc.* 2011;19:691–695.

35. Sri-Ram K, Robinson AHN. Arthroscopic assessment of the syndesmosis following ankle fracture. *Injury.* 2005;36: 675-678.

36. Ogilvie-Harris DJ, Reed SC. Disruption of the ankle syndesmosis: Diagnosis and treatment by arthroscopic surgery. *Arthroscopy.* 1994;10:561–568.

CHAPTER 19

Posterior Ankle Arthroscopy and Hindfoot Endoscopy/Tendoscopy

Florian Nickisch   Frank R. Avilucea
Phinit Phisitkul   Brad D. Blankenhorn

INTRODUCTION

The posterior ankle and hindfoot is a complex region with diverse pathology affecting several important structures that are in close proximity to each other. Due to the location of some lesions, open surgical treatment can lead to substantial morbidity requiring extensive rehabilitation.[1] Posterior hindfoot endoscopy is a minimally invasive approach that minimizes soft tissue trauma, decreases patient discomfort and morbidity, and speeds rehabilitation compared to open surgery. It offers excellent access to the posterior aspect of the tibiotalar joint, the posterior facet of the subtalar joint, and the majority of the posterior periarticular structures.

INDICATIONS

Posterior hindfoot arthroscopy often allow for both intra- and extra-articular pathology to be efficiently addressed. Surgery is generally indicated for patients with recalcitrant pain that substantially interferes with activities of normal living. Common intra-articular indications include treatment of posterior osteochondral lesions of the ankle joint, debridement of ankle or subtalar arthritis without substantial malalignment, loose body excision, synovectomy, Achilles tendon pathology, and the treatment of intraosseous talar ganglia. The surgical indications for the treatment of these lesions through a posterior arthroscopic approach are the same as for an open approach. Not only does posterior arthroscopy ease access to lesions that would be difficult to reach via an open approach, it also decreases the wound healing risks for surgical treatment of patients with soft tissue issues that would otherwise be a contraindication to surgery.

CONTRAINDICATIONS

Our surgical technique is to place patients in the prone position for posterior hindfoot arthroscopic surgery. A patient with respiratory or medical comorbidities that preclude safe prone positioning would not be a candidate for a posterior arthroscopic approach.

PATIENT POSITIONING

Posterior hindfoot arthroscopy is performed in the prone position. Before positioning on the operative table, general endotracheal anesthesia is induced, a thigh tourniquet is applied, and appropriate perioperative antibiotics are administered. The patient is then positioned prone on the operative table with the distal third of the tibia extended past the end of the table (Fig. 19–1). This allows for unrestricted ankle and subtalar motion as well as appropriate positioning of the fluoroscopy unit. The contralateral knee is then flexed to 90 degrees and stabilized against a post attached to the table (Fig. 19–1). A safety strap is positioned around the patient in a manner that provides countertraction, and the operative extremity is prepped and draped in a sterile fashion.

After draping, a 1.8-mm wire can be placed in the tuberosity of the calcaneus, which allows for skeletal traction and joint distraction. The wire is attached to a tension bow and traction device (Fig. 19–2). A sterile drape is placed over the traction device (Fig. 19–3). The fluoroscopy unit is then brought next to the end of the table around the patient's hindfoot and positioned to obtain a lateral view (Fig. 19–3). This allows for hands-free fluoroscopic guidance for establishing portals for optimal access to either the posterior ankle or subtalar joints.

SURGICAL APPROACH

First described in 2000, a two-portal endoscopic approach remains the technique we most often employ to access the posterior ankle and hindfoot.[2,3] The advantage of a two-portal technique with the patient in the prone position, is the working space available between the Achilles tendon and the posterior aspect of the tibiotalar or subtalar articulation. Moreover, this position is ergonomic for the surgeon and skeletal distraction may be easily applied.

Landmarks on the hindfoot that are essential for proper portal placement include the medial and lateral malleoli, the lateral and medial border of the Achilles tendon, and the sole of the foot. As noted, a 1.8-mm traction pin is placed into the calcaneal tuberosity from a medial to lateral direction to avoid injuring the medial

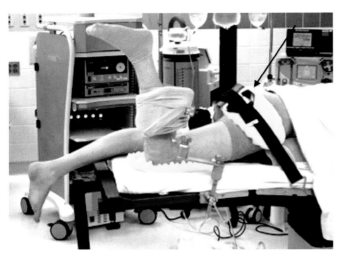

Figure 19–1. Patient positioning for posterior hindfoot arthroscopy. The patient is brought down the table until the distal third of their tibia extends beyond the end of the table. This facilitates access with the mini C-arm. The contralateral knee is flexed 90 degrees and held with a leg holder. The safety strap over the gluteal region provides counter traction (*arrow*).

neurovascular structures (Fig. 19–2). For patients with pathology of the posterior ankle joint, skeletal traction is recommended to distract the joint.[4] This allows for easier introduction of arthroscopic instruments. Skeletal traction is less helpful for distracting the posterior facet of the subtalar joint; nevertheless, placing a small amount of tension on the foot and ankle through skeletal traction stabilizes the foot and ankle and aids in instrument placement.

Judicious use of fluoroscopy is employed to confirm proper portal location before making incisions. The

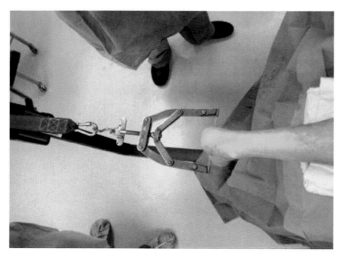

Figure 19–2. Placement of a calcaneal traction pin allows for distraction of the tibiotalar joint or stabilization of the subtalar joint. A sterile drape is placed over the traction device once it is in place.

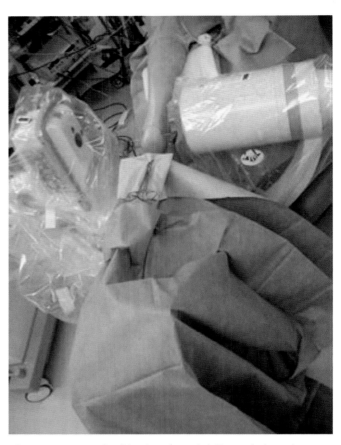

Figure 19–3. Positioning the mini C-arm below the operative leg allows for hands-free fluoroscopic assistance throughout the procedure.

direction of the portal placement depends on the location of the structures that need to be accessed. Portals are made just medial and lateral to the Achilles tendon. Using fluoroscopic guidance, a spinal needle is used to distend either the tibiotalar or subtalar joint. The medial and lateral borders of the Achilles tendon are then palpated and 1-cm parallel skin incisions flanking the tendon are created (Fig. 19–4). The incisions are made through only skin to avoid damage to subcutaneous nerves, in particular the sural nerve on the lateral aspect of the Achilles tendon.

Beginning at the lateral portal, a straight hemostat is used to bluntly dissect through the subcutaneous layer while aiming toward the web space between the first and second toe. For intra-articular procedures the hemostat is advanced through the joint capsule. A trocar for a 2.7-mm arthroscope is then inserted into this incision and an arthroscope is introduced. The surgeon must remain cognizant of the close proximity of the sural nerve to the posterolateral portal (3 to 12 mm).[5,6] Fluoroscopy is used as necessary to ensure instruments do not stray into areas containing neurovascular structures during the procedure.

Establishment of a posteromedial portal is accomplished in a similar fashion. In approaching the posteromedial hindfoot, it is important to remain cognizant of

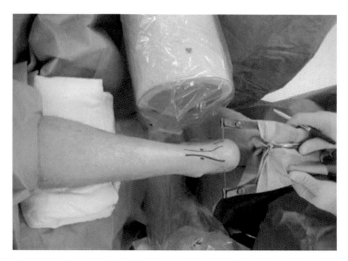

Figure 19–4. Medial and lateral portals placed on either side of the Achilles tendon. These portals may be localized using a spinal needle and fluoroscopy. The position is dependent on the structures that are going to be accessed during the procedure.

crucial medial structures. Care is taken to direct the subcutaneous tissue dissection laterally to avoid injury to the medial structures. All arthroscopic instruments should remain lateral to the flexor hallucis longus (FHL) tendon.

When approaching extra-articular structures, saline is injected around the structure to distend potential spaces and create a working area. A blunt instrument is then used to further expand this space until enough room is present to place the arthroscope. Once the arthroscope is in place, a second portal is established and the working space is expanded using the arthroscopic shaver.

COMMON CONDITIONS TREATED WITH POSTERIOR ANKLE ARTHROSCOPY

Debridement and Microfracture of Osteochondral Lesions

One of the most common indications for posterior ankle arthroscopy is debridement and microfracture of a talar osteochondral lesion. Posterior ankle arthroscopy allows

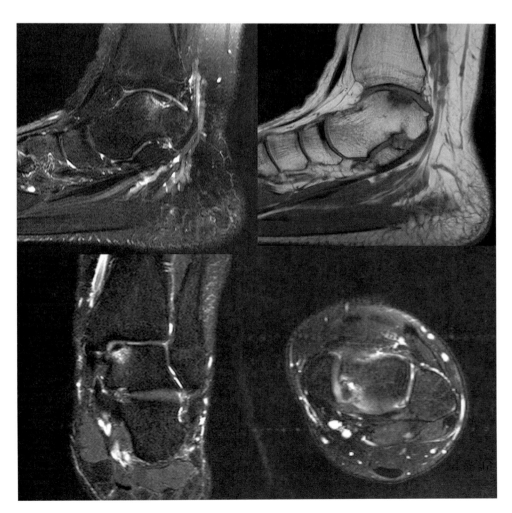

Figure 19–5. Magnetic resonance imaging of an ankle with a symptomatic posterior osteochondral defect (OCD). Posterior arthroscopy allows for improved access to this lesion for debridement compared to anterior arthroscopy.

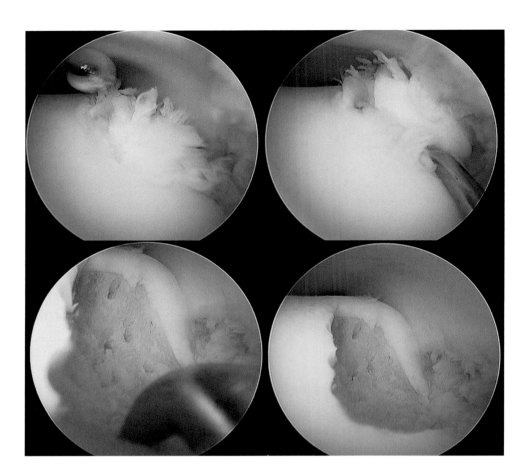

Figure 19–6. Arthroscopic views of the posterior OCD seen in Figure 19–5. After the lesion is debrided of all loose cartilage and nonviable bone, an arthroscopic pick is used to stimulate healing.

for access to lesions that cannot be easily reached from traditional anterior arthroscopic portals. Osteochondral lesions located posterior to the midcoronal line of the medial malleolus are typically accessible through posterior arthroscopic portals (Fig. 19–5). Loose cartilage fragments and necrotic bone are debrided and microfracture of the lesion is conducted in a similar manner as anterior arthroscopic debridement using a combination of curettes and arthroscopic instruments (Fig. 19–6). Once all nonviable tissue has been debrided, an arthroscopic pick is used to perforate the underlying bone. This will facilitate fibrous cartilage healing (Fig. 19–6). No studies have been conducted to specifically examine the outcomes of osteochondral lesions undergoing posterior debridement and microfracture, but these lesions are expected to behave similarly to lesions debrided by anterior arthroscopy. Debridement of painful impinging osteophytes emanating from the subtalar or posterior tibiotalar joint can be debrided in a similar fashion.

Postoperatively, patients are placed in a short leg splint until the surgical wounds have healed. After approximately 2 weeks, sutures are removed and the patient is placed in a removable boot. Ankle and subtalar range of motion is started at this point. Patients remain nonweight bearing for a total of 6 weeks, after which

progressive weight bearing is initiated and range of motion and strengthening is advanced.

Debridement of Posterior Ankle Impingement With/Without Excision of the Os Trigonum and Release the Flexor Hallucis Longus (FHL) Tendon

Posterior ankle impingement can be related to soft tissue impingement or secondary to a symptomatic os trigonum. Posterior arthroscopy allows for a minimally invasive approach to debridement and release of these posterior structures. For soft tissue impingement alone, the majority of debridement is performed in an extra-articular space. Arthroscopic portals are created in a similar fashion to typical hindfoot posterior arthroscopy, except a space is made in the posterolateral soft tissues posterior to the ankle and subtalar joints using fluoroscopic assistance before entering the joint capsule (Fig. 19–7). Once a space is established, dissection is carried in a lateral to medial fashion until the tendon of the FHL is identified. No dissection is carried medial to this tendon to prevent injury to the medial neurovascular structures (Fig. 19–8). Once the medial border of the arthroscopic

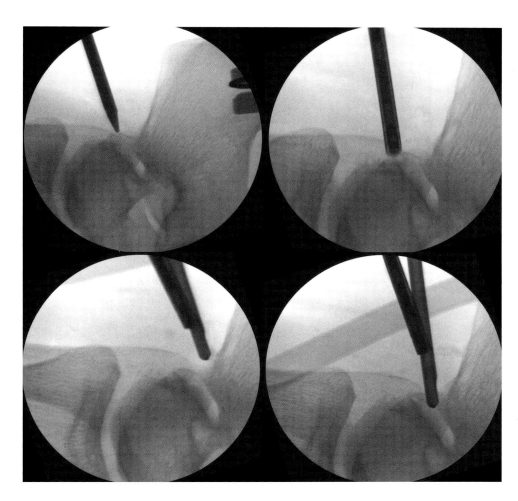

Figure 19–7. Fluoroscopic views of the creation of a posterior extra-articular working space to allow for the debridement of posterior tibiotalar impingement.

space is defined, the posterior joint capsule of the subtalar and tibiotalar joints is debrided (Fig. 19–8). Posttraumatic posterior arthrofibrosis of ankle or subtalar joint is debrided in a similar fashion. If a Stieda process of the talus is present and felt to be symptomatic, debridement can be extended to include the posterior portion of the talus. This is debrided using an arthroscopic burr or shaver (Fig. 19–8).

If an os trigonum is present and is felt to be symptomatic, a similar posterior extra-articular space is created using triangulation and fluoroscopic assistance. Using an arthroscopic shaver the soft tissue surrounding the os is removed (Fig. 19–9). Using a Freer elevator, the os trigonum is released from its attachment to the talus (Fig. 19–9). The tibiotalar and subtalar joints are also inspected. The bony os is then removed from the posteromedial portal (Fig. 19–9). This portal is recommended for removal to prevent injury to the sural nerve, which is in close proximity to the posterolateral portal.

Postoperatively, patients are placed in a posterior splint until wound healing. Sutures are removed approximately 2 weeks after the operation. At that point, range of motion and progressive weight bearing is initiated.

Previous studies have shown favorable outcomes for posterior ankle impingement treated with a posterior arthroscopic approach. In a retrospective study of 30 patients with posterior ankle impingement treated with arthroscopic debridement, Galla and Lobenhoffer[7] showed an improvement in VAS score from 7.2 to 1.3 with 79% of patients returning to their preoperative level of sport activity. However, in this study two patients developed infections, two patients had sural nerve neuropraxia, and two patients required open revision decompression due to persistent pain.[7] In a similar study, Noguchi et al.[8] treated 12 patients with posterior impingement arthroscopically and had an improvement in AOFAS hindfoot score improved from 68.0 to 98.3 points. In this study all patients returned to sport activity in 5.9 weeks and only one patient displayed a transient sural nerve neuropraxia.

In patients with stenosing tenosynovitis of the FHL tendon the tenosynovium is carefully debrided starting proximal and lateral. Once the FHL tendon is well visualized posterior to the ankle and subtalar joint, the dissection is carried distally, releasing the tendon sheath from the lateral aspect of the calcaneus. With the arthroscopic instruments remaining lateral to the tendon complete release of

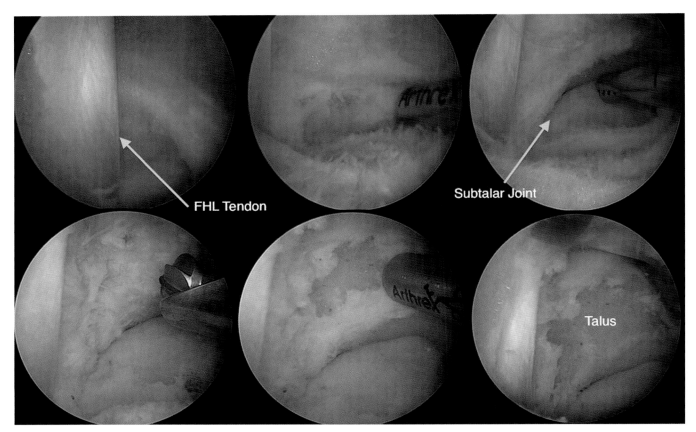

Figure 19–8.   Arthroscopic views of the posterior capsule of the tibiotalar and subtalar joints. The tendon of the FHL is identified as the most medial border of the arthroscopic working space. The capsule is then debrided revealing the posterior tibiotalar and subtalar joints. If there is concern for impingement of the posterior talus, this can be removed with an arthroscopic burr.

the tendon sheath can usually be safely performed until the tendon courses under the sustentaculum tali.

Noninsertional Achilles Tendinopathy

The authors prefer to use van Dijk technique to debride paratenon adhesions and to denervate the intratendinous lesions as well as Maffulli technique to allow revascularization and repair of the tendon.[9–11]

A 4.0-mm arthroscope is used for this procedure. In the prone position, endoscopic debridement is performed using proximal medial and distal lateral portals (Fig. 19–10). The arthroscopic trocar is inserted from the distal lateral portal created just distal and lateral to the tendon enlargement. Blunt dissection is performed using the arthroscopic trocar to break down the adhesion in the space between the paratenon and the tendon. A 3.5-mm full-radius shaver is inserted from the proximal medial portal created proximal and medial to the tendon enlargement. The instruments are interchanged through both portals for a complete debridement. Any fibrotic tissue binding the tendon sheath to the tendon is debrided under direct visualization.

Percutaneous tenotomy is performed with a no. 11 blade in longitudinal planes without endoscopic visualization (Fig. 19–11A). Each tenotomy is made from a stab incision posterior to the tendon enlargement. To assist with the cut, the ankle is ranged into dorsiflexion and plantarflexion. Five longitudinal tenotomies are made creating a pattern similar to "number 5" on a dice over the enlarged portion of the Achilles tendon (Fig. 19–11B). The patient is allowed to bear full weight on the operated limb using a boot. The boot is weaned off at 4 to 6 weeks.

Endoscopic Calcaneoplasty for Haglund Deformity

The authors perform an endoscopic calcaneoplasty only in select cases without an ossification or intratendinous spur at the Achilles insertion as these pathologies are not adequately addressed endoscopically. The ideal patient usually has tenderness only with mediolateral palpation anterior to the Achilles tendon insertion without direct posterior tenderness.

The patient is placed in prone position with a thigh tourniquet. Medial and lateral portals as described by van Dijk et al.[12] are made at the superior border of

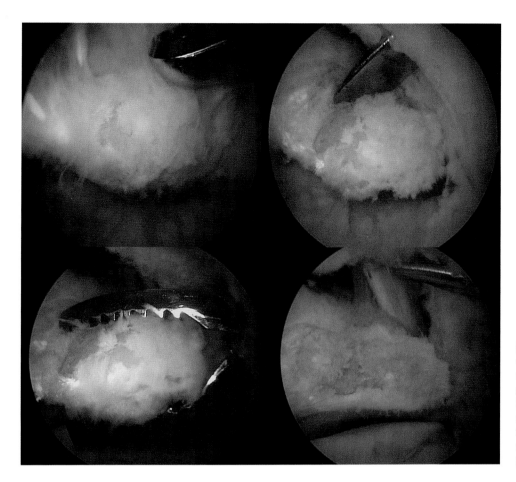

Figure 19–9. Arthroscopic views of a symptomatic os trigonum. Using a shaver, the soft tissue surrounding the os is removed. A Freer elevator is used to release the os from the talus. The bony fragment is then removed through the medial portal.

the calcaneal tuberosity on both sides of the Achilles insertion. A thorough synovectomy and retrocalcaneal bursectomy is performed with a 4-mm shaver and the bony prominence is debrided with a 4-mm barrel burr. All bony prominences especially on the medial and lateral aspects are thoroughly removed. The adequacy of debridement and absence of impingement is evaluated as the ankle is moved into full dorsiflexion. Optionally, the amount of bone excision can be checked with lateral fluoroscopic images. The patient can start full weight bearing and ankle range-of-motion exercise right away. Normal activities may be resumed at 4 to 6 weeks.

This technique has been adopted by Jerosch et al.[13] who report their results in a series of 164 patients. At an average follow-up of 4 years, 155 patients demonstrated good–excellent Ogilvie–Harris score. Three patients with poor results had an ossified area at the Achilles tendon insertion.

Posterior Intraosseous Talar Ganglion

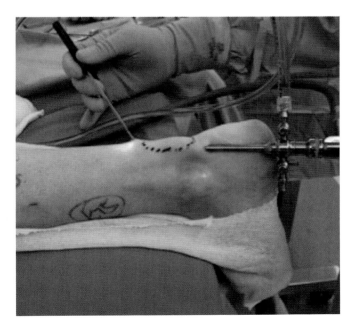

Figure 19–10. Endoscopic treatment in a patient with left Achilles noninsertional tendinopathy.

Although they are rare, posterior intraosseous abnormalities can be reached easily using a posterior arthroscopic

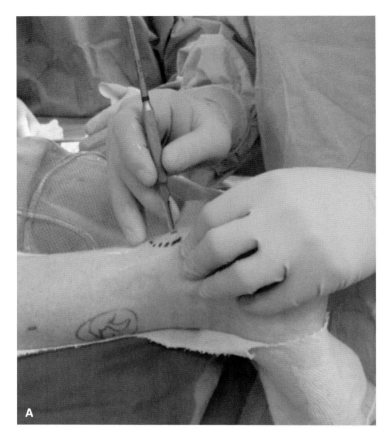
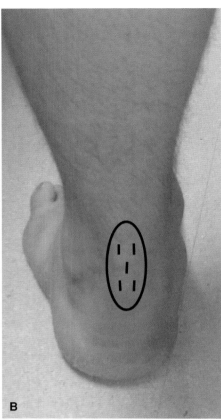

Figure 19–11. **A:** Percutaneous longitudinal tenotomy is performed with a no.11 blade. **B:** The incisions are made in the "5" pattern from a playing card.

approach (Fig. 19–12). The posterior portals are created in the usual fashion and the soft tissues over the posterior tibiotalar and subtalar joints are debrided, exposing the posterior talus (Fig. 19–13). After identification, the intraosseous abnormality is accessed using a curette or arthroscopic shaver (Fig. 19–13). The area is debrided to bleeding bone and if appropriate, packed with bone graft (Fig. 19–13).

If the lesion is felt to be stable, the patient is immobilized postoperatively until the surgical wounds are healed and sutures are removed. Protected weight bearing and range-of-motion exercises are initiated after wound healing. If the bony integrity is felt to be compromised, weight bearing is delayed until healing has adequately progressed.

COMPLICATIONS

Due to the lack of visualization, neurologic injury is the most common complication reported. Recent work by Nickisch et al.[14] reports on 186 consecutive patients who underwent hindfoot endoscopy to treat various pathologies. In this study, there was an overall 8.5% complication rate with neurologic injury being the most common

complication. Four patients were found to have plantar numbness, and three had findings consistent with sural nerve dysesthesia. In these seven patients, five had resolution of the aforementioned neurologic findings. Other reported complications in this series included Achilles contracture (4), chronic regional pain syndrome (2), and superficial infection (2), all of which resolved.[14] Sural nerve neuropraxia was also a complication found in other studies.[7,8]

Several technical recommendations to minimize sural nerve injury can be made. Only the skin should be incised with a scalpel while establishing the posterolateral portal. The incision should be made at the lateral border of the Achilles tendon and blunt dissection of subcutaneous tissue should follow. Minimizing torque on arthroscopic instruments also minimizes the risk of neuropraxia in subcutaneous nerves.

Within the deep tissues, identification of the FHL is paramount to help prevent iatrogenic injury to the adjacent posteromedial neurovascular structures. As it is generally safe to proceed with dissection lateral to FHL, a shaver should be utilized from a lateral to medial direction until the FHL tendon is identified. Lastly, there are anatomic variations reported. Phisitkul and Amendola[15] describe two cases where the so-called, "false FHL," or

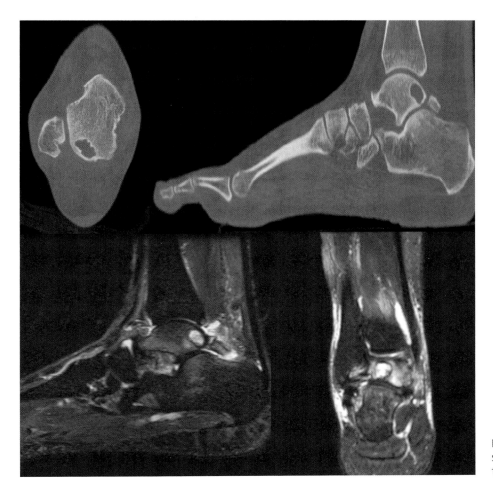

Figure 19–12.   MRI and CT scans showing a symptomatic posterior talar ganglion cyst.

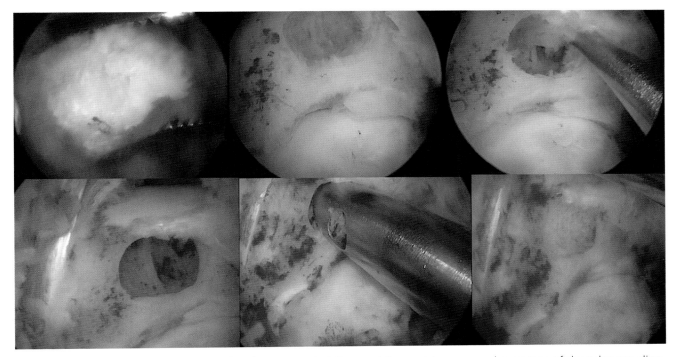

Figure 19–13.   Arthroscopic pictures showing removal of the overlying os trigonum and exposure of the talar ganglion cyst. The cyst was debrided and packed with bone graft.

peroneocalcaneus internus muscle was identified. This muscle may be found directly posterior to FHL and immediately superficial to the tibial neurovascular bundle. Due to the proximity of the peroneocalcaneus internus muscle to the posteromedial neurovascular structures, it is paramount to be aware of this anatomic variant to prevent inadvertent injury to crucial structures. Once a medial tendon structure is identified, flexion and extension of the great toe is very useful to ensure the structure is the FHL tendon. If there is no movement of the tendon with great toe motion, a "false FHL" tendon may be present, and a very careful evaluation anterior to the "false FHL" tendon should be completed until the FHL tendon is identified.

REFERENCES

1. Abramowitz Y, Wollstein R, Barzilay Y, et al. Outcome of resection of a symptomatic os trigonum. *J Bone Joint Surg Am*. 2003;85-A(6):1051–1057.
2. Acevedo JI, Busch MT, Ganey TM, et al. Coaxial portals for posterior ankle arthroscopy: An anatomic study with clinical correlation on 29 patients. *Arthroscopy*. 2000;16(8):836–842.
3. van Dijk CN, Scholten PE, Krips R. A 2-portal endoscopic approach for diagnosis and treatment of posterior ankle pathology. *Arthroscopy*. 2000;16(8):871–876.
4. Beals TC, Junko JT, Amendola A, et al. Minimally invasive distraction technique for prone posterior ankle and subtalar arthroscopy. *Foot Ankle Int*. 2010;31(4):316–369.
5. Sitler DF, Amendola A, Bailey CS, et al. Posterior ankle arthroscopy: An anatomic study. *J Bone Joint Surg Am*. 2002;84-A(5):763–769.
6. Tryfonidis M, Whitfield CG, Charalambous CP, et al. Posterior ankle arthroscopy portal safety regarding proximity to the tibial and sural nerves. *Acta Orthop Belg*. 2008;74(3):370–373.
7. Galla M, Lobenhoffer P. Technique and results of arthroscopic treatment of posterior ankle impingement. *Foot Ankle Surg*. 2011;17(2):79–84.
8. Noguchi H, Ishii Y, Takeda M, et al. Arthroscopic excision of posterior ankle bony impingement for early return to the field: Short-term results. *Foot Ankle Int*. 2010;31(5):398–403.
9. Maffulli N, Binfield PM, Moore D. Surgical decompression of chronic central core lesions of the Achilles tendon. *Am J Sports Med*. 1999;27(6):747–752.
10. Steenstra F, van Dijk CN. Achilles tendoscopy. *Foot Ankle Clin*. 2006;11(2):429–438, viii.
11. Maffulli N, Longo UG, Oliva F, et al. Minimally invasive surgery of the achilles tendon. *Orthop Clin North Am*. 2009;40(4):491–498, viii-ix.
12. van Dijk CN, van Dyk GE, Scholten PE, et al. Endoscopic calcaneoplasty. *Am J Sports Med*. 2001;29(2):185–189.
13. Jerosch J, Sokkar S, Dücker M, et al. [Endoscopic calcaneoplasty (ECP) in Haglund's Syndrome. Indication, surgical technique, surgical findings and results.] *Z Orthop Unfall*. 2012;150(3):250–256.
14. Nickisch F, Barg A, Saltzman CL, et al. Postoperative complications of posterior ankle and hindfoot arthroscopy. *J Bone Joint Surg Am*. 2012;94(5):439–446.
15. Phisitkul P, Amendola A. False FHL: A normal variant posing risks in posterior hindfoot endoscopy. *Arthroscopy*. 2010;26(5):714–718.

Subtalar Joint Arthroscopy and Arthroscopically Assisted Subtalar Arthrodesis

Lijkele Beimers   C. Niek van Dijk

INDICATIONS

Subtalar joint arthroscopy may be applied as a diagnostic and therapeutic tool. Diagnostic subtalar arthroscopy may be used for complaints of persistent pain, swelling, stiffness and locking of the subtalar joint area. Therapeutic indications for subtalar joint arthroscopy include debridement of chondromalacia, removal of impingement, excision of osteophytes, lysis of adhesions with posttraumatic arthrofibrosis, and the removal of loose bodies of the subtalar joint (Table 20–1). Other therapeutic indications are debridement and drilling of osteochondritis dissecans, retrograde drilling of cystic lesions, and removal of a symptomatic os trigonum. Subtalar joint arthrodesis is indicated for the treatment of primary degenerative, inflammatory, and posttraumatic subtalar arthritis. In addition, subtalar arthrodesis can be performed with neuropathic conditions, end stage posterior tibial tendon dysfunction, and symptomatic congenital talocalcaneal coalition.

There is increasing interest in arthroscopically assisted subtalar joint arthrodesis. For arthroscopically assisted subtalar joint arthrodesis it is necessary that no severe deformity of the joint or hindfoot exist. Visualization and instrumentation of the subtalar joint is often very difficult in these cases. With severe bone loss in the hindfoot where bone grafting is necessary, arthroscopically assisted subtalar joint arthrodesis is not considered the treatment of choice. Furthermore, repair of previously failed open subtalar joint fusions should not be done arthroscopically. Contraindications to subtalar arthroscopy include infection of the joint or soft tissues surrounding the joint, severe edema, poor skin quality, and an impaired vascular status.

PATIENT POSITIONING

In 2000, a two-portal posterior approach for hindfoot and subtalar arthroscopy was introduced.[1] The patient is placed in the prone position on the operating table with a tourniquet inflated around the thigh. A triangular pad is placed under the lower leg to provide unconstrained motion of the ankle joint during surgery. The foot must hang slightly over the edge of the operating table to allow dorsiflexion of the ankle joint. A lateral support is placed against the ipsilateral hip to allow tilting of the operating table (Fig. 20–1). Image intensification using a mobile C-arm is mandatory for confirmation of correct placement of the lag screws with arthroscopically assisted subtalar joint arthrodesis.

SURGICAL TECHNIQUE

The procedure is carried out in an outpatient surgery setting under general or spinal anesthesia. The two portals that are used for subtalar joint arthroscopy are the standard posterolateral and posteromedial portals for hindfoot endoscopy.[1] Important anatomical landmarks that should be identified before making the portals are the lateral malleolus, the lateral border of the Achilles tendon at the level of the lateral malleolus, and the medial border of the Achilles tendon. First, the posterolateral portal is created at the level or slightly above the tip of the lateral malleolus, approximately 5 mm lateral to the Achilles tendon (Fig. 20–2A). It is obligatory to have the sole of the foot in the neutral position with respect to the lower leg before incising the skin. After making the longitudinal skin incision laterally, the medial skin incision is made approximately 5 mm medial to the Achilles tendon at the same height as the lateral skin incision (Fig. 20–2B). Starting laterally, a mosquito clamp is used to dissect through the subcutaneous layer. The foot is now in the relaxed (slightly plantar-flexed) position. The mosquito clamp should point anteriorly, in the direction of the web space between the first and second toe (Fig. 20–3A). When the tip of the mosquito clamp touches the bone, it is exchanged for a 4.5-mm arthroscope trocar and obturator combination. By palpating the bone in the sagittal plane with the tip of the blunt trocar, the level of the ankle joint and subtalar joint often can be identified with the prominent posterior talar process between the joints. The trocar remains extra-articular at the level of the ankle joint. The obturator is then exchanged for a 30-degree 4-mm diameter arthroscope. The direction of view is routinely to the lateral side. At this time, the arthroscope is still outside the joint with its tip in the

TABLE 20–1. Indications for Subtalar Joint Arthroscopy

	Good indications	No indications
Subtalar joint pathology	Isolated subtalar joint osteoarthritis, consider an arthroscopically assisted subtalar joint arthrodesis	Previously failed subtalar joint fusion, severe bone loss and hindfoot deformity with malalignment
	Talocalcaneal coalition, consider an arthroscopically assisted subtalar joint arthrodesis	Severe bone loss and hindfoot deformity with malalignment
	Treatment of cystic lesions, intraosseous talar ganglions	
	Loose bodies and osteophytes	
Extra-articular pathology	Os trigonum or hypertrophic processus posterior tali, soft tissue posterior ankle impingement	

fatty tissue overlying the capsule. Subsequently, the posteromedial portal is created just medial to the Achilles tendon. Through the medial skin incision a mosquito clamp is inserted and contacts the arthroscope shaft just anterior to the Achilles tendon (Fig. 20–3B). When the clamp touches the shaft, the shaft is then used as a guide to slide the tip of the mosquito clamp toward the ankle joint. The tip of the mosquito clamp has to stay in contact with the arthroscope trocar all the way down to the ankle joint at which point bony resistance is encountered (Fig. 20–3C). Normal saline is used for irrigation, however, Ringer solution can also be used. The arthroscope is now pulled back a fraction and tilted slightly until the tip of the mosquito clamp comes into view of the arthroscope (Fig. 20–3D). The clamp is used to spread the extra-articular soft tissues in front of the arthroscope. The mosquito clamp is exchanged for a 4.5 mm diameter full-radius shaver through the posteromedial portal. Again, the arthroscope shaft is used to guide the shaver toward the ankle and subtalar joint. The tip of the shaver is directed in a lateral and slightly plantar direction toward the lateral aspect of the subtalar joint. Now the fatty tissue overlying the capsule of the posterior subtalar compartment is debrided using the shaver. The shaver blade should be facing toward the bony surfaces. After removal of the capsule of the subtalar joint, the posterior compartment of the subtalar joint is visualised. The shaver is then retracted and the arthroscope is moved anteriorly through the opening in the crural fascia to visualize the posterolateral aspect of the subtalar joint (Fig. 20–4A–E). Once the subtalar joint is identified, the opening in the deep crural fascia is enlarged to increase the working area in the hindfoot. At the level of the ankle joint, the posterior tibiofibular and posterior talofibular ligaments are recognized. The posterior talar process can be freed from the soft tissue using the full-radius shaver. This is followed by identification of the flexor hallucis longus (FHL) tendon medially. The FHL tendon is an important anatomic landmark in hindfoot endoscopy as the posteromedial neurovascular bundle is located medially from the FHL tendon. Therefore, the FHL tendon is always located first, before addressing any ankle or subtalar pathology. After removal of the thin joint capsule of the ankle joint, the intermalleolar and inferior transverse ligament can be lifted up to enter and inspect the ankle joint. In most cases, it is not possible to introduce the 4-mm arthroscope into the posterior subtalar joint. However, the posterior subtalar joint can be adequately visualized from its margins without entering the joint. Intra-articular pathology can be treated under direct view looking from outside-in using small arthroscopic instruments. Distraction of the subtalar joint can be accomplished during surgery using the noninvasive ankle distractor or through manual traction by the assistant. Because of potential complications (i.e., infection, nerve injury, and fractures of the talus/calcaneus) the use of the invasive joint distraction techniques is not recommended.

ARTHROSCOPICALLY ASSISTED SUBTALAR JOINT ARTHRODESIS

Arthroscopic subtalar joint arthrodesis was intended to yield less morbidity, preserve the blood supply, and

Figure 20–1. Patient positioning for subtalar joint arthroscopy and arthroscopically assisted arthrodesis. The patient is in the prone position. A tourniquet is applied around the thigh. The ankle is placed just distal from the end of the operating table to allow ankle joint motion during surgery. A small triangular cushion supports the lower leg. A lateral hip support allows safe tilting of the patient to the ipsilateral side if required.

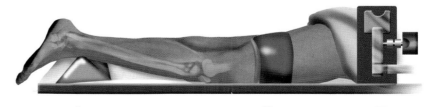

I   II   III

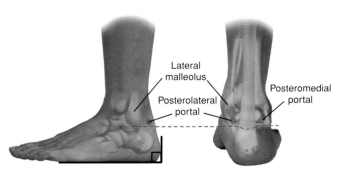

Figure 20–2. Lateral (**A**) and medial (**B**) views of the ankle and hindfoot illustrating portal placement for subtalar joint arthroscopy with the patient in the prone position. Important anatomical landmarks are the foot sole, the Achilles tendon, and the tip of the lateral malleolus. With the foot in the neutral position (foot sole 90 degrees with respect to the lower leg), a line is drawn from the tip of the lateral malleolus to the Achilles tendon parallel to the sole of the foot. This line is extended over the Achilles tendon to the medial side. The posterolateral portal is located proximal to and 5 mm anterior to the intersection of both lines. The posteromedial portal is located at the same height as the posterolateral portal, also 5 mm anterior from the medial border of the Achilles tendon.

preserve proprioception and neurosensory input.[2] In arthroscopically assisted subtalar joint arthrodesis, the posterior subtalar joint is fused using the posterior two-portal hindfoot endoscopy technique with the patient in the prone position. The two standard posterior portals for hindfoot endoscopy are created in the same manner as described above. After local capsulotomy, the posterior subtalar joint is identified. This is followed by identification of the FHL tendon medially. Next release of the flexor retinaculum from the posterior talar process is performed using the arthroscopic punch to establish better access to the posterior subtalar joint. Via the posterior portals, the articular cartilage is removed from the posterior subtalar joint using ring curettes. To open up the posterior subtalar joint and create an increased working space, a blunt trocar is introduced in the subtalar joint through an accessory anterolateral sinus tarsi portal (Fig. 20–5). A small skin incision is made at the level of the sinus tarsi. A spinal needle is introduced and directed toward the tip of the lateral malleolus. The arthroscope is used to check the position of the needle. A large blunt trocar (4.0 mm diameter) is inserted through the sinus tarsi portal and is maneuvered toward the posterior facet of the subtalar joint (Fig. 20–6). The blunt trocar is put in the posterior subtalar joint from a lateral position. As the blunt trocar is almost parallel to the posterior subtalar joint, the sideward movement prevents the trocar of gouging the subchondral bone. With the assistant holding the blunt trocar in place, all the cartilage is removed from the posterior facet of the subtalar joint using ring curettes. The portals can be switched if necessary. After

complete removal of the articular cartilage, the subchondral bone is entered to expose the vascular cancellous bone. The subchondral bone plate is partially removed with a burr. Using a small chisel, multiple 2-mm deep longitudinal grooves are made in the subchondral cancellous bone of the talus and calcaneus. A vertical skin incision is made at posterior heel for introduction of two cannulated lag screws off the weight-bearing surface of the calcaneus. Using the C-arm image intensifier 6.5-mm lag screws are placed across the posterior subtalar joint (Fig. 20–7A–D). The length of the two screws can be estimated using the preoperative weight-bearing lateral radiographs of the ankle. Before drilling, it is important to check the correct alignment of the hindfoot (approximately 5 degrees of valgus). The assessment of correct hindfoot alignment by eyeballing is facilitated by having the patient in the prone position. Biomechanical and finite element analysis of screw position in subtalar joint arthrodesis showed that a double diverging screw configuration confers the highest compression, the greatest torsional stiffness, and the least joint rotation.[3,4] The position of the lag screws is also important; one screw in the talar neck and the other screw in the medial dome of the talus is optimal. Countersinking the screw heads in the dorsal cortex of the calcaneus prevents posterior screw head prominence. Coaptation of the posterior subtalar surfaces can be checked arthroscopically when tightening both the screws. No bone grafting is used. The skin is closed using 3-0 nonresorbable Ethilon sutures. A plaster cast is applied to the lower leg.

PORTAL SAFETY

Investigators studied the safety of posterior portals for hindfoot endoscopy in anatomic specimens. The posterolateral portal presents the lowest risk of neurovascular injury in the hindfoot. According to Feiwell and Frey, the sural nerve is located at a mean distance of 6 mm (0 to 12 mm) and the small saphenous vein at 9.5 mm (2 to 18 mm) from the posterolateral portal.[5] Sitler found a mean distance of 3.2 mm (0 to 8.9 mm) and 4.8 mm (0 to 11.0 mm) for the sural nerve and small saphenous vein respectively.[6] The tibial nerve, the posterior tibial artery, and the medial calcaneal nerve are in close proximity to the posteromedial portal (Table 20–2). Based on the anatomic studies it appears that the posterior portals for hindfoot and subtalar arthroscopy are relatively safe with little risk of injuring the posterior neurovascular structures. It should be kept in mind that the distances measured between the neurovascular structures and the posterior portals have a direct relationship with the height of the portal placement. Lijo et al.[7] found that a posteromedial portal that was placed 1 cm more proximal was on average 2.9 mm closer in proximity to the medial neurovascular bundle. Using MRI imaging in healthy volunteers, Urgüden et al.[8] confirmed that neurovascular structures recede away from the posterior portals of hindfoot arthroscopy distally.

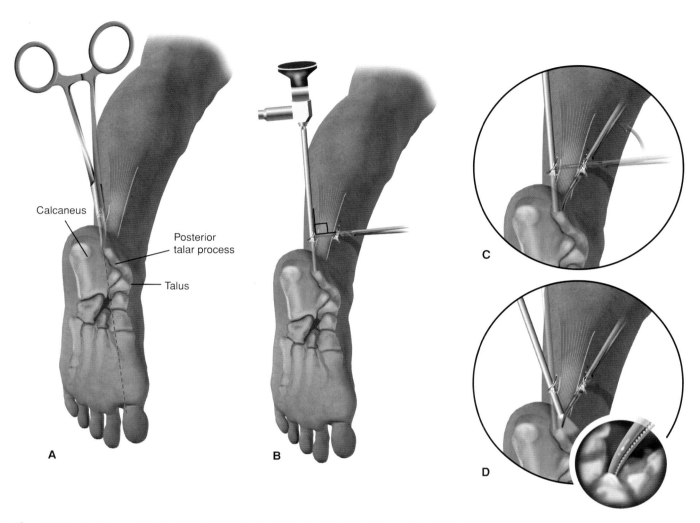

Figure 20–3. **A:** Introduction of mosquito clamp in the direction of the first web space. **B:** Arthroscope laterally and introduction of mosquito clamp medially. **C:** Arthroscope used as a guide for the mosquito clamp. **D:** Tilting the arthroscope laterally to visualize the tip of the mosquito clamp and the shaver.

Figure 20–4. Crural fascia penetration and visualization of the posterolateral subtalar joint. (**A**) Identification of proper starting point for tissue clearance. (**B**) Retraction of the arthroscope to allow arthroscopic shaving to commence. (**C**) Clearance of the posterior crural fascia with the arthroscopic shaver. (**D**) Retraction of the shaver to allow (**E**) arthroscopic investigation of the posterolateral subtalar joint.

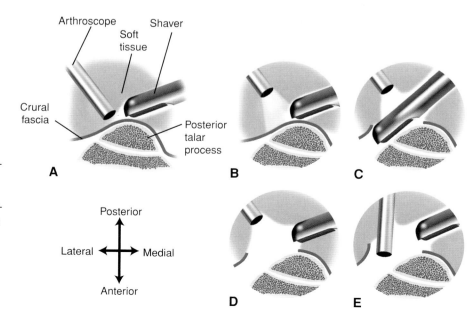

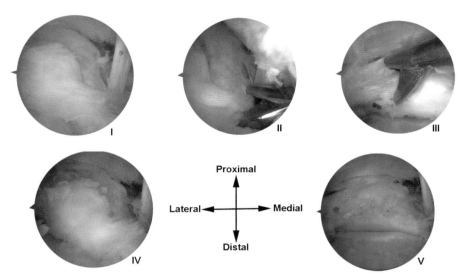

Figure 20–5. Extra-articular views of a left ankle, illustrating some surgical steps for an endoscopic removal of a painful os trigonum. The arthroscope is introduced through the posterolateral portal and the shaver through the posteromedial portal. (**I**) After removal of the Rouviere ligament and the crural fascia, the ankle and subtalar joints, the os trigonum, and the flexor hallucis longus tendon can be identified. The ligaments that attach to the os trigonum on the dorsomedial side that are shown in this view are the flexor retinaculum and the posterior talocalcaneal ligament. (**II**) The attachment of the flexor retinaculum on the medial side of the os trigonum is released using an arthroscopic end biter. (**III**) The posterior talofibular ligament attachment to the lateral side of the os trigonum should also be partially released for removal of the os trigonum. (**IV**) Release of the posterior talocalcaneal ligament attachment to the os trigonum over the dorsal aspect of the os is completed. The os can then be removed with an arthroscopic grasper or morselized using an arthroscopic shaver. (**V**) Endoscopic hindfoot view after removal of the os trigonum.

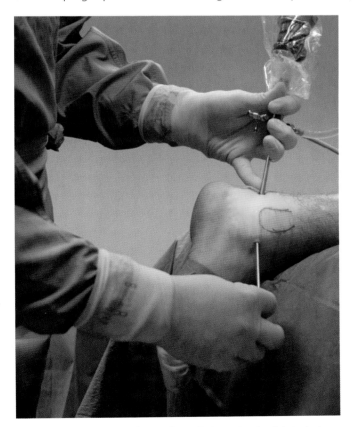

Figure 20–6. For distraction of the subtalar joint during arthroscopically assisted subtalar arthrodesis, a blunt trocar is positioned in the accessory sinus tarsi portal.

COMPLICATIONS

Severe intraoperative complications using the posterior two-portal hindfoot endoscopy technique, such as iatrogenic damage of the neurovascular structures are rare and have not been observed by the authors. In addition, there are few reports with serious complications following hindfoot or subtalar arthroscopy and this fact underlines the safety of the posterior two-portal technique as described.[11–14] In Galla's series of 30 patients treated with hindfoot endoscopy for posterior ankle impingement, one superficial and one deep wound infection occurred.[15] The deep infection at the lateral portal can be considered a serious complication as it was treated by repetitive surgical debridement. Although very satisfying results were achieved with the arthroscopic treatment, Galla reported that two of the 30 patients (6.6%) complained about impaired sensitivity of the sural nerve. Van Dijk also reported on the possibility of an area of hypoesthesia of the heel pad with the use of the hindfoot endoscopy technique in his patient series (<2%).[11] Pitfalls during arthroscopically assisted subtalar joint arthrodesis include difficulties with removing all the cartilage from the posterior subtalar joint. A reason can be that it is difficult to obtain sufficient subtalar joint distraction with associated limitation of the working space. The solution for this is the use of the blunt trocar positioned in to the subtalar joint. The use of an invasive ankle distractor is not recommended because it is complicated and has the risk of fracturing the tibia or

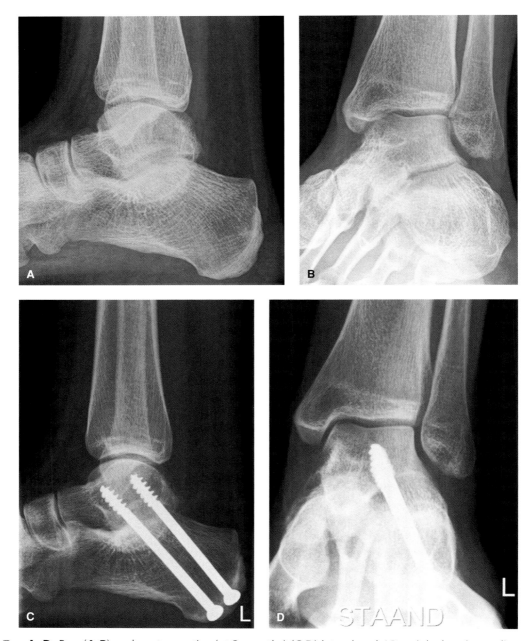

Figure 20–7. **A–D:** Pre- (**A,B**) and postoperative (at 3 months) (**C,D**) lateral and AP weight-bearing radiographs of a patient with a symptomatic talocalcaneal coalition treated with an arthroscopically assisted subtalar arthrodesis.

TABLE 20–2. Posteromedial Portal Safety in Posterior Subtalar Joint Arthroscopy

Reference	Tibial nerve	Posterior tibial artery	Medial calcaneal nerve
Mouilhade et al.[9]	Average distance was 6.8 mm (95% CI: 4.4 to 9.2 mm)		
Urgüden et al.[8]	13.3 ± 4.6 mm		
Lijoi et al.[7]	13.3 (11–17)	17.3 (15–21)	14.7 (8–20)
Sitler et al.[6]	6.4 (0–16.2)	9.6 (2.4–20.1)	17.1 (19–31)
Mekhail et al.[10]	Tibial neurovascular bundle: 10 mm (at least 8 mm)		
Feiwell and Frey[5]	7.5 (0–13)	12.6 (3–20)	2.5 (0–6)

TABLE 20–3. Problems and Complications		
Problem/Complication	Frequency	How to prevent—what's to do?
Temporary hypoesthesia heel pad/scar numbness	<2%[11]	Use the standard safe technique for making the posterolateral and posteromedial portals
Deep or superficial wound infection	Estimated <1%	Routine prophylactic antibiotics are only given when using hardware (screws in subtalar fusion), if necessary surgical debridement should be carried out with deep wound infection
Complex regional pain syndrome (type 1)	Unknown	CRPS treatment protocol
Nonunion of subtalar joint arthrodesis	None	In case of an earlier arthroscopically assisted subtalar joint arthrodesis, a second attempt can be done with patient informed consent. Bone grafting can be performed through the portals

calcaneus. In the case of difficulties with entering the subtalar joint due to a hypertrophic posterior talar process, the surgeon may reduce the process by using a small chisel. Malpositioning of the screws can result in the need for a reoperation. Postoperative problems include nonunion of the subtalar arthrodesis and screw head irritation (Table 20–3). The screws are not routinely taken out after bony consolidation of the subtalar joint arthrodesis. However, in the case of screw head irritation they can be removed.

REHABILITATION PROTOCOL

After completing the subtalar joint arthroscopy, the portals are closed with 3-0 nonabsorbable sutures. A compression dressing is applied from the toes to the midcalf. This dressing is removed the following day and the patient is encouraged to start range of motion exercises of the ankle and foot. The leg should be elevated for 2 to 3 days following surgery. The patient is allowed to ambulate with the use of crutches. Weight bearing is permitted as tolerated by the patient. The sutures are removed approximately 10 days after the procedure. When the joint swelling has completely resolved, the patient can be referred to a physical therapist for exercises and rehabilitation. Normally, the patient should be able to return to full activities at 8 to 12 weeks postoperatively.

In the case of an arthroscopically assisted subtalar joint arthrodesis, a nonweight bearing lower leg cast is provided for 4 to 6 weeks. At 6 weeks following surgery, AP and lateral weight bearing ankle radiographs are made. With radiographic signs of union of the subtalar arthrodesis, the patient is allowed full weight bearing in a walker boot for another 4 weeks. Postoperative radiographs should also routinely be taken at 3 months and 6 months.

OUTCOME

Three reports are available in the literature on arthroscopically assisted posterior subtalar joint arthrodesis using either a two- or three-portal technique with the patient in the prone position.[16–18] The largest series of patients was reported by Lee; out of 16 patients nonunion occurred in one case because of deep infection.[17] Infection was controlled after screw removal and curettage of the screw holes and fusion was successfully achieved. In the series of Albert et al. a total of 10 arthroscopically assisted subtalar arthrodesis were performed successfully.[18] Mean average AOFAS scores improved from 47 to 78 postoperatively.[16] No complications were noted related to the technique. With the posterior two-portal ankle and subtalar joint arthroscopy procedure with the patient in the prone position, a safe and time-efficient treatment modality has become available to treat subtalar pathology with proven excellent clinical results. It should be mentioned that subtalar arthroscopy is an advanced endoscopic procedure. Surgeons not familiar with endoscopic surgery are advised to practice on cadaveric material before treating patients.

REFERENCES

1. Van Dijk CN, Scholten PE, Krips R. A 2-portal endoscopic approach for diagnosis and treatment of posterior ankle pathology. *Arthroscopy.* 2000;16(8):871–876.
2. Tasto JP. Arthroscopic subtalar arthrodesis. *Techniques in Foot and Ankle Surgery.* 2003;2(2):122–128.
3. Chuckpaiwong B, Easley ME, Glisson RR. Screw placement in subtalar arthrodesis: A biomechanical study. *Foot Ankle Int.* 2009;30(2):133–141.
4. Lee JY, Lee YS. Optimal double screw configuration for subtalar arthrodesis: A finite element analysis. *Knee Surg Sports Traumatol Arthrosc.* 2011;19(5):842–849.
5. Feiwell LA, Frey C. Anatomic study of arthroscopic portal sites of the ankle. *Foot Ankle.* 1993;14(3):142–147.
6. Sitler DF, Amendola A, Bailey CS, et al. Posterior ankle arthroscopy: An anatomic study. *J Bone Joint Surg Am.* 2002;84-A(5): 763–769.
7. Lijoi F, Lughi M, Baccarani G. Posterior arthroscopic approach to the ankle: An anatomic study. *Arthroscopy.* 2003;19(1): 62–67.
8. Urgüden M, Cevikol C, Dabak TK, et al. Effect of joint motion on safety of portals in posterior ankle arthroscopy. *Arthroscopy.* 2009;(12):1442–1446.

9. Mouilhade F, Oger P, Roussignol X, et al. Risks relating to posterior 2-portal arthroscopic subtalar arthrodesis and articular surfaces abrasion quality achievable with these approaches: A cadaver study. *Orthop Traumatol Surg Res.* 2011;97(4):396–400.

10. Mekhail AO, Heck BE, Ebraheim NA, et al. Arthroscopy of the subtalar joint: Establishing a medial portal. *Foot Ankle Int.* 1995;16(7):427–32.

11. Van Dijk CN. Hindfoot endoscopy. *Foot Ankle Clin.* 2006; 11(2):391–414, vii.

12. Jerosch J, Fadel M. Endoscopic resection of a symptomatic os trigonum. *Knee Surg Sports Traumatol Arthrosc.* 2006;14(11):1188–1193.

13. Scholten PE, Sierevelt IN, Van Dijk CN. Hindfoot endoscopy for posterior ankle impingement. *J Bone Joint Surg Am.* 2008;90-A(12):2665–2672.

14. Willits K, Sonneveld H, Amendola A, et al. Outcome of posterior ankle arthroscopy for hindfoot impingement. *Arthroscopy.* 2008;24(2):196–202.

15. Galla M, Lobenhoffer P. Technique and results of arthroscopic treatment of posterior ankle impingement. *Foot Ankle Surg.* 2011;17(2):79–84.

16. Beimers L, de Leeuw PA, van Dijk CN. A 3-portal approach for arthroscopic subtalar arthrodesis. *Knee Surg Sports Traumatol Arthrosc.* 2009;17(7):830–834.

17. Lee KB, Park CH, Seon JK, et al. Arthroscopic subtalar arthrodesis using a posterior 2-portal approach in the prone position. *Arthroscopy.* 2010;26(2):230–8.

18. Albert A, Deleu PA, Leemrijse T, et al. Posterior arthroscopic subtalar arthrodesis: Ten cases at one-year follow-up. *Orthop Traumatol Surg Res.* 2011;97(4):401–405.

CHAPTER 21

Arthroscopy of the Hallux MTP Joint

C. Christopher Stroud

INDICATIONS

Arthroscopy of the first MTP joint is a useful component within the Foot and Ankle Surgeon's armamentarium[1-13] First described by Watanabe in 1972,[1] this procedure has been infrequently described in the literature. Published outcomes comparing open versus the arthroscopic technique are almost nonexistent. However, the procedure offers the benefits of minimally invasive surgery noted in other joints, that is, less postoperative pain, scarring and swelling, all of which enable the patient to recover more quickly from the procedure and rehabilitate the injured joint. Although the joint is small and the range of indications for the procedure are somewhat limited, the technique is beneficial in certain situations.

Indications for first MTP arthroscopy include loose body removal; debridement procedures for synovitis, gouty arthritis, or PVNS; debridement or microfracture of osteochondral lesions; intra-articular fracture reduction; cheilectomy for hallux rigidus; and capsular releases for arthrofibrosis.[2,3] The procedure has also been reported for use in arthrodesis of the first MTP joint.[4,5] The technique does have a learning curve. However, when utilized appropriately, the patient benefits from the more limited surgical approach.

PATIENT POSITIONING

The patient is positioned supine on a standard operating room table. The patient's foot and ankle are anesthetized with a local or regional block supplemented with general anesthesia if desired. Traction is not normally utilized but can be helpful if joint entry is difficult. Noninvasive traction can be accomplished with the use of sterile finger traps (Fig. 21–1). The traps can be suspended from a pulley system with or without weight attached. Alternatively, an assistant can provide the necessary joint distraction to enter the joint. Invasive traction can involve the use of a mini external fixation device with one pin in the proximal metatarsal and the other pin in the distal aspect of the proximal phalanx, however, manipulation of the joint will then be made more difficult. A supramalleolar pneumatic or Esmarch tourniquet is used to aid in hemostasis. In the former case, it is generally inflated to 250 mm Hg (or 100 mm Hg above the systolic blood pressure). Instruments required during the procedure include a small joint arthroscope (2.7 mm, 30 and 70 degree), syringe with saline, small joint shaver (2.7 mm), probe, an array of small joint basket forceps, graspers and scissors, and angled ringed curettes (Fig. 21–2).

SURGICAL APPROACHES

In general, two arthroscopic portals are utilized, the dorsomedial and the dorsolateral portals. These portals lie on either side of the extensor tendon apparatus at the level of the joint line (Fig. 21–3). An accessory third portal has been described[6] and is located directly medially. Because most individuals have a slight physiologic valgus at the MTPJ, the dorsomedial portal is established first, as this side of the joint is relatively wider. Initially, the first metatarsophalangeal joint is insufflated with approximately 5 cc of saline. Then, a scalpel is used to incise the skin. Knowledge of the anatomy of the dorsocutaneous sensory nerve branch is requisite. This nerve lies over the dorsomedial aspect of the first metatarsal head just above the midline medially (Fig. 21–3). A mosquito clamp is used to spread down to the capsule. A blunt obturator is used to perforate the joint capsule and to enter the joint itself. The 30-degree, 2.7-mm arthroscope is then inserted. Inflow and is provided at a pressure of approximately 20 mm Hg. A 22G needle can be used to provisionally establish the lateral portal (Fig. 21–4). Outflow is also accomplished through the camera via a rotating bridge setup. A small joint (2.7 mm or smaller) shaver is introduced to clear debris and to aid in joint visualization (Fig. 21–5). The portals are used interchangeably throughout the procedure and it is not uncommon to repeatedly switch sides to accomplish the desired view.

REDUCTION/OPERATIVE TECHNIQUES

Joint inspection: The inspection begins with an examination of the joint. Similar to the ankle examination, a serial point examination of the joint should first be accomplished.[7] First evaluate the medial gutter and capsular attachment while inspecting for hypertrophic synovium or loose bodies. Thereafter, move the camera lens to inspect the superomedial aspect of the metatarsal head followed by the central and dorsal articular surface followed by the superolateral aspect of the metatarsal head. Evaluate and note the presence of osteophytes about the dorsal aspect of the metatarsal head as well as their size and extent. Inspect the lateral gutter and capsular attachment. Move back medially and repeat the examination of the articular surface of the proximal phalanx, moving

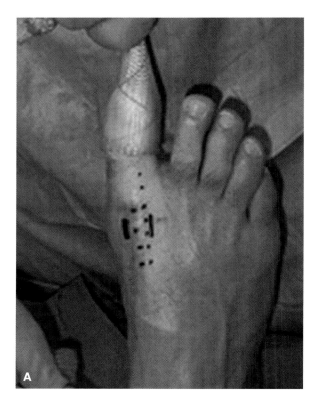
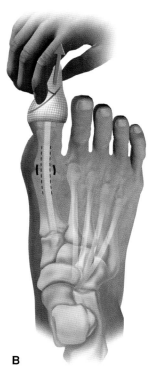

Figure 21–1. **(A)** Photograph and **(B)** illustration showing noninvasive traction accomplished with the use of sterile finger traps. The location of dorsomedial and dorsolateral portals are indicated by lines over the joint line. The location of the EHL tendon is indicated by the area between the dashed lines.

superiorly and laterally with the camera to view the central and lateral aspect. Osteophytes, cartilage loss, and loose bodies are addressed.

The portals can then be switched to examine the joint from the lateral side if inadequate visualization is realized, again noting abnormalities previously mentioned. Introducing the camera through the direct medial portal is helpful to evaluate the plantar aspect of the joint in this

sequence: the proximal plantar capsule as it attaches to the metatarsal head and sesamoids; the sesamoids themselves; the central/plantar aspect of the metatarsal head; the sesamoid-phalangeal ligaments and flexor hallucis brevis attachments to the proximal phalanx.

In general, visualization of the plantar aspect of the joint can be improved with slight plantarflexion of the joint by an assistant, while inspection of the dorsal aspect of the joint is aided with the use of slight dorsiflexion of the joint.

Loose body removal: Loose fragments of cartilage and/or bone are best removed with the use of small joint graspers and shavers or a mosquito clamp (Fig. 21–6).

Cartilage loss/chondroplasty/microfracture: Slight flexion of the great toe coupled with traction performed by an assistant can aid in addressing cartilage defects (Fig. 21–7). The area can be debrided with the use of small joint basket forceps or scissors. Small, angled, ringed curettes are useful to create a stable cartilage rim. A small joint awl or 0.45 K-wire is used to make perforations into the subchondral bone, spaced 1 to 2 mm apart to stimulate marrow infiltration.

Cheilectomy[13]: Once the joint has been debrided of loose material and visualization has been optimized, a small freer elevator can be used to define the amount of overriding osteophytes. A small 3.0-mm round or oval burr is then inserted. With the camera in the dorsomedial portal, begin the bone resection 3 mm from the superior aspect of the joint, progressing lateral to medial. Pause intermittently to clear the joint of bone debris that can

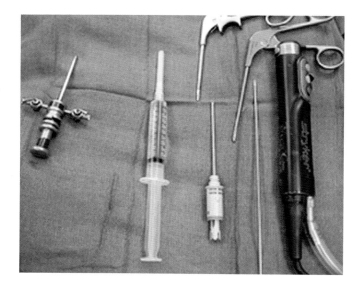

Figure 21–2. An array of small joint instruments will be useful during the procedure.

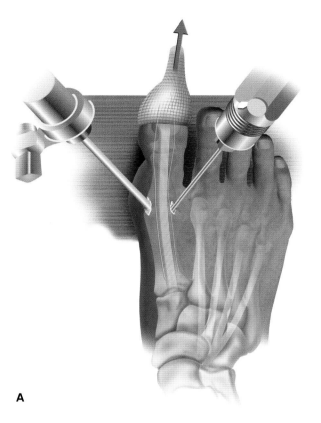

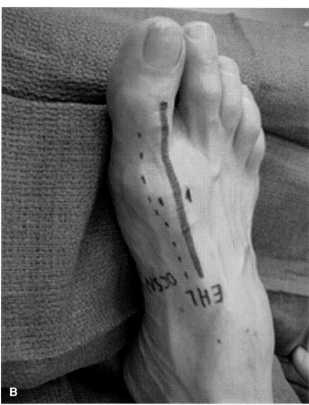

Figure 21–3. **(A)** Illustration and **(B)** Photograph outlining the two dorsal portals. The dorsocutaneous sensory nerve branch and EHL tendon are indicated in photograph by the dashed line and the long solid line, respectively. The location of the arthroscopy portals are shown by the short solid lines.

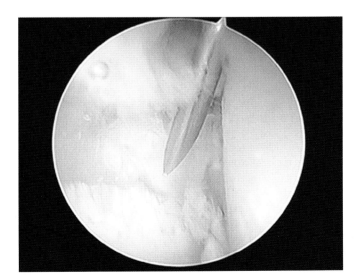

Figure 21–4. Arthroscopic photograph demonstrating localization of the lateral portal with a 22G needle being inserted form the dorsum of the joint. The metatarsal head is to the left in this image. Direction of the needle and thus portal placement can also be used to note the best angle to address osteochondral lesions if present.

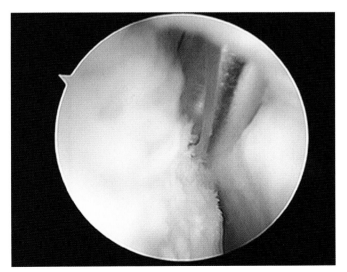

Figure 21–5. Arthroscopic photograph showing debridement of hypertrophic synovium at the dorsal aspect of the joint. The proximal phalanx is located at the right of the image while the metatarsal head is at the left. The arthroscopic shaver is coming in from the dorsum of the joint.

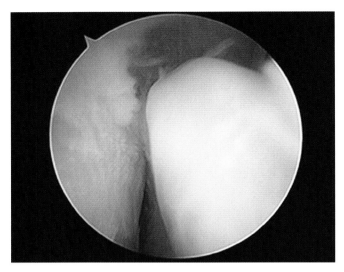

Figure 21–6. Arthroscopic photograph noting the presence of a loose body in a patient with unexplained pain at the MTP joint. Preoperative radiographs were unable to appreciate this abnormality and it was identified and addressed at arthroscopy.

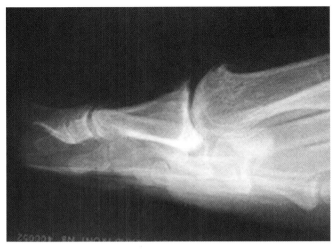

Figure 21–8. Radiograph showing the extent of dorsal spurring of the metatarsal head which will need to be addressed at the time of arthroscopy.

obscure visualization. At this point that the surgeon must be patient, as this portion of the procedure often requires more time than a standard open approach. Remember to slope the amount of resection more inferior distally in order to decompress the joint and remove the mechanical "block" to great toe dorsiflexion. Up to one-third of dorsal joint surfaces can be safely removed to complete the procedure (Fig. 21–8). The camera and instrument portals may be switched to allow bone resection along the entire perimeter of the dorsal joint surface. Repeat the procedure addressing the proximal phalangeal side of the joint. A small beaver blade or hooked electrocautery unit may be used to address medial and/or lateral capsular contracture. The blade can be introduced under direct arthroscopic visualization, and used to incise the capsule. With the camera in the superomedial portal, the small beaver blade is directed to the plantarmedial joint capsule. A 70-degree 2.7-mm joint scope can be used to visualize this acute angle. The incision is carried from plantar to dorsal until the blade cannot be seen. The portals are switched to repeat the capsular incision from the opposite side. Alternatively, a hooked electrocautery unit can be used. Care should be taken to note the position of the extensor hallucis longus tendon dorsally and neurovascular bundle laterally so as to not injure these structures. The instruments are then removed and range of motion measured. It is unusual to obtain the full motion that occurs with an open procedure, but at least 45 degrees of hallux dorsiflexion and plantarflexion should be accomplished at the completion of the procedure. Intraoperative fluoroscopy can be used to judge the amount of bony resection.

Arthrofibrosis: This condition can be encountered in a number of different situations. It may be seen following a cheilectomy in which the motion obtained intraoperatively has not been regained in the postoperative period. It also

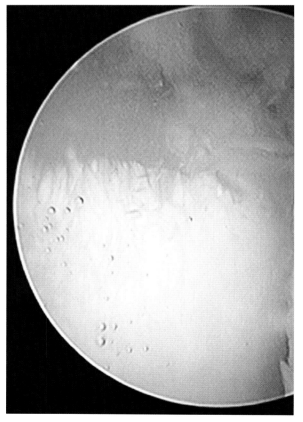

Figure 21–7. Arthroscopic photograph noting the presence of an osteochondral lesion on the metatarsal head. The edges of the lesion will need to be debrided with a ringed curette to create a stable lesion.

may be seen following nonsurgical treatment for a turf toe or other injury to the metatarsophalangeal ligament complex. Addressing contracture of this joint has not been well reported but the arthroscopic approach seems reasonable, as it is used to address contractures in other joints such as adhesive capsulitis of the shoulder or postoperative knee flexion contracture following various procedures on this joint.[9] Once the diagnostic examination has been performed, a hooked electrocautery unit is inserted into the joint from either portal. At low frequency, the device is used to release the capsular contracture at the level of the joint and is done in small layers using smooth hand motions. At the completion of the procedure, the joint is manipulated to ensure adequate range of motion.

Arthrodesis: Using the previously mentioned arthroscopic portals including the accessory medial portal, it has been reported that 94% to 97% of the articular surface on both sides of the joint can be denuded.[6] Additionally, the use of a central plantar portal can be used to completely denude the plantar aspect of the joint,[8] although the flexor hallucis longus tendon is at risk. Again, using a combination of the burr and shaver, the articular cartilage is removed and subchondral bone perforated. Once the joint has been adequately prepared, the instruments are removed and the position of arthrodesis is inspected. Mini C-arm fluoroscopy is used at this point to ensure proper position of the joint and adequate bony apposition. Two 4.0 partially threaded cancellous screws are then placed percutaneously.[12] This procedure frequently requires 50% more time than the traditional open approach with significant surgeon patience required.

Summary of results: Most studies published to date have noted significant improvement in preoperative symptoms. Good to excellent results have been noted in 64% to 95% of patients at 2 to 24 months follow-up.[2,7,10,11,13] Best results have been noted in mild–moderate hallux rigidus, debridement/microfracture procedures, and arthrodesis. Significant joint disease treated with an arthroscopic debridement procedures have resulted in substantially suboptimal outcomes. Arthrodesis is favored in this patient population.

COMPLICATIONS

Complications are few and include wound healing problems, sensory nerve injury, tendon injury, iatrogenic cartilage damage, inadequate bony resection, or capsular releases resulting in postoperative pain and stiffness.

Wound healing issues: The soft tissue around the joint is thin and pliable. Significant swelling can occur with the procedure. Care should be taken to inspect the skin during the procedure to note potential healing problems. Care should be taken to ensure the pump flow rate is not too high during the procedure to avoid fluid extravasation and resultant soft tissue edema. Torquing of instruments in the small portals should be minimized to avoid unnecessary trauma to the instruments,

skin, and subcutaneous tissues. Procedure time should be carefully monitored and the arthroscopic procedure aborted and converted to an open procedure if needed. Skin closure should be performed with Nylon suture as commonly used absorbable sutures may not be able to resist the swelling and bleeding that may occur postoperatively. The tourniquet should be deflated prior to closure to ensure hemostasis. While postoperative antibiotics are not routinely used, they may be considered given the nature of the area and the general risk of contamination noted in foot procedures.

Nerve injury: The medial dorsocutaneous nerve, which is the terminal branch of the superficial peroneal nerve, is at risk with the dorsomedial portal and effort must be made to avoid injury to this structure. Injury to the superficial dorsolateral sensory nerve branch is also at risk with the superolateral portal. The dorsocutaneous sensory nerve branch and the dorsolateral sensory nerve branch lie an average of 3.4 and 4.0 mm away from these portals, respectively. In general these portals can be created safely if careful attention is paid to this anatomy.[6] The deep peroneal nerve lies within the first interdigital space. Injury to this structure can result in neuropathy.

Iatrogenic cartilage damage: The procedure is technically challenging and time-consuming. Slow, gentle movements with the camera and camera lens and careful placement of the scope when introduced into the joint will aid in a reduction of this complication. A reasonable assessment of the surgeons' arthroscopic skills is required to perform the procedure well.

Tendon injury: Knowledge of the course of the extensor hallucis longus and brevis tendon is essential to avoid injury to these structures.

Postoperative stiffness: An inadequate bony resection will result in failure to improve motion postoperatively. Defining landmarks and estimating the amount of hypertrophic bone to be removed before and during the procedure is helpful to avoid this complication.

REHABILITATION PROTOCOL

The patient's foot is sterilely dressed with a compressive wrap and the patient remains nonweight bearing until the first postoperative visit at 7 to 10 days. At that time, if the wounds are well healed and the swelling has diminished, progressive weight bearing as tolerated is allowed.

If an arthrodesis has been performed, the patient can be advanced to heel or lateral border of the foot weight bearing for the remainder of the first 6 weeks. Range of motion of the ankle, subtalar joint, and particularly the first MTP joint begins at that time. Once soft tissue and/or bony healing is complete, the patient begins heating the foot with a warm water bath or shower, immediately followed by patient administered, aggressive active range of motion and active-assisted range-of-motion exercises.

For debridement procedures and cheilectomy, the patient is instructed to manually manipulate the great toe emphasizing dorsiflexion, as this typically is the most difficult motion to regain. At the completion of at least three sets of 10 range-of-motion exercises, the patient is instructed to ice the toe for 10 minutes. Progressive weight bearing as tolerated exercises are continued until the patient can ambulate without the use of assisted devices. For arthrodesis procedures, full weight bearing will begin once bony consolidation on radiographs is noted. In cheilectomy and debridement procedures, full range of motion is expected by 6 weeks postoperatively. Soft tissue edema and residual swelling may take approximately 12 weeks for resolution. A formal course of physical therapy is typically not needed, however, if the patient demonstrates residual contracture or is experiencing significant postoperative pain, this can be prescribed.

OUTCOME

The arthroscopic procedure typically results in less pain and swelling than the standard open procedure. Narcotic requirements are less and the patients generally feel that they can regain motion quicker with this approach. There is a paucity of literature to evaluate this technique however and detailed outcome studies are lacking.

REFERENCES

1. Watanabe M. *Selfox-arthroscope (Watanabe No. 24 arthroscope) (monograph)*. Tokyo, Teishin Hospital; 1972: 46–53.
2. Debnath UK, Hemmady MV, Hariharan K. Indications for and technique of first metatarsophalangeal joint arthroscopy. *Foot Ankle Int.* 2006;27(12):1049–1054.
3. Bartlett DH. Arthroscopic management of osteochondritis dissecans of the first metatarsal head. *Arthroscopy.* 1988;4:51–54.
4. Stroud CC. Arthroscopic arthrodesis of the ankle, subtalar and first metatarsophalangeal joint. *Foot Ankle Clin.* 2002;7:135–146.
5. Carro LP, Vallina BB. Arthroscopic-assisted first metatarsophalangeal joint arthrodesis. *Arthroscopy.* 1999;15:215–217.
6. Vaseenon T. Arthroscopic debridement for first metatarsophalangeal joint arthrodesis with a 2-versus 3-portal technique: A cadaveric study. *Arthroscopy.* 2010;26(10): 1363–1367.
7. Ferkel Rd. Great toe arthroscopy. In: Whipple TL, ed. *Arthroscopy, the foot and ankle*. Philadelphia, PA: Lippincott-Raven; 1996:255–272.
8. Carreira D. Arthroscopy of the hallux. *Foot Ankle Clin.* 2009;14:105–113.
9. Lui TH. Arthroscopic release of first metatarsophalangeal arthrofibrosis. *Arthroscopy.* 2004;22(8):901–906.
10. van Dijk CN, Veenstra KM, Nuesch BC. Arthroscopic surgery of the metatarsophalangeal first joint. *Arthroscopy.* 1998;14:851–855.
11. Davies MS, Saxby TS. Arthroscopy of the first metatarsophalangeal joint. *J Bone Joint Surg Br.* 1999;81(2):203–206.
12. Carro LP, Vallina BB. Arthroscopic-assisted first metatarsophalangeal joint arthrodesis. *Arthroscopy.* 1999;15(2): 215–217.
13. Iqbal MJ, Chana GS. Arthroscopic cheilectomy for hallux rigidus. *Arthroscopy.* 1998;14(3):307–310.
14. Frey C, van Dijk CN. Arthroscopy of the great toe. *Instr Course Lect.* 1999;48:343–346.

CHAPTER 22

Hallux Valgus Correction with a Suture-Button Construct

Jeremy T. Smith   *Christopher P. Chiodo*

INDICATIONS

The decision-making process for the surgical treatment of any hallux valgus deformity is complex. Numerous factors must be taken into consideration. These include degree of deformity, presence of arthritis, joint congruency, articular deformity, soft tissue balance, and the exact location of the deformity. While the specifics and subtleties of various surgical options are complex, certain general principles have traditionally guided treatment decisions. These include treating arthritic joints with a fusion, avoiding procedures that cause incongruence, and using a more powerful corrective procedure for larger deformities. For nonarthritic and noncongruent hallux valgus, mild deformities have been traditionally treated with either a distal soft tissue release or a distal metatarsal osteotomy. As the intermetatarsal (IM) angle increases, more powerful proximal osteotomies are indicated.[1]

The addition of a metatarsal osteotomy to correct an elevated IM angle adds a degree of complexity to hallux valgus correction. Along with this complexity comes added potential morbidity. Potential complications associated with a first metatarsal osteotomy include metatarsal shortening, malunion, delayed union, nonunion, avascular necrosis, and fixation failure. Metatarsal shortening has been associated with the development of lateral metatarsalgia. After chevron osteotomy, metatarsal shortening has been shown to range from 2 mm to 8 mm.[2–4] Other metatarsal osteotomy procedures have also been associated with shortening of up to 11 mm.[4,5]

Recently, suture-button fixation between the first and second metatarsals has been introduced as an alterative to metatarsal osteotomy. This procedure has several distinct advantages. These include a smaller incision, earlier weight bearing, and avoidance of metatarsal shortening as well as the other potential complications associated with metatarsal osteotomy.

The indications for hallux valgus correction with a suture-button construct are still being defined. In general, the technique is indicated primarily for deformities with an incongruent metatarsal-phalangeal joint, with a sufficiently increased IM angle.[6] We agree with Holmes that it is possible to use this technique even in patients with an IM angle of greater than 15 degrees.[6] In these patients, however, the flexibility of the IM deformity is as important as the magnitude of the increased IM angle. While the historical literature has investigated the concept of dorsal-plantar instability of the first tarsometatarsal joint,[7–9] little attention has been paid to the transverse (medial–lateral) flexibility of the deformity. This is surprising given the traditional emphasis on flexible versus rigid deformity with regard to deformity correction in other parts of the body.

To this end, a more advanced hallux valgus deformity may be effectively treated with a suture-button device if the deformity demonstrates adequate flexibility. Flexibility is in the transverse plane and can be elicited with gentle compression of the first metatarsal head toward the second. Often, the true flexibility of the deformity is not apparent until distal release of the contracted lateral first metatarsophalangeal joint soft tissue structures has been

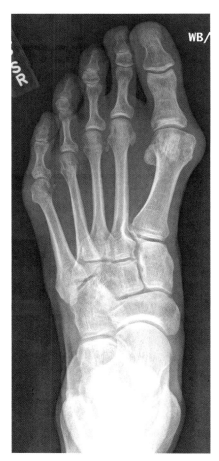

Figure 22–1. Proximal intermetatarsal facet between first and second metatarsals with hallux valgus deformity. This patient was treated with a proximal metatarsal osteotomy, not a suture-button construct.

performed. As such, the surgeon may consider consenting patients with advanced deformity for suture-button fixation and also for proximal metatarsal osteotomy.

PITFALLS/CONTRAINDICATIONS

Certain anatomic variations may inhibit adequate translation through this joint. An IM facet between the lateral base of the first metatarsal and medial base of the second metatarsal can limit reduction of the 1 to 2 IM angle (Fig. 22–1).[10–12] Another potential anatomic block to reduction is an os intermetatarseum.[13] The presence of these anatomic variants has been shown to occur in 8% of feet.[14] Additional contraindications to suture-button fixation include the presence of arthrosis and a congruent deformity. As noted, a rigid IM deformity is also a contraindication.

PATIENT POSITIONING

The patient is placed supine on the operating room table. A peripheral nerve block is used for the majority of

patients. Folded blankets are placed under the ipsilateral hip and buttock to bump the operative extremity such that the toes are pointing toward the ceiling. A platform of folded blankets is placed under the operative extremity, elevating the foot to facilitate intraoperative imaging and medial exposure. A thigh or supramalleolar Esmarch tourniquet may be used.

SURGICAL APPROACH AND TECHNIQUE

As with most procedures for hallux valgus, correction of the deformity requires distal release of the contracted lateral soft tissue structures. These structures include the adductor hallucis tendon, the transverse IM ligament, the metatarsal-sesamoid ligament, and the lateral joint capsule. A dorsal longitudinal incision is made over the first IM web space. Dissection is carried down through the deep fascia of the foot to the level of the metatarsal heads. A small Weitlaner retractor is placed between the first and second metatarsal heads to apply tension to the adductor hallucis and transverse IM ligament. The adductor tendon is then sharply transected. A Freer Elevator is then used to open the plane directly deep to the IM ligament and this ligament is transected. Care is taken to protect the deep neurovascular bundle. The metatarsal-sesamoid ligament is then fully released and the soft tissue release completed by sharply opening the lateral metatarsophalangeal joint capsule from the lateral sesamoid to the dorsum of the joint. The lateral sesamoid/flexor hallucis brevis complex should be left in continuity to prevent postoperative hallux varus. A gentle medially directed force is then applied to the hallux while stabilizing the first metatarsal to ensure that the lateral structures have been adequately released and the metatarsal head reduces over the sesamoids. At times, a small capsular band between the metatarsal-sesamoid and capsular release prevents complete reduction of the metatarsal head over the sesamoids. If this is the case, this capsular band is transected to achieve reduction. The surgeon should be able to readily "sweep" a Freer Elevator from the metatarsal-sesamoid articulation to the metatarsal-phalangeal articulation. Flexibility of the IM deformity is then reassessed by applying a laterally directed force to the first metatarsal at the level of the metatarsal head.

A 4-cm midline longitudinal incision is then made at the medial aspect of the first metatarsophalangeal joint, extending from 3 cm proximal to the medial eminence to 1 cm distal. Dissection is carried down to the level of the medial joint capsule. Care is taken to protect the dorsal medial cutaneous nerve. The dorsal and plantar flaps are retracted and a capsulotomy is made sharply (Fig. 22–2). While various capsulotomies have been described, we have found that a longitudinal capsulotomy readily facilitates appropriate medial soft tissue tensioning. The metatarsophalangeal joint is now visualized and assessed for cartilage

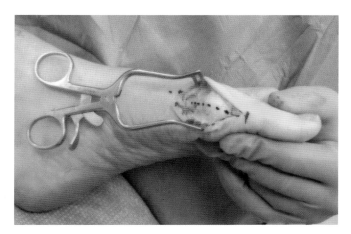

Figure 22–2. A longitudinal medial capsulotomy is made to expose the medial eminence.

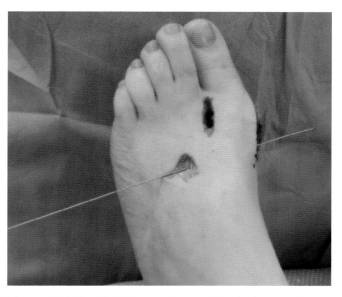

Figure 22–4. A 1.1-mm suture-guidewire is passed from lateral to medial.

injury. The medial eminence is then removed beginning approximately 1 mm medial to the sagittal sulcus (Fig. 22–3). Excessive medial eminence resection may lead to joint instability and postoperative hallux varus.

Once adequate IM flexibility has been confirmed, suture-button fixation is performed. Our current technique involves passing the suture-button construct from lateral to medial. A 1-cm longitudinal incision is made at the lateral border of the second metatarsal proximal to the second metatarsal head–neck junction. If present, we prefer that this be proximal to the thin diaphyseal isthmus. The lateral aspect of the second metatarsal is then exposed and a 1.1-mm suture-passing guidewire is drilled from lateral to medial, bisecting both the second and first metatarsals from dorsal to plantar (Fig. 22–4). The optimal exit point on the first metatarsal is just proximal to the medial eminence to ensure a strong diaphyseal cortex on which the metallic button rests (Fig. 22–5). Guidewire placement is confirmed fluoroscopically (Fig. 22–6).

The suture-button construct is then threaded through the loop on the guidewire and passed from lateral to medial through the metatarsals (Fig. 22–7). The lateral button is guided into place such that it sits flush against the second metatarsal (Fig. 22–8). The medial button is placed by cutting one limb of the looped suture and then threading the button onto both suture limbs. A medial knot secures the suture-button construct (Fig. 22–9).

Hallux alignment is assessed by tensioning the medial capsulotomy and suture-button device. Based on surgeon preference, these may be tensioned simultaneously to confirm alignment. If so, a single capsular figure-of-eight knot is placed to temporarily hold capsular tension. Either the dorsal or plantar capsular flap is advanced proximally depending upon which orientation of tissue achieves

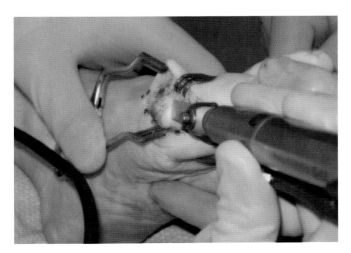

Figure 22–3. The medial eminence is removed, beginning 1 mm medial to the sagittal sulcus.

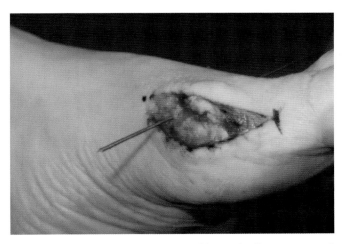

Figure 22–5. The guidewire should exit the first metatarsal just proximal to the medial eminence, bisecting the first metatarsal from dorsal to plantar.

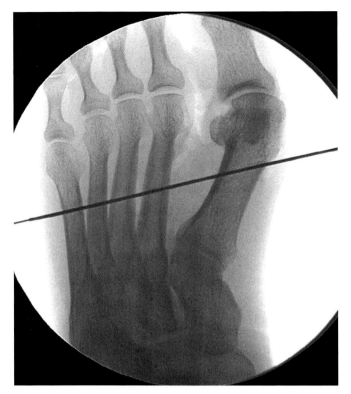

Figure 22–6. The guidewire placement is evaluated fluoroscopically.

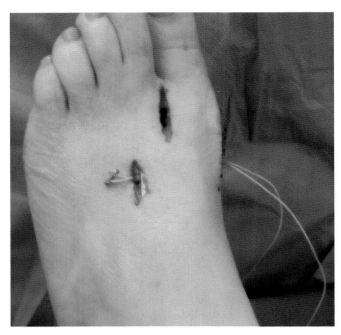

Figure 22–8. The lateral button is guided into place to sit flush against the second metatarsal.

better correction. The suture-button device is then tensioned to laterally translate the first metatarsal and correct the IM angle. A single half hitch is laid flat against the medial button and held with a snap. The alignment of the hallux is then confirmed fluoroscopically. Changes can be made to the first metatarsal position by adjusting the tension on the suture-button construct and similarly to the metatarsophalangeal joint by adjusting the capsular advancement. Once satisfactory alignment has been achieved, the snap is removed from the suture and three additional half hitches are laid down against the medial button. The suture is then cut sharply and the knot is tamped down to avoid knot prominence. The medial capsular repair is then completed with suture. Alignment is again confirmed fluoroscopically (Fig. 22–10).

Of note, with an adequate lateral release as well as removal of the medial directed force that the base of the proximal phalanx exerts on the metatarsal head in the

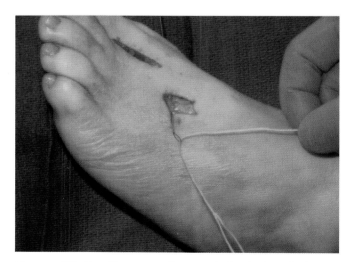

Figure 22–7. The suture-button device is threaded through the loop on the guidewire and passed from lateral to medial through the metatarsals.

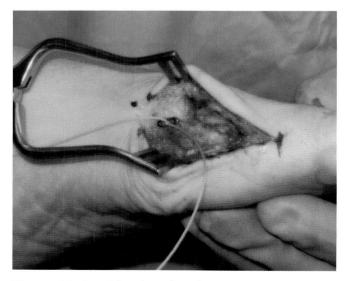

Figure 22–9. After threading the medial button, a medial knot will close the suture-button construct.

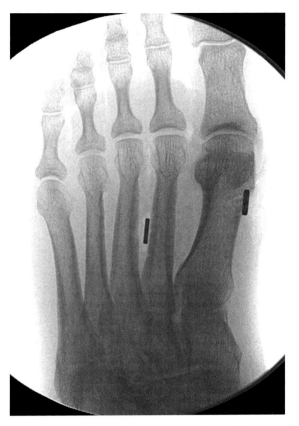

Figure 22–10. The alignment is confirmed fluoroscopically after the suture-button construct has been tightened and the medial capsule has been repaired.

pathologic state, the suture-button construct serves to maintain the IM correction, rather than obtain it. If anything greater than minimal effort is needed to obtain a correction after lateral release an osteotomy should be considered.

COMPLICATIONS

As with other techniques of hallux valgus correction, potential complications of this procedure include infection, metatarsophalangeal joint fibrosis, recurrence, hallux varus, failure of fixation, and peripheral nerve injury. A distinct advantage of the suture-button construct technique is that potential complications associated with a metatarsal osteotomy are avoided, specifically malunion, delayed union, nonunion, metatarsal head avascular necrosis, and metatarsal shortening.

In the largest series of suture-button hallux valgus correction published to date, the single complication reported from 44 cases was a recurrence of deformity.[15] There are several reports of second metatarsal fracture at the site of the lateral suture button.[6,16–18] Potential causes of this complication include placing the drill hole too close to the neck of the second metatarsal or failing to drill centrally from the plantar to dorsal aspects of the metatarsal.[6] This

complication occurred when using an older technique with a cannulated 2.7-mm drill. Using a 1.1-mm suture-passing guidewire eliminates the need for over drilling and minimizes the risk of second metatarsal fracture.

REHABILITATION PROTOCOL

Surgical incisions are closed in layers with absorbable suture. Our preference is to use a 3-0 absorbable monofilament suture for the subdermal layer and then a 3-0 nylon suture for skin closure. A gauze bolster is placed between the first and second toes and additional gauze strapping is used to protect the correction. A soft dressing is then applied. Patients are typically permitted to immediately weight bear on the heel in a postoperative shoe. If additional procedures have been performed, weight-bearing restrictions may be modified. The surgical dressing is changed 10 to 14 days postoperatively and sutures are removed. The hallux is taped to maintain correction for an additional 4 weeks. Heel weight bearing is maintained until 6 weeks postoperatively. Wide toe-box shoes are encouraged.

OUTCOME

Kayiaros et al. reported the outcomes of 44 cases using a suture-button device at an average of 6 months postoperatively.[15] In this series, the average hallux valgus angle improved from 32.2 to 15.2 degrees, the first IM angle improved from 14.6 to 8.2 degrees, and the distal metatarsal articular angle improved from 17.0 to 9.6 degrees. The average American Orthopaedic Foot & Ankle Society (AOFAS) forefoot score improved from 45.4 to 84.7. The authors of this study concluded that this technique is capable of maintaining correction while allowing early weight bearing.

A series of 36 cases, published in the Spanish orthopaedic literature also used a suture button device. They reported an average postoperative hallux valgus angle of 10.0 degrees and an IM angle of 4.8 degrees with a follow-up of 24 months. AOFAS score improved from 47.7 preoperatively to 88.0 postoperatively.[18]

Although limited, current data suggest that suture-button fixation for hallux valgus can be a useful tool in a patient with a mild, moderate, or even a flexible severe deformity. Proper patient selection is important, with specific attention paid to the presence of arthritis, metatarsophalangeal joint congruency, degree of deformity, and IM flexibility. Larger series with longer follow-up are needed to further evaluate this novel technology.

REFERENCES

1. Coughlin MJ, Mann RA, Saltzman CL. *Surgery of the foot and ankle.* 8th ed. Philadelphia, PA: Mosby; 2007.
2. Hirvensalo E, Bostman O, Tormala P, et al. Chevron osteotomy fixed with absorbable polyglycolide pins. *Foot Ankle.* 1991;11:212–218.

3. Mann RA, Donatto KC. The chevron osteotomy: A clinical and radiographic analysis. *Foot Ankle Int.* 1997;18:255–261.
4. Pring D. Chevron or Wilson osteotomy: A comparison and follow-up. *J Bone Joint Surg Am.* 1985;67:671–672.
5. Fokter SK, Podobnik J, Vengust V. Late results of modified Mitchell procedure for the treatment of hallux valgus. *Foot Ankle Int.* 1999;20:296–300.
6. Holmes G. Correction of hallux valgus deformity using the mini tightrope device. *Tech Foot Ankle Surg.* 2008;7:9.
7. Butson AR. A modification of the Lapidus operation for hallux valgus. *J Bone Joint Surg Br.* 1980;62:350–352.
8. Johnson KA, Kile TA. Hallux valgus due to cuneiform-metatarsal instability. *J South Orthop Assoc.* 1994;3:273–283.
9. Faber FW, Kleinrensink GJ, Verhoog MW, et al. Mobility of the first tarsometatarsal joint in relation to hallux valgus deformity: Anatomical and biomechanical aspects. *Foot Ankle Int.* 1999;20:651–656.
10. Lapidus PW. The author's bunion operation from 1931 to 1959. *Clin Orthop.* 1960;16:119–135.
11. Mann RA. Hallux valgus. *Instr Course Lect.* 1986;35:339–353.
12. Tuslow W. Metatarsus primus varus or hallux valgus? *J Bone Joint Surg.* 1925;7:98–108.
13. Mann RA, Coughlin MJ. Hallux valgus–etiology, anatomy, treatment and surgical considerations. *Clin Orthop Relat Res.* 1981;157:31–41.
14. Coughlin M. Hallux valgus: Demographics, radiographic assessment and clinical outcomes. A prospective study. Paper presented at 21st Annual Meeting of the American Orthopaedic Foot and Ankle Society; Boston, MA: July 2005.
15. Kayiaros S, Blankenhorn BD, Dehaven J, et al. Correction of metatarsus primus varus associated with hallux valgus deformity using the arthrex mini tightrope: A report of 44 cases. *Foot Ankle Spec.* 2011;4:212–217.
16. Kemp TJ, Hirose CB, Coughlin MJ. Fracture of the second metatarsal following suture button fixation device in the correction of hallux valgus. *Foot Ankle Int.* 2010;31:712–716.
17. Mader D. Bilateral second metatarsal stress fractures after hallux valgus correction with the use of a tension wire and button fixation system. *J Foot Ankle Surg.* 2010;49:488. e15–e19.
18. Cano-Martinez J. Tratamiento del Hallux valgus moderado con sistema mini TightRope®: Técnica modificada. *Rev Esp Cir Ortop Traumatol.* 2011;55:1.

CHAPTER 23

Hallux Valgus Correction—SERI Technique

Sandro Giannini   Francesca Vannini

INTRODUCTION

Most procedures involving bone that exist for hallux valgus correction may be divided in two major subgroups: proximal osteotomies and distal osteotomies.[1] Historically, proximal osteotomies were used for correction of major deformities where the 1–2 intermetatarsal angle (IMA) is greater than 15 to 20 degrees, while distal metatarsal osteotomies have been indicated in cases of mild to moderate deformity with an IMA as large as 15 to 20 degrees.[1] The versatility and reliability of the distal osteotomies has led to a wider application of these procedures. Distal osteotomies are capable of correcting all the altered parameters typical of hallux valgus, such as hallux valgus angle (HVA), IMA, distal metatarsal articular angle (DMAA), and to derotate the metatarsal head in order to address the pronation of the hallux, or to reduce concomitant stiffness by shortening the first metatarsal.[2–10]

Current trends for distal osteotomies are to perform them through smaller operative wounds, with less tissue damage and shorter operative times; all to achieve more rapid recovery.[2,11]

Less invasive techniques were pioneered by New, who in 1983 described a percutaneous technique for the correction of hallux valgus (personal communication). This technique was popularized by Bösch[12] by using an osteotomy similar to Hohmann's,[13] but with single Kirschner wire (K-wire) fixation as previously described by Lamprecht and Kramer.[14] This percutaneous technique led to a substantial decrease in surgical trauma, since no soft tissue procedure is required. Aspects considered disadvantages of the procedure include the need for a C-arm, since direct visualization is not obtained as well as the use of a power burr, which inevitably produces a slight shortening of the metatarsal, due to the thickness of the tool. Nevertheless these have been used with satisfactory results.[11]

The minimally invasive hallux valgus correction SERI (Simple Effective Rapid Inexpensive)[2] is not a new technique because it uses an osteotomy and a stabilization method already described. The transverse osteotomy is made immediately proximal to the metatarsal head, as described by Hohmann,[13] Wilson,[15] and Magerl.[14] This is performed through a small incision that need to be no larger than 1 cm, as suggested by Kramer[16] and by Bösch.[12] There is no need for a tangential resection of

the prominence or open lateral release, since manual stretching of the abductor tendon is usually sufficient to obtain HV angle correction. Obviation of these steps substantially reduces the amount of time necessary to perform it. Its high efficacy derives from the unique combined characteristics of simplicity, versatility, and good stability of the construct all while being minimally invasive.[2,17] Finally it is inexpensive due to the reduced surgical time and simple fixation device used (single K-wire).

INDICATIONS

The SERI technique is appropriate for correction of mild to moderate reducible deformity when the HVA is up to 40 degrees and the IMA is up to 20 degrees.

The operation is may be used if the metatarsophalangeal joint is either incongruent or congruent or with increased DMAA, and if mild degenerative arthritis is present (up to grade 2 of the Regnault classification).[18]

Specific contraindications of the SERI technique are severe deformity with the IMA more than 20 degrees, severe degenerative arthritis or stiffness of the metatarsophalangeal joint, and severe instability of the cuneometatarsal or metatarsophalangeal joint.

PREOPERATIVE PLANNING

The preoperative plan includes acquiring a complete history of the patient, and a physical and radiographic examination. The severity of the prominent medial eminence and the hallux valgus deformity should be evaluated by pushing the metatarsal head laterally with one hand and simultaneously the great toe medially with the other hand. Stability of the metatarsophalangeal and cuneometatarsal joints must be assessed. Combined rotational deformity of the great toe or callosities under the external metatarsal heads must be considered, as well as any associated deformities of the lesser toes.

A standard radiographic examination, including anteroposterior and lateral weight-bearing views of the forefoot, allows the assessment of the arthritis and congruency of the joint; measurement of the HVA, IMA, and DMAA. Therefore, planning of the operation is performed in terms of the obliquity of the bone cut, the

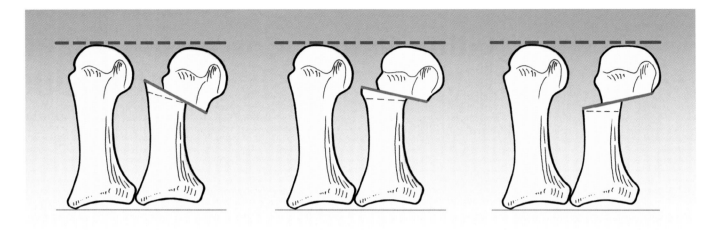

A

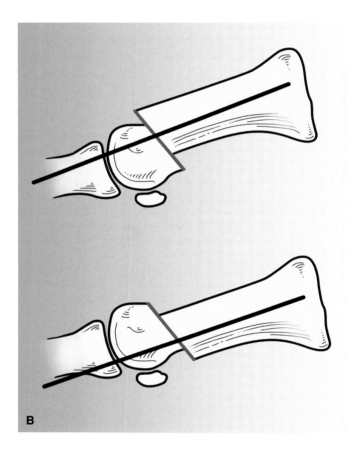

B

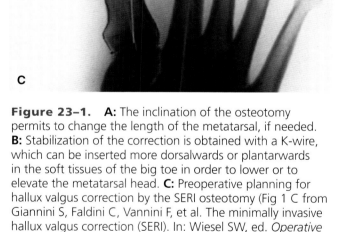

C

Figure 23–1. **A:** The inclination of the osteotomy permits to change the length of the metatarsal, if needed. **B:** Stabilization of the correction is obtained with a K-wire, which can be inserted more dorsalwards or plantarwards in the soft tissues of the big toe in order to lower or to elevate the metatarsal head. **C:** Preoperative planning for hallux valgus correction by the SERI osteotomy (Fig 1 C from Giannini S, Faldini C, Vannini F, et al. The minimally invasive hallux valgus correction (SERI). In: Wiesel SW, ed. *Operative techniques in orthopaedic surgery.* Philadelphia, PA: Wolters Kluwer Health; 2010, with permission).

extent of the medial-lateral or dorsal-plantar dislocation of the metatarsal head and the correction of the DMAA (Fig. 23–1A–C).

PATIENT POSITIONING

The patient is positioned on a radiolucent operating table in the supine position. Intraoperative imaging in two projections should be obtainable in particular during the

period the technique is being adopted. With experience, the use of fluoroscopy is unnecessary.

TECHNIQUE

The operation is usually performed under local or block anesthesia using ropivacaine 7.5 mg per mL. An Esmarch bandage or tourniquet may be optionally used at the ankle level.

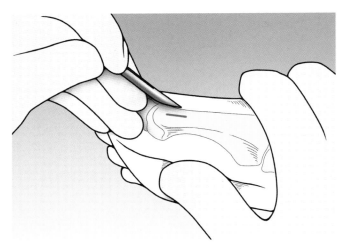

Figure 23–2. Surgical technique. A 1 cm medial incision at the neck of first metatarsal is practised.

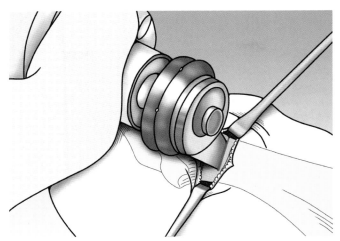

Figure 23–4. Osteotomy of the neck of first metatarsal is performed.

Normally, when the deformity is manually reducible, a lateral soft tissue release is not needed because release of tension is achieved with the lateral offset of the metatarsal head itself. If the deformity is not reducible, a manual stretching of the adductor hallucis is performed, gently easing the big toe into a varus position. Otherwise, especially in younger patients, the detachment of the adductor hallucis tendon may be obtained through a percutaneous tenotomy by sliding the scalpel adjacent to the lateral side of the metatarsal head toward the base of the proximal phalanx.

A 1 cm medial incision is made just proximal to the medial eminence through the skin, subcutaneous tissue, down to the bone.

The soft tissues are separated dorsal and plantar and retracted by two small retractors 5 mm in width (Figs. 23–2 and 23–3).

The medial wall of metatarsal neck is now well evident and the osteotomy is performed using a standard

microsagittal saw with a 0.4-mm blade thickness (Fig. 23–4).

With a small osteotome, the head is mobilized.

The inclination of the osteotomy in the mediolateral direction is perpendicular to the foot axis (i.e., the long axis of the second metatarsal bone) if maintenance of the length of first metatarsal bone is desired.

A 2-mm K-wire is inserted, using a wire collette passing through the incision, into the soft tissue adjacent to the medial cortex of the metatarsal head proximal to distal subcutaneously along the longitudinal axis of the great toe (Fig. 27–5).

The K-wire exits at the medial tip of the toe, about 3 to 4 mm from the lateral border of the nail, it is withdrawn distally (Fig. 23–6A) and retracted so the proximal tip is just distal to the osteotomy (Fig. 23–6B).

The correction is obtained by using a small grooved lever placed along the medial cortex within the metatarsal

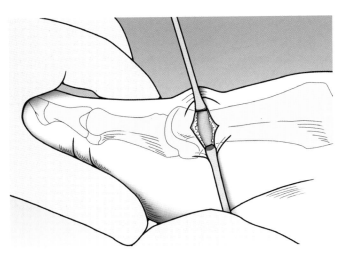

Figure 23–3. Soft tissues are retracted.

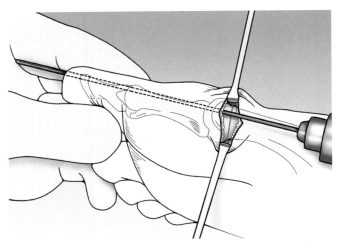

Figure 23–5. A K-wire is inserted proximal to distal in soft tissue of the first toe.

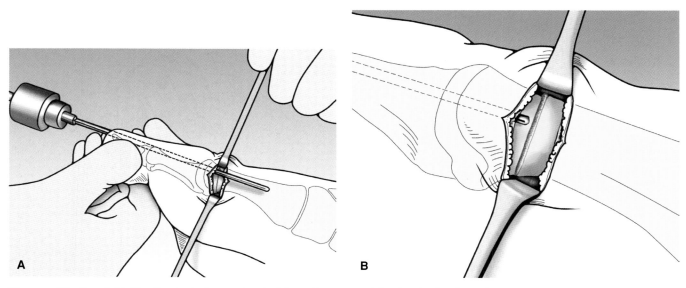

Figure 23–6. **A,B:** The K-wire is then retracted from the apex of the toe to the line of osteotomy.

shaft to lateralize the metatarsal head, along the osteotomy site (Fig. 23–7A,B).

If the pronation of the first metatarsal bone is present, the correction is obtained with a derotation of the hallux to the neutral position (Fig. 23–8).

Stabilization of the correction is obtained advancing the K-wire into the diaphysis in a distal to proximal direction until its proximal end reaches the metatarsal base (Fig. 23–9).

To correct an increased DMAA, the K-wire is introduced close to the medial cortex of the metatarsal diaphysis obliquely and advanced laterally as many degrees as necessary to obtain the correction plantar translation of the metatarsal head, or more rarely dorsal translation, is

obtained introducing the K-wire more superiorly, or inferiorly respectively along the metatarsal head (Fig. 23–1B).

If the proximal osteotomy site is prominent medially, a small wedge of bone is removed (Fig. 23–10).

Fluoroscopic images are obtained in AP and oblique views to confirm correct placement of the hardware and correction of the deformity.

The skin is sutured with absorbable sutures. The distal extremity of the K-wire is bent and cut at the tip of the toe.

This technique can be performed bilaterally or combined concomitantly with correction of any other associated deformity of the forefoot or hindfoot. Preoperative, early postoperative, and late postoperative radiographs of a representative patient are shown in Figure 23–11.

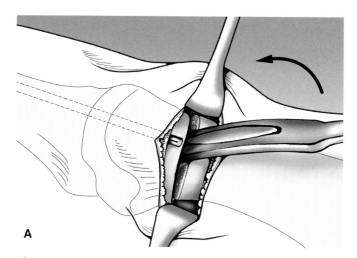
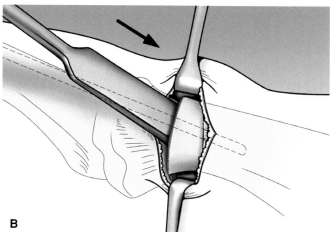

Figure 23–7. **A,B:** With a small osteotomy the metatarsal head is mobilized in order to correct the deformity.

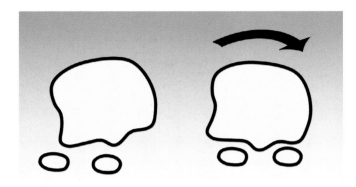

Figure 23–8. Derotation corrects the pronation of the metatarsal and reduces subluxation of sesamoids.

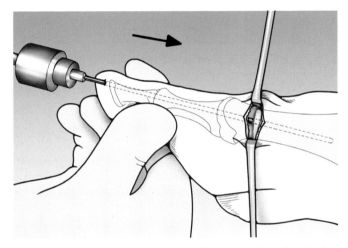

Figure 23–9. The correction is fixed inserting the K-wire distal to proximal in the diaphysis of the first metatarsal.

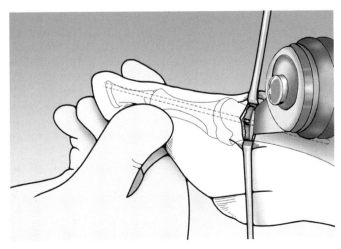

Figure 23–10. The corner of the metatarsal bone is resected by the saw.

PEARLS

- Choice of the correct site for osteotomy is simple, since the 1 cm incision should be performed immediately before the prominence of the metatarsal head and the osteotomy should be performed just before the insertion of the capsule (Fig. 23–2).
- The osteotomy is inclined in a distal-medial to proximal-lateral direction up to 25 degrees if shortening of the metatarsal bone or decompression of the metatarsophalangeal joint is necessary in case of mild arthritis. More rarely, if a lengthening of the first metatarsal bone is necessary (i.e., if the first metatarsal bone is shorter than the second or if laxity of the metatarsophalangeal joint is present), the osteotomy is inclined in a proximal-medial to distal-lateral direction as much as 25 degrees (Fig. 23–1A).
- A key point of the stability of SERI technique is inclusion of a 15-degree inclination in a distal-dorsal to proximal-plantar direction. This helps to avoid dorsal dislocation of the metatarsal head under weight bearing.
- Adjustment of the lateral displacement of the metatarsal head is performed altering the insertion of the K-wire relative to the medial eminence (If the K-wire is inserted inside the eminence itself, the lateral displacement of the head will be reduced).

PITFALLS

- An osteotomy placed too proximally in the metatarsal increases the risk of nonunion.
- An osteotomy placed too distally predisposes to osteonecrosis of the metatarsal head and arthritis of the sesamoid-metatarsal articulation.
- Excessive lateral displacement of the head, even when there is no residual contact with the metatarsal shaft, is usually still able to unite, but produces a residual shortening of the metatarsal bone.
- Insufficient lateral displacement of the metatarsal head may produce a higher recurrence rate.
- Excessive shortening of the first metatarsal can lead to overloading the lesser toes.
- Performing this technique in presence of severe arthritis or stiffness increase the risk of poor results due to occurrence of hallux rigidus.
- The use of a K-wire less than 2 mm results in a substantial decrease of the lateralizing force applied to the osteotomy (a decrease of the radius of the pin of 20% results in a reduction of 60% of the applied force).[19]

POSTOPERATIVE CARE

After surgery, a gauze compression dressing is applied. Ambulation is allowed immediately using a postoperative

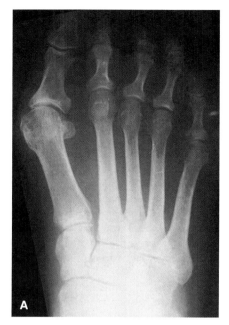 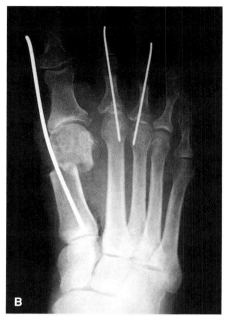 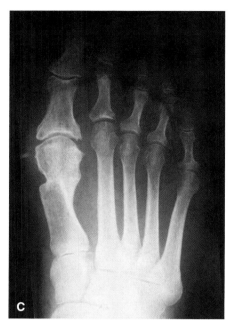

Figure 23–11. **A:** Dorsoplantar radiographs showing a hallux valgus deformity in a female patient 50 years old. **B:** Postoperative radiograph. **C:** Radiographs at 3 years of follow-up (From Giannini S, Faldini C, Vannini F, et al. The minimally invasive hallux valgus correction (SERI). In: Wiesel SW, ed. *Operative techniques in orthopaedic surgery.* Philadelphia, PA: Wolters Kluwer Health; 2010, with permission).

shoe. Foot elevation is advised when the patient is at rest. Slight bending of the K-wire seen after insertion results in a laterally directed force and contributes to the stabilization of the osteotomy. This helps maintain the correction obtained during surgery. This stabilization promotes healing of the osteotomy and in many cases allows for early weight bearing.

After 1 month, the dressing, suture, and K-wire are removed. Passive and active toe mobilization, cycling, and swimming are advised. Comfortable shoes are used initially, with a gradual return to former footwear.

COMPLICATIONS

A limited number of complications may occur intraoperatively, if attention is paid to the correct position and alignment of the osteotomy as well as to the K-wire insertion.

A mild inflammatory reaction of the skin surrounding the K-wire at the tip of the toe, may be experienced, but usually resolves in a few days. A gauze should be placed between the skin and the K-wire itself.

Nonunion is a very rare complication experienced by the authors in a negligible percentage of cases. It may occur in case of technical error, when the osteotomy is performed too proximally, or the K-wire used is of insufficient size.[20]

The most frequent complication experienced postoperatively is loss of first metatarsophalangeal joint

ROM.[17] The residual ROM is usually sufficient for a satisfactory result and may be addressed by physiotherapy.

Another possible cause of residual pain is the prominence of the corner of metatarsal bone, if it has not been adequately resected intraoperatively.

OUTCOME

Several case series are now available to document outcomes and complications of minimally invasive hallux valgus correction. Nevertheless, the studies available up to now are not homogeneous: they differ in study design, type of patients, type and level of hallux deformity, type of surgical procedures, and type of outcomes assessed. Not all data from the selected papers were available, and most papers describe low-quality (mainly level IV evidence) case series.[21]

The results regarding the first consecutive 54 feet operated in 37 patients (17 bilateral; 34 female, 3 male) were reported at a mean follow-up of 36 months by Giannini et al.[2]

Patients' mean age was 48 years (range 10 to 70). Clinical evaluation (AOFAS) and radiographic evaluation was performed preoperatively and at established follow-up.[22]

All patients except four (7.4%) declared satisfaction with the result obtained. Postoperatively the mean AOFAS score obtained was 81 points. An excellent result was obtained by 64.8% of the patients, while 18.5% had a good result, 9.2% were fair and 7.4% poor. All the osteotomies healed nicely with radiographical evidence of callus formation and metatarsal bone remodelling at 3 months, even in case of marked off set of the osteotomy. No severe complications were reported. The patients unsatisfied with the result had worsening of MTP joint arthritis or a persistence of the transfer metatarsalgia.[2]

In a series of 13 patients, Kadakia et al.[20] used a modified SERI technique performed through a longer incision, with the use of a 1.6-mm K-wire instead of a 2-mm, and an additional 1.6-mm K-wire in some of the cases. At an average of 130 days the authors reported a significant improvement in the parameters related to the HVA and IMA, but the osteotomy angulated dorsally in nine cases. One case of osteonecrosis of the metatarsal head developed in a case in which the osteotomy was performed extremely distally at the sesamoid level and one superficial cellulitis were also reported.

Lin et al.[23] reported on 31 consecutive patients (47 feet) with mild to moderate hallux valgus deformities, corrected by a distal metatarsal osteotomy through a minimally invasive approach with the same characteristics as SERI. The follow-up period was 23.7 weeks. The satisfaction rate was 90%. A statistically significant improvement of both the clinical and radiographical parameters was evident. On final weight-bearing anteroposterior foot radiographs, the mean HVA and first IMA corrections were 11.8 degrees and 6.3 degrees. Both represented statistically significant improvements ($p < 0.001$) from the preoperative values. Complications included two (4%) episodes of stiffness, six (13%) episodes of pin tract infection, and one (2%) deep infection. There were no cases with nonunion, malunion, overcorrection, transfer metatarsalgia, or osteonecrosis.

Giannini et al.[24] performed a prospective randomized study comparing linear distal metatarsal osteotomy with Scarf osteotomy in 40 patients affected by bilateral hallux valgus at 4 years follow-up. All patients were operated bilaterally, and received Scarf osteotomy on one side and SERI osteotomy on the other performed through a 1-cm skin incision under direct visual control. No statistical differences were observed in preoperative HVA, IMA, and DMMA in both groups. No complications were observed in the series, with no wound dehiscence. All osteotomies healed. At 4 years follow-up, no statistical differences were observed in HVA, IMA, and DMMA comparing Scarf with SERI at follow-up. Both techniques resulted in significant corrections of the radiographic parameters from their preoperative states. Average AOFAS score at follow-up was 87 ± 12 in Scarf and 89 ± 10 in SERI ($p < 0.07$). The authors concluded that both Scarf and linear distal metatarsal osteotomy techniques resulted in effective correction of hallux valgus. However SERI, which was performed with a shorter skin incision, more rapid surgical time, fixed with a less expensive device (one K-wire), resulted in a subjectively better clinical outcome.

Giannini et al.[24] also reported on 1,000 feet in 641 patients (359 bilateral) with hallux valgus managed by SERI. Inclusion criteria were deformity less than 40-degree HVA and IMA up to 18 degrees. All patients were checked at an average follow-up of 37 months. The mean AOFAS score was 48 degrees ± 15 degrees preoperatively and 89 degrees ± 13 degrees at follow-up ($p < 0.005$). The preoperative HVA was 32 degrees ± 8 degrees, while at follow-up it was 18 degrees ± 8 degrees ($p < 0.005$). Preoperatively, the IMA was 14 degrees ± 3 degrees, while at follow-up it was 6 degrees ± 4 degrees ($p < 0.005$); the preoperative DMMA was 21 degrees ± 9 degrees, while at follow-up it was 9 degrees ± 8 degrees ($p < 0.005$). Delayed consolidation was observed in 25 feet, but all the osteotomies finally healed. Slight stiffness of the metatarsal joint was observed in 31 feet. This study confirmed the validity of the technique in one of the largest case series presented on this topic.

Minimally invasive procedures are still not widely accepted, and doubts arise mainly from "classically" trained orthopedic surgeons. Concerns focus both on the fixation by a K-wire, rather than screws and with the theoretically higher percentage of complications. Both the literature and our experience support the validity of the K-wire as a fixation device, if correctly used.[2,11,24,25] Complications, when present, seem in most of the cases related to incorrect technique.

REFERENCES

1. Kelikian H. Hallux valgus. In: Mann RA, Coughlin MJ, eds. *Allied deformities of the forefoot and metatarsalgia.* Philadelphia, PA: WB Saunders; 1965:213–225.
2. Giannini S, Ceccarelli F, Bevoni R, et al. "Hallux valgus surgery: The minimally invasive bunion correction (SERI). *Tech Foot Ankle Surg.* 2003;2:11–20.
3. Reverdin J. De la deviation en dehors du gros orteil (hallux valgus. Vulg. "oignon" "bunions" "ballen") et de son traitement chirurgical. *Trans Int Med Congr.* 1881;2:406–412.
4. Mitchell CL, Fleming JL, Allen R, et al. Osteotomy bunionectomy for hallux valgus. *J Bone Joint Surg Am.* 1958;40-A: 41–60.
5. Austin DW, Leventen EO. A new osteotomy for hallux valgus: A horizontally directed "V" displacement osteotomy of the metatarsal head for hallux valgus and primus varus. *Clin Orthop Relat Res.* 1981;157:25–30.
6. Youngswick FD. Modifications of the Austin bunionectomy for treatment of metatarsus primus elevatus associated with hallux limitus. *J Foot Surg.* 1982;21:114–116.
7. Kalish SR, Spector JE. The Kalish osteotomy: A review and retrospective analysis of 265 cases. *J Am Podiatr Med Assoc.* 1994;84:237–249.
8. Laird PO, Silvers SH, Somdhal J. Two Reverdin-Laird osteotomy modifications for correction of hallux abducto valgus. *J Am Podiatr Med Assoc.* 1988;78:403–405.
9. Elleby DH, Barry LD, Helfman DN. The long plantar wing distal metaphyseal osteotomy. *J Am Podiatr Med Assoc.* 1992;82:501–506.
10. Grace DL. Metatarsal osteotomy: Which operation? *J Foot Surg.* 1987;36:46–50.

11. Magnan B, Pezze L, Rossi N, et al. Percutaneous distal metatarsal osteotomy for correction of hallux valgus. *J Bone Joint Surg Am.* 2005;87:1191–1199.

12. Bosch P, Markowski H, Rannicher V. Technik und erste ergebnisse der subkutanen distalen metatarsale I osteotomie. *Orthopaedische Praxis.* 1990;26:51–56.

13. Hohmann G. Symptomatische oder Physiologische Behandlung des Hallux Valgus?*Munch Med Wochenschr.* 1921;33:1042–1045.

14. Lamprecht E, Kramer J. Die metatarsale I osteotomie nach behandlung des hallux valgus. *Orthop Praxis.* 1982;8:636–645.

15. Wilson JN. Oblique displacement osteotomy for hallux valgus. *J Bone Joint Surg Br.* 1963;45:552–556.

16. Magerl F. Stabile osteotomien zur behandlung des hallux valgus und metatarsale varum. *Orthopäde.* 1982;11:170–180.

17. Giannini S, Vannini F, Faldini C, et al. The minimally invasive hallux valgus correction (S.E.R.I.). *Interact Surg.* 2007;2(1):17–23.

18. Regnauld B. Disorders of the great toe. In: Elson R, ed. *The foot: pathology, aetiology, semiology, clinical investigation and therapy.* New York, NY: Springer; 1986:269–281, 344–349.

19. Stagni R, Vannini F, Giannini S. 1st Congress of the International Foot & Ankle Biomechanics (i-FAB) community Bologna, Italy. 4–6 September 2008(Abstract published on *J Foot Ankle Research.* 2008, 1(suppl 1):O41.

20. Kadakia AR, Smerek JP, Myerson MS. Radiographic results after percutaneous distal metatarsal osteotomy for correction of hallux valgus deformity. *Foot Ankle Int.* 2007;28(3):355–360.

21. Maffulli N, Longo UG, Marinozzi A, et al. Hallux valgus: Effectiveness and safety of minimally invasive surgery. A systematic review. *Br Med Bull.* 2011;97:149–167.

22. Kitaoka HB, Alexander IJ, Adelaar RS, et al. Clinical rating systems for the ankle-hindfoot, midfoot, hallux, and lesser toes. *Foot Ankle Int.* 1994;15(7):349–353.

23. Lin YC, Cheng YM, Chang JK, et al. Minimally invasive distal metatarsal osteotomy for mild-to-moderate hallux valgus deformity. *Kaohsiung J Med Sci.* 2009;25(8):431–437.

24. Giannini S, Faldini C, Vannini F, et al. Minimally invasive distal metatarsal osteotomy for surgical treatment of hallux valgus: Clinical study of the first 1000 consecutive cases at mean 5 years follow up. *J Bone Joint Surg Br Proceedings.* 2009;91-B:143–144.

25. Giannini S, Faldini C, Vannini F, et al. Surgical treatment of hallux valgus: A clinical prospective randomized study comparing linear distal metatarsal osteotomy with scarf osteotomy. *J Bone Joint Surg Br Proceedings.* 2009;91-B:162.

CHAPTER 24

Minimally Invasive Operative Treatment of Bunionette Deformity with Percutaneous Distal Metatarsal Osteotomy

Jin Woo Lee   Woo Jin Choi

INDICATIONS

Bunionette or "tailor's bunion" is a painful lateral prominence of the fifth metatarsal head, leading to a chronic bursitis overlying the lateral side of the fifth metatarsal head. Conservative treatment with wide toe box shoes, semirigid shoe inserts, metatarsal pads, metatarsal bars, and stretching of the shoes may relieve the symptoms.[1] Operative management is indicated when nonoperative treatments can no longer control symptoms and when the patient has special demands, particularly in sports.[1] The indication for performing a percutaneous distal osteotomy is the same as that for performing a distal osteotomy with an open technique. Mild to moderate bunionette deformities may be corrected with this technique. The percutaneous procedure has evolved from the traditional open techniques that depend on stabilization with a Kirschner wire (K-wire) for hallux valgus[2-5] and was standardized by Bösch et al.[6,7] Giannini et al.[8] recently presented a new minimally invasive technique of percutaneous distal metatarsal osteotomy, the characteristics of which can be summarized with the abbreviation "S.E.R.I" (simple, effective, rapid, inexpensive), for correction of bunionette deformity.

PATIENT POSITIONING

The patient is placed in supine position on a radiolucent operating table (Fig. 24–1). The foot is kept internally rotated with a small sandbag under the ipsilateral hip. The operation is usually performed using regional anesthesia and a tourniquet is used. Skin preparation and draping is performed with standard technique. Portable C-arm image intensifier television fluoroscopy is necessary to identify the correction of deformity and the pin position.

SURGICAL APPROACHES

A lateral incision of 1 cm is made just proximal to the lateral eminence of the fifth metatarsal head through the skin and subcutaneous tissue, down to bone. The soft tissue is separated dorsally and plantarly, and held by two small retractors. The lateral wall of the metatarsal neck is now visualized (Fig. 24–2).

REDUCTION TECHNIQUES

The complete osteotomy usually is made using a small blade oscillating saw from lateral to medial side with the obliquity oriented from plantar proximal to dorsal distal with an angle of approximately 30 degrees (Fig. 24–3). The key points of the technique are the inclinations of the osteotomy in the medial-lateral and dorsal-plantar direction, the displacement of the head in the medial-lateral and dorsal-plantar direction, and the rotation of the metatarsal head according to the types of deformity.[8] The plane of the osteotomy in the lateral to medial direction is perpendicular to the fourth ray if the length of fifth metatarsal bone must be maintained. The osteotomy may be directed from distal to proximal up to 25 degrees, if shortening of fifth metatarsal bone is necessary in cases of mild arthritis. More rarely, if a lengthening of the fifth metatarsal bone is necessary the plane of the osteotomy is inclined in a proximal-distal direction approximately 15 degrees.

To control the dorsal translation of the metatarsal head with weight bearing the osteotomy is normally inclined about 30 degrees in distal-dorsal to proximal-plantar directions (Fig. 24–4). The adjustment of the lateral-medial position of the metatarsal head is performed by introducing the K-wire superficial with regard to the lateral eminence. The adjustment of the plantar-dorsal position of the metatarsal head is obtained introducing the K-wire in the upper or lower aspect, with regard to the long axis of the metatarsal head. If supination of the fifth metatarsal bone is present, the correction is obtained with derotation of the lesser toe to the neutral position.

FIXATION

The fifth metatarsal head is mobilized with a small osteotome. A 1.8-mm K-wire is inserted into the soft tissue

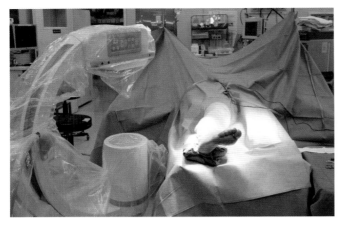

Figure 24–1. Patient positioning and imaging setup.

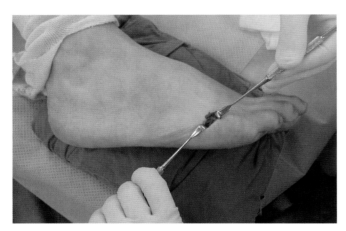

Figure 24–2. Skin incision and exposure of the lateral cortex.

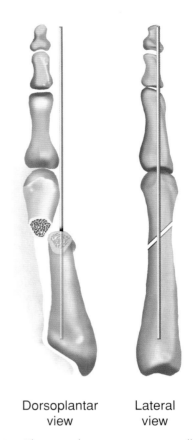

Dorsoplantar view   Lateral view

Figure 24–4. The complete osteotomy usually is made using a small blade oscillating saw from lateral to medial with the obliquity oriented from plantar proximal to dorsal distal with an angle of approximately 30 degrees.

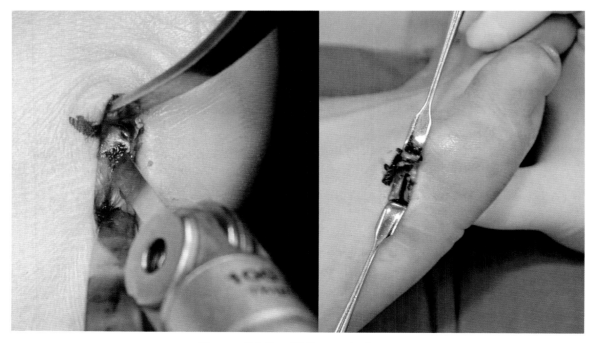

Figure 24-3. Oblique osteotomy.

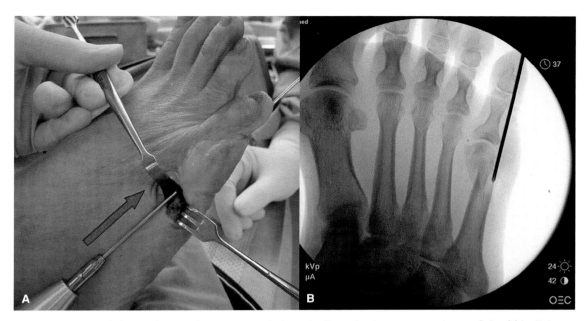

Figure 24–5.   (**A**) Inserting K-wire anterograde into the lateral subcutaneous tissue of the fifth digit. (**B**) Wire advanced to the osteotomy and ready to be driven retrograde back into the fifth metatarsal shaft.

adjacent to the bone in a proximal to distal direction along the longitudinal axis of the fifth toe (Fig. 24–5). The K-wire exits at the lateral distal fifth toe, about 5 mm from lateral border of the nail and is retracted with the drill to the proximal end of the osteotomy (Fig. 24–6). Using a small grooved lever to pry the osteotomy, the correction is obtained by medial displacement of the metatarsal head. Medial transposition of the capital fragment must be done carefully, as overcorrection with less bone contact might lead to malunion or medial

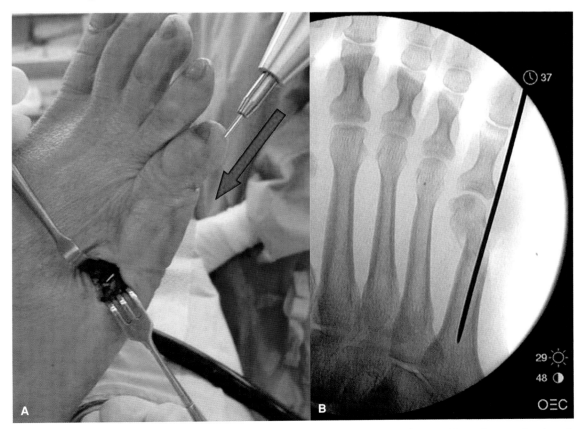

Figure 24–6.   (**A**) Clinical and (**B**) fluoroscopic views of K-wire being advanced into the proximal end of osteotomy after medial displacement of the distal fragment.

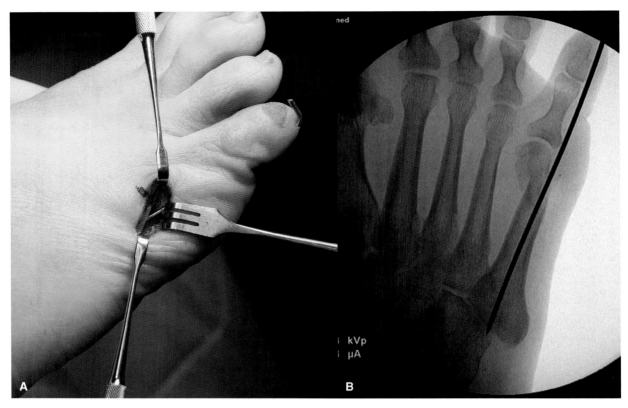

Figure 24–7. Final intraoperative (**A**) and fluoroscopic (**B**) results after fixation of the displaced osteotomy with the K-wire.

subluxation (Fig. 24–7). Stabilization of the correction is obtained by inserting the K-wire into the diaphyseal canal in a distal to proximal direction until the metatarsal base is reached. The K-wire acts as a buttress to prevent loss of position of distal fragment. If the cut edge of the metatarsal is laterally prominent, a small wedge of bone can be removed. No soft tissue procedure is necessary because sufficient displacement of the metatarsal head provides realignment of the fifth toe under the image intensifier fluoroscopy. The skin is sutured with a single 3-0 absorbable stitch (Fig. 24–8). The K-wire is bent and cut at the tip of the toe.

COMPLICATIONS

Major complications, such as nonunion, osteonecrosis, recurrent deformity, or degenerative arthritis, seem to be extremely rare and have not been observed in previous studies.[8,9] In a series of 50 consecutive symptomatic bunionette deformities treated using this technique, Giannini et al.[8] found that no major complications, such as avascular necrosis of the metatarsal head or nonunion occurred. In 12% (6 out of 50 feet) of patients, delayed unions were observed. However, none showed displacement nor increased postoperative pain. Two percent (1 out of 50 feet) of patients had skin irritation around the K-wire and 4% (2 out of 50 feet) of patients reported

symptomatic plantar callosities under the fourth metatarsal head. Legenstein et al.[9] reported pin site infection in 4 out of 77 feet. In two cases of infection, the K-wire was removed earlier than other cases. All cases of infection were treated with oral or intravenous antibiotics without complications. There was one transfer lesion under the fourth metatarsal head, which was managed with shoe inserts. In the author's experience treating 22 patients (26 feet) for bunionette deformity using this technique, there were no malunions, nonunions, or delayed unions or other perioperative complications.[10]

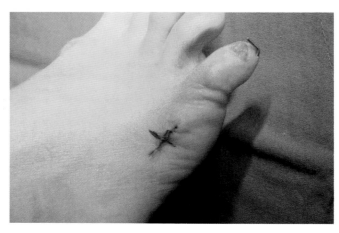

Figure 24–8. Skin closure.

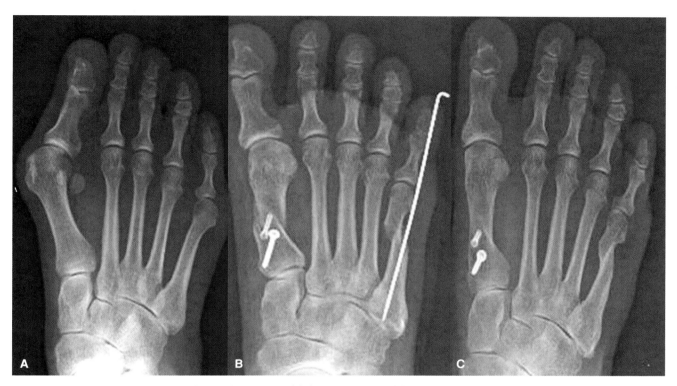

Figure 24–9. Dorsoplantar radiographic views of (**A**) preoperative, (**B**) approximately 6 weeks postoperative, and (**C**) final postoperative fifth metatarsal of a patient who underwent minimally invasive bunionette deformity correction.

REHABILITATION PROTOCOL

The patient is instructed to rest and elevate their extremity after surgery. The bulky compression dressing holding the lesser toe in a corrected position is changed the following day and at daily intervals for 2 weeks. Weight bearing to tolerance is allowed from the day of surgery on the heel and medial forefoot in a hard-soled postoperative shoe with open toe box. The sutures are removed at 2 weeks, and the K-wire is remained until 4 weeks. After the pin is removed, gentle active and passive range of motion is begun. The postoperative shoe is discontinued at 4 to 6 weeks when evidence of bone healing and stability of the osteotomy are confirmed on x-ray (Fig. 24–9).

OUTCOME

There are only a few reports available on the outcome of bunionette deformity correction with percutaneous distal metatarsal osteotomy. Giannini et al.[8] reported a series of 32 patients with 50 feet affected by symptomatic bunionette deformity. The average follow-up was 4.8 years. The average modified lesser toe American Orthopaedic Foot & Ankle Society (AOFAS) score significantly increased from 62.8 ± 15.2 to 94 ± 6.8 ($p < 0.0005$). The average fifth metatarsophalangeal angle (MPA) decreased from 16.8 ± 5.1 degrees to 7.9 ± 3.1 degrees ($p < 0.0005$). The fourth-fifth intermetatarsal angle (IMA) improved from 12 ± 1.7 degrees to 6.7 ± 1.7 degrees at the last follow-up ($p < 0.0005$).

REFERENCES

1. Koti M, Maffulli N. Bunionette. *J Bone Joint Surg Am.* 2001;83-A:1076–1082.
2. Trnka HJ, Hofmann S, Wiesauer H, et al. Kramer versus Austin osteotomy: Two distal metatarsal osteotomies for correction of hallux valgus deformities. *Orthopaed Internat Ed.* 1997;5:110–116.
3. Lamprecht E, Kramer J. Die metatarsale-I-Osteotomie nach Kramer zur behandlung des hallux valgus. *Orthop Prax.* 1982;28:635–645.
4. Kramer J. Die Kramer-Osteotomie zur behandlung des hallux valgus und des digitus quintus varus. *Operat Orthop Traumat.* 1990;2:29–38.
5. Lamprecht E, Kramer J. Die retrokapitale osteotomie nach Kramer und ihre stabitisierung ohne schraube, platte oder gips. *Z Orthop Ihre Grenzgeb.* 1984;22:607.
6. Bösch P, Markowski H, Rannischer V. Technik und erste ergebnisse der subkutanen distalen metatarsale-I-osteotomie. *Orthopa Prax.* 1990;26:51–56.
7. Bösch P, Wanke S, Legenstein R. Hallux valgus correction by the method of Bösch: A new technique with a seven-to-ten-year follow-up. *Foot Ankle Clin.* 2000;5:485–498.
8. Giannini S, Faldini C, Vannini F, et al. The minimally invasive osteotomy "S.E.R.I." (simple, effective, rapid, inexpensive) for correction of bunionette deformity. *Foot Ankle Int.* 2008;29:282–286.
9. Legenstein R, Bonomo J, Huber W, et al. Correction of tailor's bunion with the Boesch technique: A retrospective study. *Foot Ankle Int.* 2007;28:799–803.
10. Kim SY, Park KH, Lee JW. Treatment of Bunionette deformity with S.E.R.I (simple, effective, rapid, inexpensive) operation. *J Korean Foot Ankle Soc.* 2010;14(1):25–30.

CHAPTER 25

The Fibula Nail for the Management of Unstable Ankle Fractures

Paul Appleton

The traditional method of open reduction and internal fixation (ORIF) of ankle fractures has changed very little since the 1960s. Traditional ORIF may lead to complications including wound dehiscence and infection, especially in higher risk patients such as those with diabetes or immunocompromise. Bulky plates in combination with tenuous skin around the lateral malleolus has led to infection rates or wound problems as high as 30 percent in some series.[1] A technique of fibula nailing has been developed that requires minimal incisions around the ankle and much lower profile hardware.[2] Several studies have supported the use of the fibula nail and have shown complication rates to be lower than traditional ORIF.[3]

INDICATIONS

Indications for the use of the fibula nail are any displaced ankle fracture that involves the lateral malleolus. We typically do not use if for high Weber C type fractures such as those treated with syndesmotic screws alone. It can also be used for fixation of lateral malleolus fractures with an associated tibial pilon fracture. Currently available fibula nails offer the possibility of placing syndesmotic screws through the nail, which was not possible previously. One must use caution in trimalleolar ankle fractures involving a large posterior fragment, as these patterns tend to do better with direct open posterior plating. In these cases a standard or minifragment plates are used as the surgical approach the fibula has already been performed and the advantage of minimal incisions is no longer beneficial.

PATIENT POSITIONING

Patients are positioned supine on a radiolucent table with a small bump under the greater trochanter to allow easier access to the lateral ankle. A tourniquet is placed but rarely inflated. Once the operative extremity has been prepped and draped, a small stack of towels can be placed under the heel to elevate the ankle to allow easier access for gaining the entry point for the fibula nail.

SURGICAL APPROACHES

A 0.5- to 1.0-cm incision should be made just distal to the tip of the fibula (Fig. 25–1). Blunt dissection can be carried out with a small clamp to avoid injuring the peroneal tendons although they are typically located posterior and distal to the incision. A guidewire is inserted into the distal fibula just at the tip and in midsaggital line of the bone. It is important to check a lateral view to insure the entry point is not too anterior or posterior (Fig. 25–2). A cannulated drill is then passed over the K-wire to open the canal approximately 2 cm in length (Fig. 25–3). Alternatively an awl can be used to establish an entry point (Fig. 25–4).

REDUCTION TECHNIQUES

Percutaneous reduction clamps can be placed around the fracture to hold it reduced before reaming and placing the nail (Fig. 25–5). Once the fracture is reduced the fibula

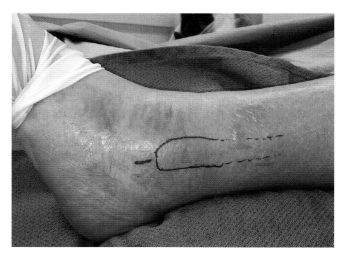

Figure 25–1. Incision for fibula nail insertion just inferior to tip of lateral malleolus.

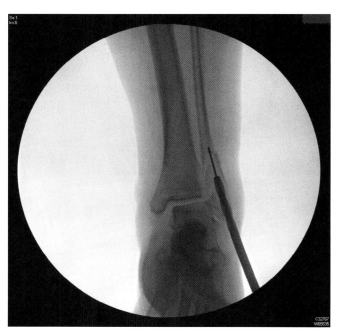

Figure 25–3. A cannulated drill is passed over the K-wire distal to the fracture.

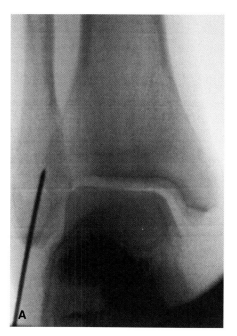

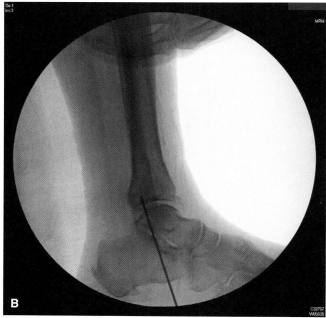

Figure 25–2. **A:** A 1.2-mm K-wire is inserted just at the tip of the lateral malleolus with the aid of intra-op fluoroscopy. **B:** The lateral view will ensure that the K-wire is in the center of the fibula.

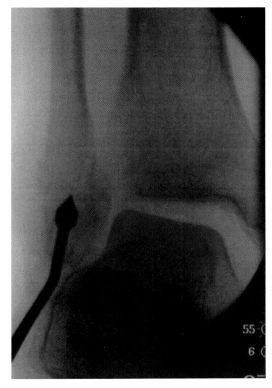

Figure 25–4.   Alternatively an awl can be used to establish an entry point for the nail.

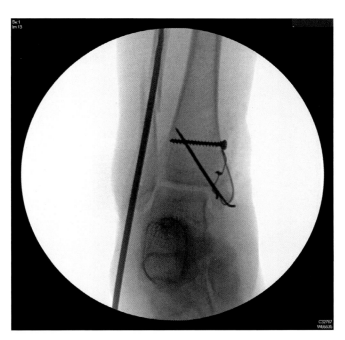

Figure 25–6.   Hand reamers are used to enable passing the fibula nail with little resistance.

canal is reamed with a 3.1-mm hand reamer (Fig. 25–6). If there is little resistance using the 3.1-mm reamer, a second 3.6-mm reamer can be used which will allow the use of the larger fibula nail (3.5 mm in diameter).

FIXATION

The fibula nail is now inserted using the percutaneous insertion guide (Fig. 25–7). One or two anterior to posterior screws are now placed through the nail. Fibula length can be assessed intraoperatively using C-arm and the

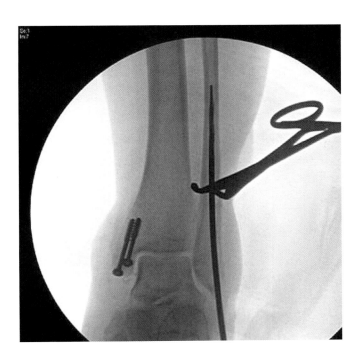

Figure 25–5.   A pointed reduction clamp can be placed percutaneously onto the fracture to hold it reduced before reaming and placing the fibula nail.

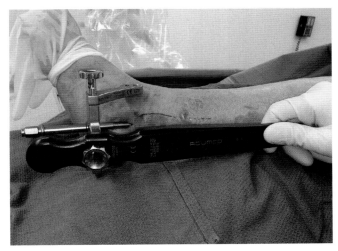

Figure 25–7.   The fibula nail is now inserted using the percutaneous locking guide.

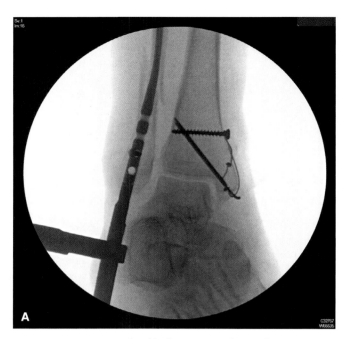

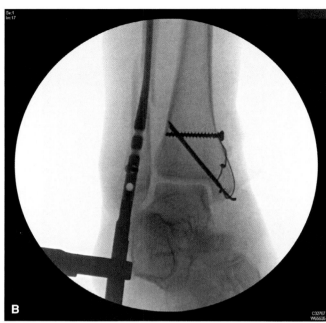

Figure 25–8.   A: The fibula remains short after the initial anterior–posterior locking screw has been placed. **B:** Longitudinal traction can be pulled on the guide lengthening the fibula prior to either syndesmotic or blocking screw placement.

assessing the talocrural angle. Obtaining intra-op images of the contralateral ankle can be helpful for comparison. If the fibula appears shortened longitudinal traction can be placed on the guide after an AP screw has been placed

(Fig. 25–8). Once length has been restored a blocking screw is placed at the proximal tip of the nail to maintain length (Fig. 25–9). Alternatively once length has been established and there is evidence of a syndesmotic widening, one or two screws can be placed through the nail to both maintain length and stabilize the syndesmosis. A temporary large pointed reduction clamp is used to hold the syndesmosis reduced prior to instrumentation (Fig. 25–10). After

Figure 25–9. A blocking screw is placed proximal to the nail through the insertion guide to prevent further shortening.

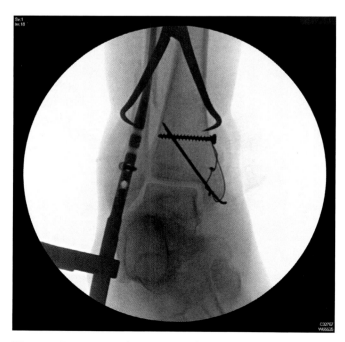

Figure 25–10. A large pointed reduction clamp can be placed percutaneously to hold the syndesmosis reduced.

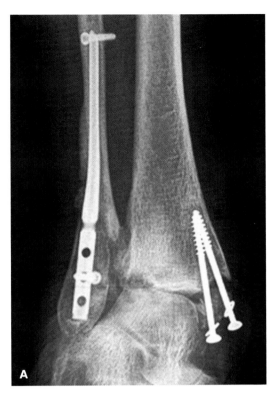
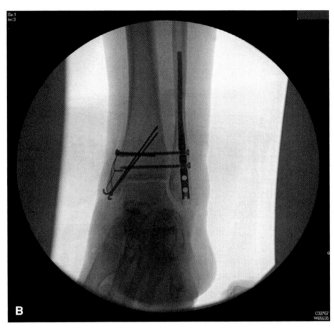

Figure 25–11.   A: Loss of fixation can occur in elderly patients with poor bone quality. **B:** We now routinely use syndesmotic screws in these patients to provide a stronger lateral construct to act more like a buttress to prevent loss of reduction.

placing the AP screw and a blocking screw at the tip of the nail, stress views are routinely taken intraoperatively to assess the syndesmosis. Any widening or talar shift warrants surgical fixation with up to two screws which can be percutaneously placed through the nail using the insertion guide. Once the nail has been secured, the surgeon can address the medial malleolus fracture if present. We have found that it can be beneficial to fix the medial malleolus fracture first as it helps restore fibula length, alignment and reduction before placing the fibula nail, but either side can be done first based on surgeon preference.

Complications: The fibular nail inserted through a percutaneous manner has been shown to have a lower complication rate when compared to formal ORIF using AO techniques. In series by Bugler et al.[4] there were no wound complications as compared to 16% in the open reduction group. Other series using the Biomet SST fibula nail reported one failure out of 35.[5] This fibula nail however did not allow the placement of syndesmotic screws through it.

In the elderly, osteoporotic patients, loss of fixation can occur with the use of the nail. Because of the poor quality bone we now routinely place syndesmotic screws in the elderly patients to allow the nail to act as a lateral buttress and have more stability to the overall ankle joint (Fig. 25–11).

REHABILITATION PROTOCOL

Upon completion of surgery, patients are placed in a standard, well-padded AO plaster splint. They return to clinic 10 to 14 days following their operation for suture removal and repeat x-rays. If there is not a syndesmotic injury, we typically place them in a removable Aircast boot and allow them to start range of motion and begin weight bearing as tolerated. If there has been a syndesmotic injury or they have diabetes or other form of neuropathy, we restrict weight bearing for up to 3 months.

OUTCOME

Several series have evaluated the Acumed fibula nail including a prospective randomized trial of 100 patients comparing the nail to traditional ORIF.[4] Bugler et al. reported significantly fewer wound complications with the fibula nail group. No infections or wound problems were reported in the fibula nail group and only one patient required a prominent locking screw to be removed; as compared to the ORIF group where eight patients (16%) developed wound infections and six elected to have their metalwork removed. The authors found that the overall cost of treatment in the fibula nail group was lower

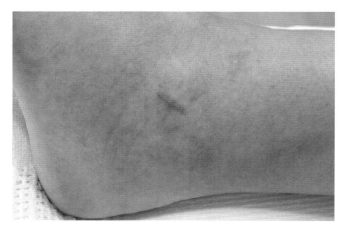

Figure 25–12. Skin incisions at 6-month postoperative visit.

than traditional ORIF despite the initial higher cost of the implant. At 1 year the fibula nail patients were also significantly more happy with the condition of their scar and had slightly (although not significantly) better Olerud and Molander ankle scores (Fig. 25–12).

CONCLUSIONS

In conclusion, we have found the fibula nail to be a viable minimally invasive technique for stabilizing displaced ankle fractures. It allows early weight bearing in nonneuropathic patients and has been found to have a lower complication rate and equivalent outcome scores to traditional ORIF.

REFERENCES

1. Lamontagne J, Blachut PA, Broekhuyse HM, et al. Surgical treatment of a displaced lateral malleolus fracture: The antiglide technique versus lateral plate fixation. *J Orthop Trauma.* 2002;16:498–502.
2. Appleton P, McQueen M, Court-Brown C. The fibula nail for treatment of ankle fractures in elderly and high risk patients. *Tech Foot Ankle.* 2006;5:204–208.
3. Bugler KE, Watson CD, Hardie AR, et al. The treatment of unstable fractures of the ankle using the Acumed fibular nail. Development of a technique. *Bone Joint Surg Br.* 2012;94(8):1107–1112.
4. Bugler, KE, White TO, Appleton PT, et al. A prospective, randomized controlled trial of a fibula nail versus standard open reduction internal fixation for fixation of ankle fractures in elderly patients. *Bone Joint Surg Br.* 2013;95 (suppl 25):8.
5. Ramasamy PR, Sherry P. The role of the fibula nail in the management of Weber type B ankle fractures in the elderly patients with osteoporotic bone: A preliminary report. *Injury.* 2001;32:477–485.

CHAPTER 26

Minimally Invasive Surgical Techniques for the Treatment of High-Energy Tibial Pilon Fractures

John P. Ketz   Roy Sanders

INTRODUCTION

High-energy tibial plafond or pilon fractures are complex injuries that involve the articular surface of the distal tibia. These articular fractures can have a wide range of patterns.[1–6] However, there is always an associated soft tissue injury, and it is often the soft tissue envelope that dictates the method and timing of fixation. Historically, acute open reduction internal fixation (ORIF) was used with some success with low-energy injuries, but poor outcomes and increased complications arose when acute fixation was used for higher-energy injuries.[1,3,6–10] External fixation techniques with no or limited internal fixation, were then tried, but these techniques did not improve outcomes and unfortunately were still associated with a high number of complications.[11–18] In an attempt to decrease complications and improve outcomes, staged treatment protocols were developed.[4,19] This concept used temporary external fixation to allow soft tissue edema to decrease until definitive ORIF could be performed. This has been the mainstay of treatment for high-energy injuries for the last twenty years. As our expertise with these fractures has improved, current trends have shifted to using multiple approaches that are even more benign to the soft tissues. These utilize direct visualization and fixation of the articular fragments in combination with minimal incisions to reconstruct the metaphyseal–diaphyseal dissociation.

INDICATIONS

There is little role for the nonoperative treatment of displaced or impacted tibial pilon fractures. It is typically reserved for truly nondisplaced fractures or for patients who have severe contraindications to surgical intervention. The goal of the surgery is not only to restore an anatomic reduction to the joint surface but to realign the mechanical alignment of the distal tibia as well. It is well understood that poor articular reductions and residual tibiotalar incongruity are poorly tolerated by patients and lead to early arthrosis of the ankle joint. There are a number of different techniques available for treatment of these injuries ranging from external fixation to open fixation, or a combination of both. The surgical management of pilon fractures depends on fracture pattern, soft tissue quality, and surgeon preference.

PREOPERATIVE ASSESSMENT

Patients are typically seen in the emergency setting and prompt reduction with splinting optimizes soft tissue management. Following splinting, formal radiographs should be obtained of the tibia and fibula as well as the ankle. A computed tomography (CT) scan may be obtained before initial stabilization with external fixation. This is more appropriate for a lower-energy pattern that may be treated acutely using percutaneous techniques. For higher-energy patterns, due to the concern of radiation exposure, CT scans should be obtained after initial external fixation. Because external fixation will realign the lower extremity, a CT thereafter will offer a much improved evaluation of the articular surface. In addition, Tornetta and Gorup[20] have shown the importance of CT scans in planning surgical incisions based on the fracture pattern.

OPERATIVE TECHNIQUES

In virtually all fractures, the first consideration is the fibula. The role of the fibula with respect to the ankle is important in that it establishes length as well as rotation. Often with a high-energy pilon fracture, there can be significant tibial metaphyseal comminution and/or a segmental defect. Because tibial length is difficult to judge, anatomic fixation of the fibula offers the best guide for definitive fixation of the tibia. Additionally, once the fibula is fixed, a stable lateral buttress of the ankle exists and this can obviate the need for lateral-based external fixation. There are a number of fixation techniques for fibular fixation including formal open reduction, percutaneous plating, intramedullary screw fixation, and intramedullary wire fixation. The authors recommend that fibular fixation only be performed by the surgeon who definitively treats the fracture. This will ensure that further incisions or treatment strategies are not compromised due to a previous incision from another surgeon.

FIBULAR FIXATION

Percutaneous Plating

The patient is placed supine on the operating table. A small 2-cm incision is placed over the posterolateral malleolus distally. The peroneal fascia is incised and the tendons are retracted posteriorly. A periosteal elevator can then be used to elevate the peroneal tendons from the posterior aspect of the fibula. A one-third tubular plate is of appropriate length is selected and passed percutaneously proximally along the posterolateral aspect of the fibula. By placing the plate beneath the peroneal fascia, the risk of injuring the superficial peroneal nerve is minimized. A separate incision is then made under fluoroscopic guidance at the proximal extent of the plate. A small tissue dissector is used to identify the plate under the peroneal fascia. The plate is stabilized proximally using 3.5-mm cortical screws. With the plate fixated proximally, attention is turned distally where the fracture is reduced using manual techniques. Next, a medial external fixator is placed across the ankle and traction applied through the ankle joint. The distal fibular fragment can be "fine tuned" through the distal based incision with the aid of pointed fracture reduction clamps. If needed, 1.6-mm K-wires can be placed through the distal fibula into the lateral aspect of the talar body or distal tibia temporarily for added fixation. Once the appropriate length and rotation of the distal fibula is confirmed, 3.5-mm cortical or 4.0-mm cancellous screws are placed distally through the plate. The wound is then irrigated and closed in layered fashion (Fig. 26–1).

Intramedullary Fixation

This technique should be reserved for transverse or short-oblique fractures of the fibula that have minimal comminution. A 1 to 2 cm incision is made over the tip of the lateral malleolus. A medial external fixator is placed across the ankle and traction applied for reduction purposes. The distal fracture segment is stabilized with a pointed reduction clamp. Inversion of the hindfoot should be applied to allow better access to the distal fibula. After drilling, an intramedullary fibular nail is passed. The nail should be placed at a minimum of 4 to 6 cm proximal to the most proximal extent of the fracture.

If a long screw is used, an additional K-wire placed distally across the fibula into the lateral aspect of the talar body is recommended to prevent rotation of the distal fragment while placing the screw. This wire must be placed away from the trajectory of the drill bit, either anteriorly or posteriorly. A 2.5-mm drill bit is placed directly on the tip of the lateral malleolus and drilled across the fracture site under fluoroscopic guidance. Countersinking should be used to minimize prominence of the screw head. The path must be tapped to prevent incarceration of the screw during insertion. A 3.5-mm screw is passed across the fracture site. As with nail insertion, the screw should be 4 to 6 cm proximal to the most proximal extent of the fracture (Fig. 26–2).

Technical tip: If difficulty is encountered passing the drill bit across the fracture site, a 1.6-mm K-wire can be placed in the medullary canal and overdrilled using a cannulated drill bit, slightly past the fracture site. The cannulated tap and counter sink can then be used to create the path for the screw. A cannulated or solid 4.0-mm cortical screw can then be inserted.

When there are associated fractures of the fibula and tibia, newer techniques for limited internal fixation can be applied. Dunbar et al.[21] advocated limited fixation of proximal tibial fracture segments using anterior, medial, and lateral based incisions. By stabilizing the tibial fracture fragment this converted the fracture from a complete articular pattern to a partial articular fracture. Thus, it simplifies the fracture pattern and allows for less-invasive definitive surgical techniques. The authors have extended

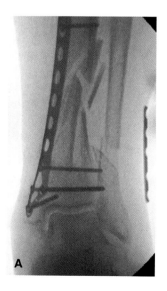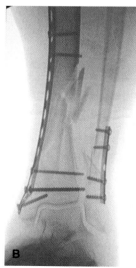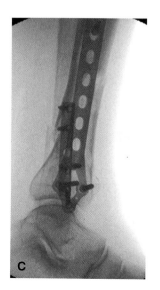

Figure 26–1. Intraoperative fluoroscopic views of percutaneous plating of a distal tibia-fibula fracture. An external fixator was used to restore the length and alignment of the fracture. (**A**) The tibia was initially percutaneously plated. Using fluoroscopy, the length of the fibular plate is then confirmed. The plate is then placed through a small incision distally and fixed proximally with a separate small incision. Final fixation as shown in (**B**) mortise and (**C**) lateral views.

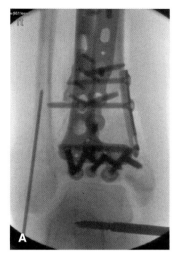 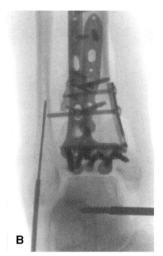 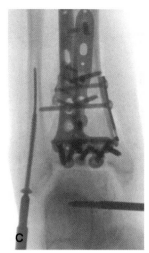 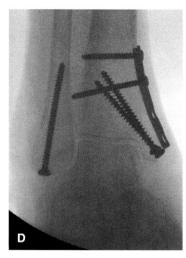

Figure 26–2. Percutaneous fixation of a distal fibula fracture. (**A**) A 1.6-mm K-wire is placed, through a small incision distally, into the fibular intramedullary canal. (**B**) The K-wire is then over-drilled and (**C**) a cannulated screw is placed across the fracture. (**D**) Alternatively, this can be performed with a solid screw using lag technique.

this technique to include fixation of the displaced posterior malleolar fracture fragment initially with fixation of the fibula, if appropriate, through a posterolateral approach. This has been the authors' preferred treatment method for high-energy injuries involving a displaced posterior malleolar fragment.[22]

Open Reduction and Fixation

The patient is bought into the operating room and placed in the prone position. A tourniquet is placed high on the extremity. The lower limb is then prepped and draped in sterile fashion. The authors routinely exsanguinate the limb with an Esmarch bandage, before inflating the tourniquet. A posterolateral incision is then made midway between the posterior border of the fibula and lateral aspect of the Achilles tendon. The length of the incision is dictated by the proximal extent of the posterior tibial fracture fragment as seen on a fluoroscopic image. Sharp dissection is carried down through skin and subcutaneous tissues. Care is taken to protect the sural nerve. Dissection is carried down to the peroneal fascia. If the fibula is fractured, the fascia is split and the tendons are retracted medially to expose the posterolateral aspect of the fibula (Fig. 26–3). The fibula is then reduced with reduction clamps. If appropriate, a lag screw is placed through the fibula and a neutralization plate applied. Often, there is significant comminution of the fibula and bridge plating is required. Care should be taken in plating the fibula to restore the proper anatomic length, alignment, and rotation. Again, this can best be performed under fluoroscopic guidance.

Operative Technique—Stage 1

Through the posterolateral incision another fascial plane is created medial to the peroneal tendons. The flexor hallucis

longus and associated soft tissue are retracted medially, exposing the entire distal and posterior aspect of the tibia. The posterior malleolar fragment typically has a metadiaphyseal spike that can be reduced to the posterior aspect of the tibial shaft, but many times this "key" is fractured and care must be taken to reposition the malleolar fragment anatomically. This reduction is critical to the success of the procedure, as subsequent anterior reconstruction will be based on the proper position of the posterior malleolus. Anatomic reduction of the posterior malleolar fragment also aids in the restoration of the integrity of the ankle syndesmosis (Fig. 26–3). A small or mini fragment plate is then applied spanning the fracture in a buttress or antiglide mode, and secured proximally with cortical screws. If screws are required distally for stability of the posterior malleolar fragment(s), unicortical screws (10 to 14 mm) should be used to prevent interference with the subsequent reduction of the anterior fragments. For this reason, small fragment locking plates are ideal (Fig. 26–4). Reduction and fixation of the posterior components creates a stable buttress for the anterior fragments to be reduced to at the time of final fixation. In essence, a complete articular fracture (OTA 43C) is converted into a partial articular fracture (OTA 43B). Following stabilization of the posterior aspect of the tibia, final images are obtained to evaluate for proper length of the posterior aspect of the tibia and fibula. At this point the wound is thoroughly irrigated and layered closure is performed. The skin is closed with interrupted 3-0 nylon sutures.

Following closure of the wound, the lower leg is flexed to 90 degrees at the knee. Two 5-mm half pins are placed proximal to the fracture site anteriorly. The pins should be placed well proximal to the estimated location of the proximal end of the plate that will be used for definitive anterior fixation. A calcaneal transfixion

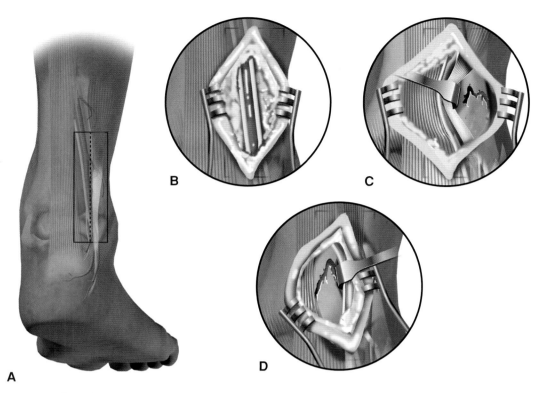

Figure 26–3.   A posterolateral incision is used for initial internal fixation in combination with external fixation. (**A**) An incision is placed between the lateral border of the Achilles tendon and the posteromedial aspect of the fibula (dotted line). (**B**) The neurovascular structures are dissected and protected. (**C**) Retracting the peroneal tendons medially allows for direct visualization and fixation of the fibula fracture. (**D**) Retracting the peroneal tendons laterally allows for exposure of the posterior malleolar fragment.

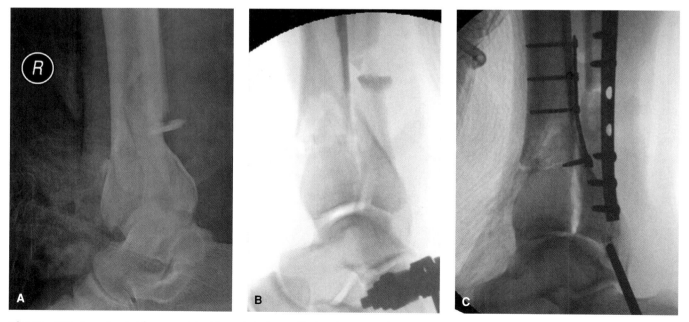

Figure 26–4.   A mini fragment locking plate is applied to buttress the posterior malleolar fragment and convert a C-type pilon fracture into a B-type. Lateral views are shown. (**A**) Injury film. (**B**) Intraoperative view after application of external fixator. (**C**) Intraoperative fluoroscopic view after placement of fibular plate and posterior tibial plate. Note that a unicortical short locking screw has been placed in the distal fragment providing stabilization without blocking anterior reduction.

pin is placed under fluoroscopic guidance to complete the simple delta frame. Additional pins in the first metatarsal or talus may be added, if needed for stability, and to prevent an equinus contracture. Bars and clamps are then placed, and gentle longitudinal traction is applied to pull the fracture out to length. Any bone fragments that are tenting the skin are manually pushed back into place to prevent pressure necrosis. The frame is then tightened. The tourniquet is released, wounds and pins are dressed and the patient is taken to the recovery room.

Postoperative Care—Stage 1

Following initial stabilization a CT scan is also recommended to visualize the articular component of the fracture. Following external fixation, the effect of ligamentotaxis will change the alignment of the articular segments. Also, if staged fixation of the fibula or tibia is to be performed, this allows for an accurate assessment of reduction. This allows the surgeon to plan for immediate or delayed strategies for revision of poorly reduced fragments. On postoperative day 2, the skin incisions are examined and the patient is started on daily pin care (50% peroxide: 50% water). The patient is typically discharged within 1 to 2 days after stage 1, and followed on a weekly basis in the outpatient clinic until the soft tissues are able to safely tolerate definitive fixation. Radiographs are checked at each visit. The definitive, second-stage surgery must be performed within 2 to 3 weeks of injury however, if the surgeon is to obtain a successful reduction of the fragments.

Operative Technique—Stage 2

The patient is placed supine with a bolster under the operative leg. The external fixation frame is removed with the pins left in place and prepped into the sterile field. The pins can be used for distraction purposes with reapplication of the external fixator or a femoral distractor. The limb is exsanguinated and the tourniquet inflated. Although an anterolateral, anteromedial (Schatzger or Tampa), or a straight anterior midline approach may be used, the authors favor the latter. This incision allows for complete visualization of the anteromedial and anterolateral surface of the distal tibia, and allows for the placement of either a medial or anterolateral "pilon" plate. It is also the authors' incision of choice if an ankle fusion or replacement is required in the future.

The anterior midline approach consists of a 4- to 6-cm incision centered over the ankle, with most of the incision proximal to the joint. After the skin incision is made, care must be taken to find and protect the superficial peroneal nerve, which crosses the wound from the lateral side, distally. The extensor retinaculum is then incised in line with the skin incision, several centimeters proximal to the ankle joint exposing the anterior tibial (AT) and extensor hallucis longus (EHL) tendons. Care must be taken to find the anterior tibial artery and deep peroneal nerve just medial to the EHL tendon at the level

of the joint. This part of the dissection is best performed using a Metzenbaum or tenotomy scissors. The neurovascular bundle should be moved laterally with the EHL, the AT should be moved medially. This exposes the ankle capsule. The exposure of the joint should be through the major tears in the soft tissue envelope. If needed, the joint capsule can be incised with a knife in a longitudinal direction, in line with the skin incision at the level of the articular surface. If the skin incision is to be extended proximally to permit plate application to the medial shaft, the incision should stay slightly lateral to the anterior tibial crest to prevent a painful scar (Fig. 26–5).

Once the fragments are identified, typically the medial malleolar fragment is manipulated so that the central impaction can be evaluated. Sequential articular reduction is then performed in a back to front manner, since the posterior aspect of the tibia has been stabilized (Fig. 26–6). If there is impaction of the posterior articular surface, reduction of this should be addressed first. Articular fragments are temporarily reduced with 1.6-mm K-wires. The joint must be reduced under direct visualization, with fluoroscopic imaging used only as an aid. This is best accomplished with the use of a femoral distractor and a head lamp. Free central osteochondral fragments can be stabilized using bioabsorbable pins or held by using the anterior fragment to wedge these pieces into place. Cancellous graft should only be used in cases of metaphyseal impaction, where a central metaphyseal defect is obvious. Local autograft from another portion of the distal tibia, allograft, or iliac autograft may also be used. The medial malleolar fragment is then reduced to "close the book", and this final reduction is held with additional 1.6-mm. K-wires or pointed reduction clamps, or a combination of the two. The metaphyseal segment can then be reduced to the tibial shaft with reduction clamps. This may be done by extending the anterior incision or by percutaneous techniques. Once the anterior tibia and its corresponding articular surface has been properly reduced, independent 2.7, 3.5, and/or 4.0 mm screws should be used to lag the fragments together. Ideally, the anterior articular fragments should be lagged into the posterior fragment.

At this point, stability between the metaphyseal and diaphyseal segments can be achieved through different plating techniques. Finally it must be reiterated that the joint must always be reduced and secured before the shaft is fixed. Even 1 mm malalignment of the shaft will translate into a fairly significant step at the articular surface. If the joint is reduced anatomically however and the shaft is malaligned by 1 to 2 degrees, this will be acceptable in the long term.

Anterior Plating

Anterolateral plating of pilon fractures is the most common method for fixation of the metaphyseal fragment to the tibial shaft. Most manufactures have precontoured plates with locking and nonlocking options for this

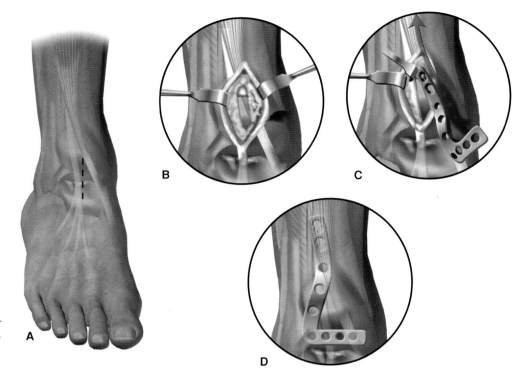

Figure 26–5. A direct anterior incision is created between the tibialis anterior (TA) and the extensor hallucis longus (EHL). The fracture is exposed and well visualized for anatomic fixation. An anterolateral plate can then be placed under the neurovascular structures and used to stabilize the diaphyseal–metaphyseal dissociation.

purpose. Using the anterior incision, the neurovascular bundle should be identified and protected. A periosteal elevator is used to separate the anterior compartment from the anterolateral aspect of the tibia. The plate is passed percutaneously through the anterior incision. The plate is placed over the distal tibial and held temporarily with 1.6-mm K-wires. Appropriate distal placement of the plate should be confirmed with direct and fluoro-

scopic visualization. Also using fluoroscopy, the trajectory of the distal screws of the plate should be assessed to confirm they will not be placed intra-articularly, especially if the surgeon is using the locking option of the plate. Before the plate is secured, proximal positioning of the plate must be evaluated to confirm that the plate is securely aligned with the tibia and not off axis (Fig. 26–7).

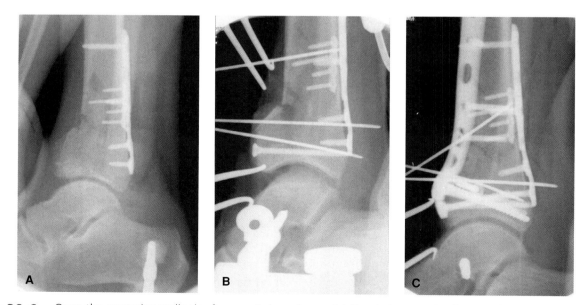

Figure 26–6. Once the posterior malleolar fragments have been stabilized, the anterior fracture fragments and articular surface can be anatomically reduced in a "back to front" fashion to a posterior buttress. Lateral intraoperative views are shown. (**A**) Application of a posterior plate. (**B**) Provisional K-wire and lag screw fixation of anterior fragments to reestablish articular surface of plafond. (**C**) Application of definitive anterior plate fixation to construct.

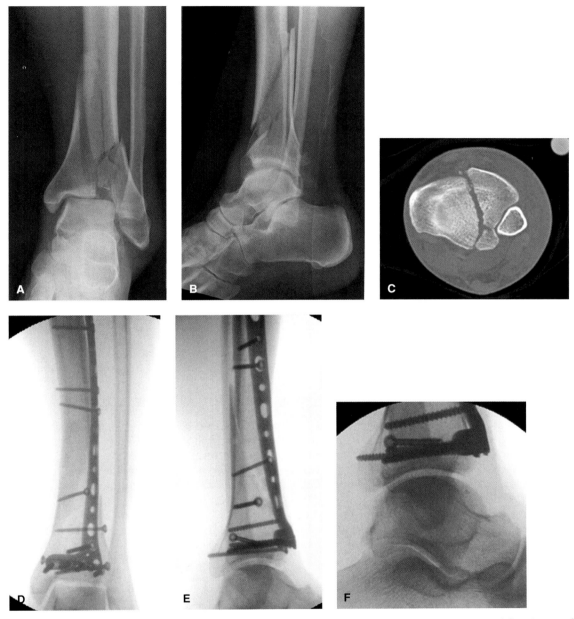

Figure 26–7.   A 48-year-old male with a distal tibial fracture dislocation treated with initial external fixation. Definitive fixation was performed using a minimally invasive anterior incision technique. Imaging of injury (**A**) AP radiographic, (**B**) lateral radiographic, and (**C**) axial CT view at plafond. Intraoperative fluoroscopic imaging after reconstruction (**D**) AP tib-fib, (**E**) lateral tib-fib, and (**F**) lateral ankle.

MEDIAL FIXATION TECHNIQUES

Screw Fixation

Isolated screw fixation is best suited for large, noncomminuted medial malleolar fragments. The fragments can be reduced anatomically through the anterior approach. Care should be taken to restore the appropriate medial clear space and anatomic reduction of the medial shoulder of the distal tibia. Temporary reduction is achieved with 1.6-mm K-wires. A small incision is made, usually less than 1 cm over the tip of the medial malleolus. Under fluoroscopic guidance, a small fragment drill bit can be passed across the fracture site and a 4.0-mm cancellous screw, 40 mm in length is placed to secure the fragment. If additional purchase is needed a cortical screw can be placed bicortically. For this application, a long pelvic drill bit (and screw) will be needed, as screw lengths can be greater than 80 mm. After screw fixation, either a medial plate or anterolateral plate is required to restore stability to the metadiaphyseal dissociation (Fig. 26–8).

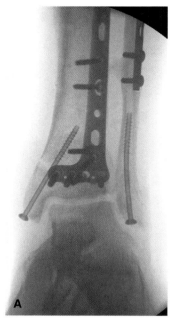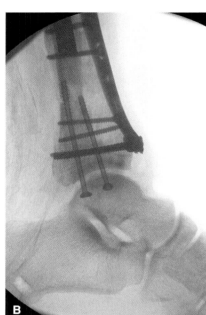

Figure 26–8.   Medial screw fixation. A 24-year-old male with a pilon fracture below a previous injury. An anterior incision was used to stabilize the articular fragments. The medial malleolar fragments were reduced and provisionally held through the anterior incision using direct visualization, while two cannulated screws were used for fixation through a small medial incision. Intraoperative (**A**) AP and (**B**) lateral fluoroscopic views.

Plating

Medial plating can be used to connect the metaphyseal fragment to the diaphysis. It can also be used in conjunction with anterolateral plating to add stability for significantly comminuted fractures through the metaphysis. Medial fragments can be reduced through the anterior incision or percutaneously. A small incision is made over the medial malleolus, starting at the tip of the medial malleolus and carrying the incision 2 to 3 cm proximally centered over the medial aspect of the tibia. Care must be taken to avoid the saphenous neurovascular structures. Once the structures are identified and protected, a periosteal elevator can be used to free the soft tissues from the medial tibia without stripping the periosteum. A medial plate can then be passed percutaneously through the incision. The plate is held distally with K-wires or a unicortical screw. A small incision is made at the proximal aspect of the plate and the plate is positioned in the center of the medial aspect of the tibia (Fig. 26–9). Screw fixation is then used proximally to secure the plate. Additional screws are placed distally through the open incision. Additional screws can then be placed through the plate using a "perfect circles" technique on lateral fluoroscopy (Fig. 26–10). The femoral distractor or external fixator frame is removed, and the ankle is taken through a range of motion under fluoroscopic control. Once a stable anatomic reduction is obtained, external fixator pins are removed, and the wound is thoroughly irrigated. The retinacular layer should be closed with 0-Vicryl sutures and a layered closure performed. The skin is closed with interrupted 3-0 nylon sutures (Fig. 26–11). Dry sterile dressings are placed over the wound and the patient is placed into a posterior, well-padded splint.

Postoperative Care—Stage 2

Postoperatively, plain radiographs and a CT scan with reconstruction images are obtained to verify joint reduction (Fig. 26–12). The limb is then placed into a removable short leg boot prior to discharge typically 2 to 3 days following surgery. Patients begin range-of-motion exercises at 10 days but are kept nonweight bearing. Sutures are removed when the wound is well healed, typically 2 to 6 weeks. Weight bearing is permitted only when the fracture is healed, based on in-office radiographs, typically at 10 to 12 weeks. Patients are followed for a minimum of 1 year, due to the high rate of complications and long-term sequelae from these devastating injuries.

COMPLICATIONS

There is a high rate of complications associated with treating pilon fractures due to a variety of factors. They occur as a result of the injury as well as operative treatment. The sequelae from the injury include stiffness, soft tissue compromise, and joint arthrosis. Some of these are largely uncontrollable as they result from the injury itself. Despite adequate reduction, arthrosis is common and rapidly progressive for high-energy injuries (Fig. 26–13). Surgical intervention may introduce complications such as pin tract infections, deep infections, nonunion, malunion, and wound complications. Adequate soft tissue management, attention to articular reduction, and limited soft tissue stripping is crucial in minimizing complications.

Initially, high rates of wound complications were noted with immediate fixation of pilon fractures, with as much as 67% wound dehiscence.[2,4,10,17] Due to these

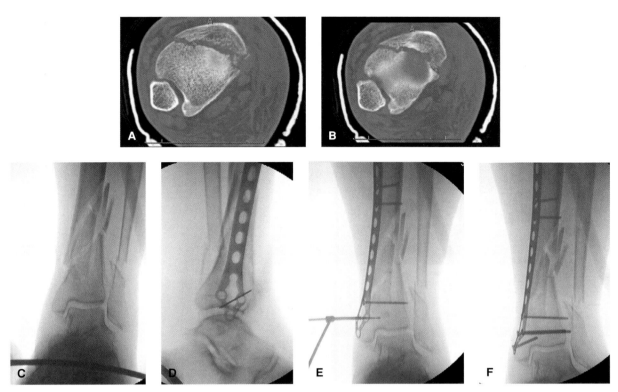

Figure 26–9.   A 38-year-old male with a "simple" intra-articular pilon fracture pattern that was treated with a minimally invasive percutaneous medial plating technique. Axial CT images of the injury (**A**) above and (**B**) within the joint. Intraoperative fluoroscopy of the ankle (**C**) AP view after application of external fixator. (**D**) Lateral view to check for proper provisional placement of plate. (**E**) AP view showing placement of screws distally after fixation proximally. (**F**) Final AP view.

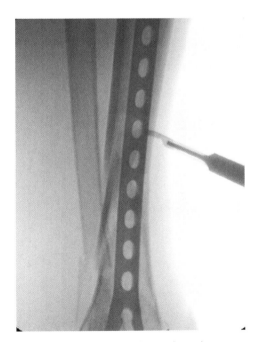

Figure 26–10.   Fluoroscopy is used to place screws through the plate. In this image a scalpel is used to localize the holes within the plate so that percutaneous screw insertion can be performed. Appropriate attention should be paid to restoring sagittal and coronal plane alignment using this technique.

high rates of wound problems, external fixation was used as definitive treatment for these fractures, with or without limited ORIF. Pin tract infections were noted to be 5% to 20%.[11–16] Aside from this, poor reductions and healing were noted with external fixators with the malunion rate noted to be between 5% to 33%.[11–16] The newer techniques that employ initial stabilization with soft tissue optimization have decreased these complication rates. The rates for wound dehiscence are 4% to 5%[4,19,23,24] and the malunion rate also decreased to 4%

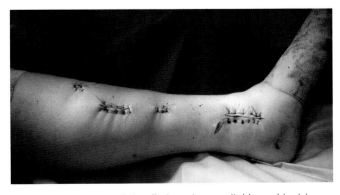

Figure 26–11.   Minimally invasive medial based incisions allow for adequate visualization and fixation of a pilon fracture, while minimizing additional soft tissue trauma.

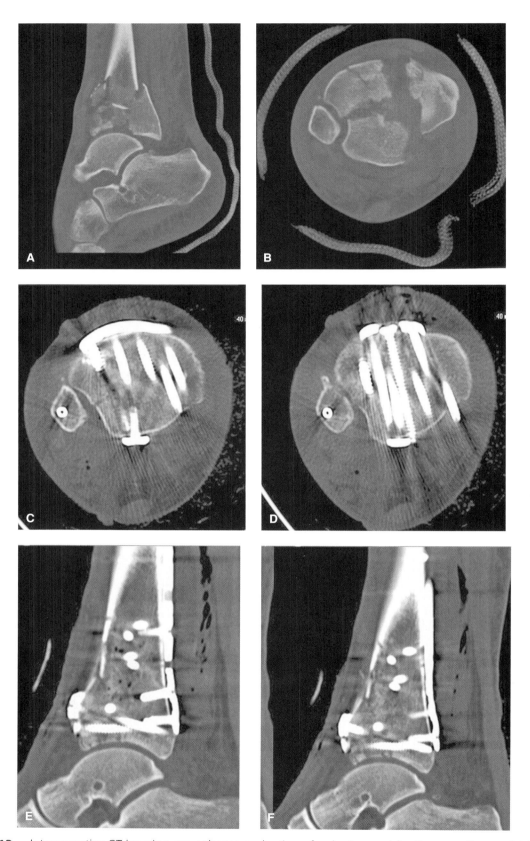

Figure 26–12. Intraoperative CT imaging can enhance evaluation of reduction and fixation over that available from intraoperative fluoroscopy. Preoperative (**A**) sagittal and (**B**) axial views of a C-type pilon fracture. Intraoperative (**C** and **D**) axial and (**E** and **F**) sagittal views after reduction and fixation of the same fracture demonstrates near anatomic alignment and excellent placement of hardware.

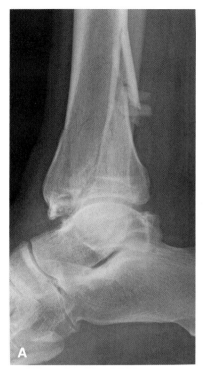
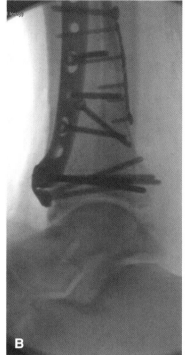
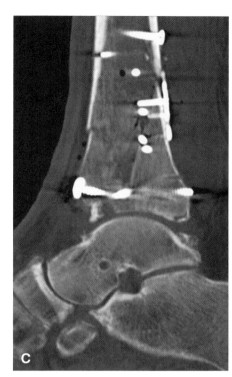

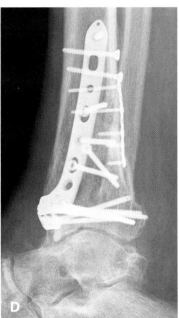

Figure 26–13.   A 56-year-old male with an OTA 43C fracture who underwent a staged protocol for fixation of his fracture. Lateral (**A**) injury radiograph and (**B**) intraoperative fluoroscopy demonstrate anatomic restoration of plafond. (**C**) Sagittal CT scan conforms this. (**D**) Despite an initial adequate reduction, he went on to rapid, progressive ankle arthrosis at 16 months following surgery.

to 5%.[4,19,22,25] Newer studies continue to show decreased rates of wound problems despite immediate ORIF and limited ORIF combined with external fixation.

OUTCOMES

Due to the historic problems with soft tissue management with these injuries, there is an emphasis on using more minimally invasive techniques. These include minimally invasive plate osteosynthesis (MIPO) and addressing the fracture with smaller fragment-specific fixation and smaller, more soft tissue friendly incisions. A combination of these techniques allows for direct inspection and reduction of the joint while minimizing the soft tissue trauma. There have been a number of recent studies evaluating the success of percutaneous plating.

Bahari et al.[26] reviewed a series of 42 pilon fractures treated with a percutaneous AO distal tibial locking plate. There were two cases of superficial infection and one deep.

Although all fractures united in acceptable alignment, articular reduction was not assessed. Lau et al.[27] reviewed a series of 48 patients that were treated with medial locking plates. There was a delayed union rate of 10%, 8% incidence of deep infection. There were a high number of patients with symptomatic hardware that required removal (48%).

Two other studies showed high rates of delayed healing using a medial distal tibial locking plate. Hazarika et al.[28] had 7 of 20 fractures heal at greater than 6 months with two nonunions. Hasenboehler et al.[29] had 4 of 30 patients heal at greater than 6 months, with one failure of fixation and two nonunions. Low soft tissue complications or infections were seen with both studies. Borens et al.[30] reviewed 17 cases in which a percutaneous nonlocking medial plate was used. All fractures healed with minimal soft tissue problems and there were no plate failures. In only four patients, medial plate fixation alone was sufficient for articular reduction, and 10 patients required an anterior arthrotomy for articular visualization. Others have advocated arthroscopically assisted reduction as well. Percutaneous plating without arthrotomy is most successful for lower-energy fractures with little to no joint displacement.

The authors have presented a series of patients who were treated with initial fibular fixation and limited posterior tibial fixation (PL group) with external fixation for high-energy injuries(AO-OTA 43 C2 and C3). These were compared to a cohort of patients treated with a standard anterior approach (A group). Definitive fixation was performed through a small anterior incision with additional medial fixation, if indicated. In that small series there were no wound healing complications and all fractures healed. Articular reduction was assessed using CT scans: seven patients had <1 mm of articular incongruity with two having 1 to 2 mm. Patients who underwent initial limited tibial fixation had improved outcome scores using the AOFAS hindfoot score, Maryland Foot Score (MFS), and SF-36. Also, at a minimum of 2 years follow-up, no patients in the PL group required additional salvage procedures compared to two in the anterior group.[22]

Pilon fractures are difficult to manage and treatment strategies have changed as knowledge has been gained in this area. Soft tissue management is paramount in avoiding complications. Anatomic reduction of the articular surface is key in the fixation of pilon fractures and direct visualization is needed, specifically for higher-energy patterns. Smaller, more soft tissue friendly incisions with fragment-specific fixation are important for success in dealing with these fractures. Percutaneous techniques are useful in minimizing soft tissue trauma. However, articular reduction should not be compromised when using these techniques.

REFERENCES

1. Bourne RB, Rorabeck CH, Macnab J. Intra-articular fractures of the distal tibia: The pilon fracture. *J Trauma.* 1983; 23(7):591–596.

2. Grose A, Gardner MJ, Hettrich C, et al. Open reduction and internal fixation of tibial pilon fractures using a lateral approach. *J Orthop Trauma.* 2007;21(8):530–537.

3. Helfet DL, Koval K, Pappas J, et al. Intraarticular "pilon" fracture of the tibia. *Clin Orthop Relat Res.* 1994;(298): 221–228.

4. Sirkin M, Sanders R, DiPasquale T, et al. A staged protocol for soft tissue management in the treatment of complex pilon fractures. *J Orthop Trauma.* 1999;13(2):78–84.

5. Egol KA, Wolinsky P, Koval KJ. Open reduction and internal fixation of tibial pilon fractures. *Foot Ankle Clin.* 2000;5(4): 873–885.

6. Babis GC, Vayanos ED, Papaioannou N, et al. Results of surgical treatment of tibial plafond fractures. *Clin Orthop Relat Res.* 1997;(341):99–105.

7. Bourne RB. Pylon fractures of the distal tibia. *Clin Orthop Relat Res.* 1989;(240):42–46.

8. Ovadia DN, Beals RK. Fractures of the tibial plafond. *J Bone Joint Surg Am.* 1986;68(4):543–551.

9. Ruedi TP, Allgower M. The operative treatment of intra-articular fractures of the lower end of the tibia. *Clin Orthop Relat Res.* 1979;(138):105–110.

10. Teeny SM, Wiss DA. Open reduction and internal fixation of tibial plafond fractures. Variables contributing to poor results and complications. *Clin Orthop Relat Res.* 1993;(292): 108–117.

11. Anglen JO. Early outcome of hybrid external fixation for fracture of the distal tibia. *J Orthop Trauma.* 1999;13(2): 92–97.

12. Barbieri R, Schenk R, Koval K, et al. Hybrid external fixation in the treatment of tibial plafond fractures. *Clin Orthop Relat Res.* 1996;(332):16–22.

13. Bone L, Stegemann P, McNamara K, et al. External fixation of severely comminuted and open tibial pilon fractures. *Clin Orthop Relat Res.* 1993;(292):101–107.

14. Marsh JL, Bonar S, Nepola JV, et al. Use of an articulated external fixator for fractures of the tibial plafond. *J Bone Joint Surg Am.* 1995;77(10):1498–1509.

15. Marsh JL, Nepola JV, Wuest TK, et al. Unilateral external fixation until healing with the dynamic axial fixator for severe open tibial fractures. *J Orthop Trauma.* 1991;5(3):341–348.

16. Tornetta P, 3rd, Weiner L, Bergman M, et al. Pilon fractures: Treatment with combined internal and external fixation. *J Orthop Trauma.* 1993;7(6):489–496.

17. Wyrsch B, McFerran MA, McAndrew M, et al. Operative treatment of fractures of the tibial plafond. A randomized, prospective study. *J Bone Joint Surg Am.* 1996;78(11): 1646–1657.

18. Dickson KF, Montgomery S, Field J. High energy plafond fractures treated by a spanning external fixator initially and followed by a second stage open reduction internal fixation of the articular surface–preliminary report. *Injury.* 2001;32 Suppl 4:SD92–SD98.

19. Patterson MJ, Cole JD. Two-staged delayed open reduction and internal fixation of severe pilon fractures. *J Orthop Trauma.* 1999;13(2):85–91.

20. Tornetta P, 3rd, Gorup J. Axial computed tomography of pilon fractures. *Clin Orthop Relat Res.* 1996;(323):273–276.

21. Dunbar RP, Barei DP, Kubiak EN, et al. Early limited internal fixation of diaphyseal extensions in select pilon fractures:

Upgrading AO/OTA type C fractures to AO/OTA type B. *J Orthop Trauma.* 2008;22(6):426–429.

22. Ketz J, Sanders R. Staged posterior tibial plating for the treatment of Orthopaedic Trauma Association 43C2 and 43C3 tibial pilon fractures. *J Orthop Trauma.* 2012;26(6):341–347.

23. White TO, Guy P, Cooke CJ, et al. The results of early primary open reduction and internal fixation for treatment of OTA 43.C-type tibial pilon fractures: a cohort study. *J Orthop Trauma.* 2010;24(12):757–763.

24. Boraiah S, Kemp TJ, Erwteman A, et al. Outcome following open reduction and internal fixation of open pilon fractures. *J Bone Joint Surg Am.* 2010;92(2):346–352.

25. Thordarson DB. Complications after treatment of tibial pilon fractures: prevention and management strategies. *J Am Acad Orthop Surg.* 2000;8(4):253–265.

26. Bahari S, Lenehan B, Khan H, et al. Minimally invasive percutaneous plate fixation of distal tibia fractures. *Acta Orthop Belg.* 2007;73(5):635–640.

27. Lau TW, Leung F, Chan CF, et al. Wound complication of minimally invasive plate osteosynthesis in distal tibia fractures. *Int Orthop.* 2008;32(5):697–703.

28. Hazarika S, Chakravarthy J, Cooper J. Minimally invasive locking plate osteosynthesis for fractures of the distal tibia–results in 20 patients. *Injury.* 2006;37(9):877–887.

29. Hasenboehler E, Rikli D, Babst R. Locking compression plate with minimally invasive plate osteosynthesis in diaphyseal and distal tibial fracture: a retrospective study of 32 patients. *Injury.* 2007;38(3):365–370.

30. Borens O, Kloen P, Richmond J, et al. Minimally invasive treatment of pilon fractures with a low profile plate: preliminary results in 17 cases. *Arch Orthop Trauma Surg.* 2009;129(5):649–659.

CHAPTER 27

Minimally Invasive Operative Treatment of Displaced Intra-Articular Calcaneal Fractures via the Sinus Tarsi Approach

Lew C. Schon   Samuel B. Adams   Alan Yan

INDICATIONS

Displaced intra-articular calcaneal fractures are difficult to treat. Historically, operative intervention was abandoned secondary to wound healing complications and poor internal fixation techniques. With the advent of modern plating techniques in the 1980s, operative intervention regained popularity as it allows anatomic restoration of the subtalar joint and the height, width, and length of the bone. By doing so it increases the potential to provide improved functional outcome. Contemporary literature has demonstrated positive clinical and cost-effectiveness outcomes in most patient populations.[1–3]

Several surgical approaches have been described, of which the extended lateral approach has been most reported upon.[4,5–10] While this approach is very utilitarian, allowing direct reduction of the lateral wall, and with further dissection, visualization of the posterior facet and calcaneocuboid joints, it is plagued by wound complications which have reported rates as high as 30%.[11,12]

Alternative limited lateral surgical approaches have been described. In 1948, Palmer described a curved incision below the lateral malleolus for direct exposure to the subtalar joint.[13] Later, Essex-Lopresti adopted a similar sinus tarsi incision to elevate depressed joint fragments.[14] Gupta, reported on a modification of Palmer's approach, in which a straight incision was made 1 cm distal to the fibula in the direction of the fourth metatarsal base. Of 32 operatively treated fractures, there was only one case of postoperative wound complication related to the incision.[15] Hospodar et al. described a similar approach using a 3- to 4-cm straight incision 1 to 1.5 cm distal to the tip of the fibula and roughly perpendicular to the fibula. Although there were only 16 patients in this series, there were no wound complications.[16]

Similarly, we advocate a limited sinus tarsi approach. This approach allows direct visualization of the posterior facet and angle of Gissane while minimizing damage to already traumatized soft tissues. This approach can be extended proximally to address peroneal tendon dislocations or tears, talus or fibular fractures, ligamentous or syndesmotic pathology or distally to visualize the calcaneocuboid joint. Direct reduction of the posterior facet is achieved and a lateral plate is placed subcutaneously that allows reduction of the calcaneal tuberosity to the posterior facet. Additional percutaneous screws can be placed as needed. The indications for using this approach are similar to the extended lateral approach. We employ the sinus tarsi approach on Sanders type II to IV fractures. Because of the limited dissection with this approach, we do not typically wait for swelling to subside before surgical intervention. Additionally, diabetes and smoking are not contraindications.

PATIENT POSITIONING

The patient is placed in the supine position on a radiolucent operating table. We routinely use a deflatable "beanbag" positioning device to achieve a partial or full lateral position. The down-leg should be padded to protect bony prominences and the common and superficial peroneal nerves. A thigh tourniquet or lower leg Esmarch is used at the surgeon's discretion (Fig. 27–1).

SURGICAL APPROACH

A standard approach to the sinus tarsi is performed. The incision is made along a line connecting the tip of the fibula to the base of the fourth metatarsal and just dorsal to the peroneal tendons. The length of the incision is based on the surgeon's familiarity with this technique and the need for exposure of the various components of the injury. Typically, the incision is 5 to 8 cm in length. We recommend a slightly longer incision early in the learning curve (Fig. 27–2, Fig. 27–3). Sharp dissection is carried through the skin (Fig. 27–3). Dissecting scissors should be used to navigate through the connective tissues. Insert deep retractors early to avoid skin damage. Occasionally a dorsal communicating branch of the sural nerve is identified in the wound. This should be dissected, retracted plantarly, and protected throughout the procedure. Incise the capsule to the subtalar joint in line with the incision and dorsal to the peroneal tendon sheath. A stack of folded towels is placed under the medial ankle to suspend the calcaneus off the OR table. This facilitates disimpaction of the talus from the calcaneus.

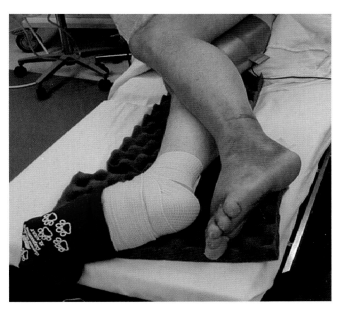

Figure 27–1. Positioning for calcaneal fracture fixation using the sinus tarsi approach. The patient is positioned in the lateral decubitus position with the down-leg common peroneal nerve padded to prevent compression neuropathy.

The sinus tarsi is entered and the fracture hematoma is evacuated. A small laminar spreader with teeth is then inserted between the head–body junction of the talus and the calcaneus at Gissane angle (Fig. 27–4). At times there is too much comminution to effectively push on the calcaneus. In these cases, sharply cut fibers of the inferior extensor retinaculum, anterior capsule of the posterior facet, and even a portion of the interosseous ligament. This will allow a deeper insertion of the laminar spreader which greatly improves the ability to visualize the posterior facet. Carefully insert a wide periosteal of Cobb elevator along the lateral wall of the calcaneus, deep to the peroneal tendons and superficial to all lateral wall fragments. Maneuver the elevator in a posterior and plantar direction. Occasionally, the peroneal tendon sheath is opened and the peroneal tendons are retracted plantarly. Mobile peroneal tendons allow for better tissue protection

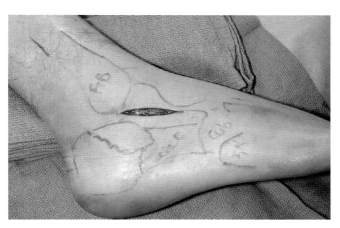

Figure 27–3. Skin incision with surface anatomy features demarcated. The incision extends from just distal to the tip of the fibula toward the base of the fourth metatarsal.

throughout the case and provide better access to the far posterior aspect of the posterior facet during "rafting" screw placement (discussed later). If there is anterior comminution, carry the dissection anteriorly until the calcaneocuboid joint is visualized by lifting off the extensor digitorum brevis from the bone.

With the lamina spreader in place between the plantar aspect of the lateral talar neck and Gissane angle of the calcaneus, the posterior and middle facet can be visualized with its associated fracture fragments. Use a scalpel and a small rongeur to remove the ligaments and the fat from the sinus tarsi. Irrigate the joint. Continue the intra-articular debridement if the medial facet is not visualized.

FRACTURE REDUCTION

Place a Key or Freer elevator into the fracture plane between the depressed fracture fragments of the posterior

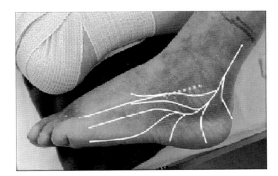

Figure 27–2. Skin incision for sinus tarsi approach. *Dotted yellow line* indicates location of incision. *White lines* indicate the sural nerve and its potential branches.

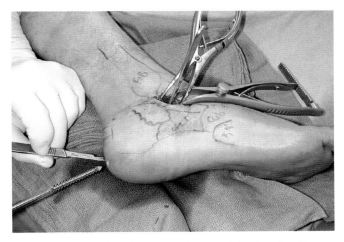

Figure 27–4. Laminar spreaders used to visualize the posterior facet. An incision is being made for Schanz pin insertion into the heel.

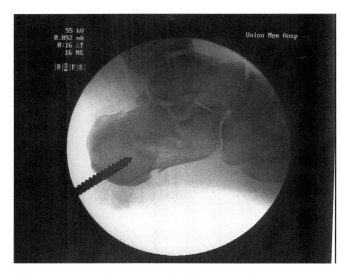

Figure 27–5. Intraoperative fluoroscopy image demonstrating ideal placement of the Schanz pin into the calcaneal tuberosity.

facet and the nonarticular portion of the calcaneus and elevate them. Typically this is a posterior rotational reduction in the sagittal plane. If the piece does not rotate, disimpact the bone underneath it. At times this fragment is impacted posteriorly into the calcaneal tuberosity and needs to be released by going behind the peroneal tendons. Similarly the sagittal plane between the posterior facet fragments requires dissection. At this point, a 5-mm Schanz pin is placed into the tuber. Check an image to insure that the pin only goes into the posterior piece and does not bind into any other fragments (Fig. 27–5). Next, using a T-handle Jacob's chuck on the Schanz pin distract the tuberosity from the sustentacular piece and the facet fragment (Fig. 27–6). In the void where the now elevated

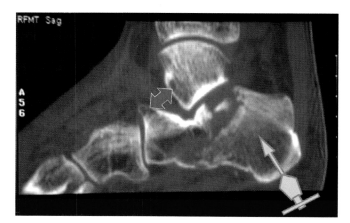

Figure 27–6. Schanz pin and Laminar spreader application. Cartoon demonstrates the axis of distraction applied through the laminar spreader *(double red arrow)* and Schanz pin insertion into calcaneus *(yellow arrow)*. A stylized T-handle Jacobs chuck is depicted as attached to the Schanz pin.

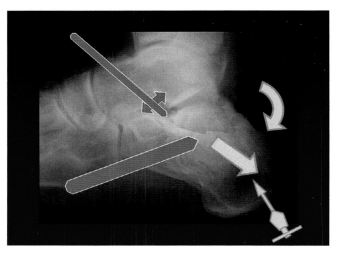

Figure 27–7. Periosteal elevator use with Schanz pin and laminar spreader in joint reduction. Traction is applied on the Schanz pin *(thick yellow arrow)* with the heel suspended from the table. The laminar spreader *(double red arrow)* is used between the shoulder of the talus and the calcaneus. The Schanz pin *(thin yellow arrow)* is attached to a stylized T-handle Jacobs chuck. The freer *(thin blue line)* lifts up the posterior facet piece and the larger periosteal elevator *(thick blue line)* is used through the impaction void or through fracture plane in conjunction with the Schantz pin to separate the sustentacular piece from the posterior tuberosity piece and reduce the tuberosity *(curved yellow arrow)*.

posterior facet sat and/or through lateral wall comminution planes, insert a periosteal elevator underneath the facet and between the sustentaculum and the posterior tuberosity. The elevator is now rotated and manipulated to further separate the fragments. Thus, with this final move the sustentacular piece, the facet pieces, the tuberosity, and the body are all free to move. The tuberosity fragment is typically shortened and in varus. Therefore, apply a plantar and valgus directed force through the Schanz pin (Fig. 27–7). Conversely if the fragment is in valgus, distraction and varus is needed. It can be helpful to accentuate the deformity in varus or valgus before shifting into the final reduction. At the same time, an elevator through the posterior facet fracture line can be used to help free the tuberosity fragment from the sustentaculum fragment.

Using the sustentaculum tali as the constant fragment, reduce the remaining posterior facet fracture fragments to the sustentaculum tali progressing medial to lateral. Typically the calcaneal tuberosity is wedging between these fragments and can block optimal reduction. Therefore an assistant should be applying the reduction maneuver to the Schanz pin, as the sagittal fractures of the facet pieces are compressed into anatomic reduction under direct visualization. At times longitudinal traction with supination and pronation of the midfoot/hindfoot will aid in the final reduction. Abduction and adduction manipulation of the foot can also be of help. Traction forces on the heel and forefoot are in line with their longitudinal axis against the

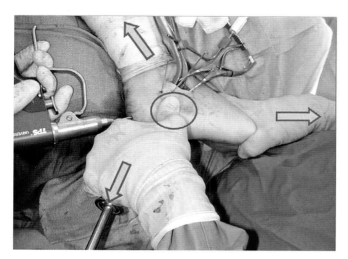

Figure 27–8. Intraoperative reduction maneuver with traction on the foot and heel. The joint reduction is visualized and the fragments compressed together. Guidewires are inserted from lateral to medial holding the reduced joint fragments. A third (pictured) and fourth wire are placed from the tuberosity into the sustentacular piece and the lateral facet piece. *Yellow arrows* indicate lines of applied traction.

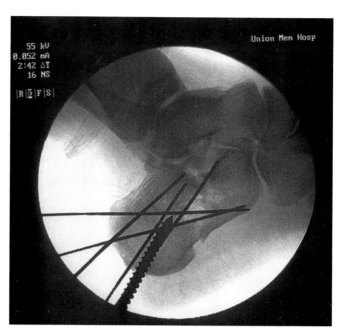

Figure 27–9. Intraoperative lateral fluoroscopic view after K-wire provisional reduction of calcaneus fracture.

held leg (Fig. 27–8). Place one or two guide wires from the lateral facet piece to the more medial fragments. Place provisional Kirschner or guide wires from the tuberosity into the sustentaculum and then another into the posterior facet more laterally. As needed, restore Gissane angle and place longitudinally directed Kirschner or guide wires from the tuberosity into the posterior facet and anterior process. Confirm the reduction with intraoperative fluoroscopic Harris heel and lateral views. Anterior comminution can be reduced now or later with guide wires perpendicular to the plane (Fig. 27–9).

FRACTURE FIXATION

Often, we place 2.7- to 4.0-mm lag screws in the subchondral bone of the posterior facet. These act as "rafting" screws similar to fixation of a tibial plateau fracture and are intended to be placed outside of a plate. They should obtain purchase in the sustentaculum tali.

If using a lateral plate, slide the plate into the pocket between the lateral wall and soft tissues (Fig. 27–10–Fig. 27–12). Often an additional pass with a periosteal elevator is needed to deepen the pocket posteriorly and inferiorly. Many manufacturers have a handle that threads into the plate to aid in plate placement. Confirm the plate position with fluoroscopy and manual palpation. Secure the plate to bone using bicortical nonlocking screws. It is important to reduce the plate directly to bone to minimize peroneal tendon irritation. As needed, place additional posterior locking or nonlocking screws into the plate. Screw placement outside of the sinus tarsi incision is

performed through a small posterior incision that is parallel to the peroneal tendons and sural nerve. Next, reduce any anterior comminution using Kirschner or guide wires and place the anterior plate screws. Additional small- or mini-fragment screws are necessary in cases of severe comminution. If there is extensive comminution of the body of the calcaneus with loss of structural continuity, a hybrid locking/ nonlocking plate may be helpful.

If not using a plate, axially directed 3.5- to 4.5-mm cannulated screws from posterior to anterior capturing the appropriate fracture fragments can be placed over the

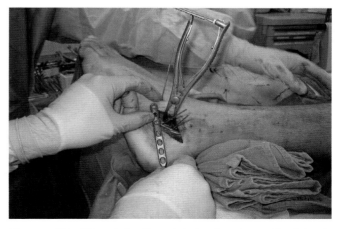

Figure 27–10. A fixation plate is placed over the lateral heel to confirm proper size. This plate is a more standard straight plate that does not give purchase options into the posterior facet.

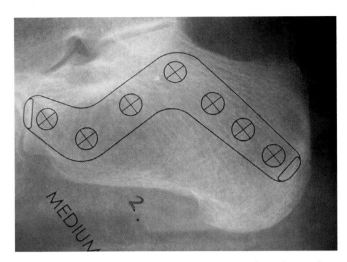

Figure 27–11. Radiographic templating for calcaneal fracture-specific fixation plate.

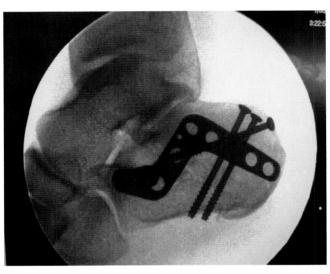

Figure 27–13. Intraoperative fluoroscopic lateral image of calcaneus after plate and screw fixation.

previously inserted guide wires. Depending on the fracture, these screws may be partially threaded or fully threaded with or without lagging. Some plate systems require the use of a small separate incision plantar and posterior to the sural nerve, to insert the most posterior screws into the plate. Apply bone graft as needed into voids. Typically this is not necessary. Confirm fracture reduction and hardware placement with fluoroscopy. Often 6 to 10 screws are used with or without a plate (Fig. 27–13, Fig. 27–14).

CLOSURE

Perform copious irrigation and control hemostasis. The deep tissues and subtalar joint capsule can be closed with 2-0 absorbable sutures. Close the skin with subcutaneous 4-0 absorbable suture and 4-0 nonabsorbable stitches

on the surface. The senior author routinely supplements fracture healing with concentrated bone marrow aspirate. Approximately 60 cc of bone marrow aspirate is drawn from the iliac crest early in the procedure. Using various systems that typically involve a specialized chamber and centrifugation, the platelet rich portion of the aspirate is obtained. The resultant concentrated aspirate is injected outside of the incision deep into the fractured bone fragment after closure to prevent leakage. We do not routinely place a drain. A well-padded splint is applied with the ankle in neutral dorsiflexion.

POSTOPERATIVE RECOVERY

The patient should return at 10 to 14 days after surgery. The splint is removed and the patient is placed in a boot brace

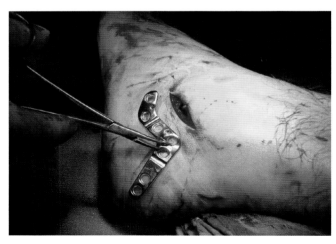

Figure 27–12. Intraoperative templating for calcaneal fracture-specific fixation plate shown in Figure 27–11. Fluoroscopic imaging with plate placed on the lateral heel can aid in confirming proper implant size.

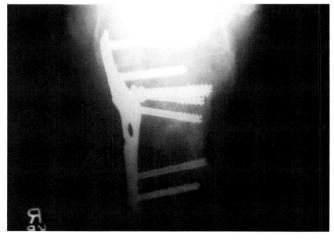

Figure 27–14. Intraoperative fluoroscopic Harris view of calcaneus after plate and screw fixation.

or cast but remains nonweight bearing while walking. The boot brace is advantageous for early ankle range of motion, which is encouraged in dorsiflexion, plantar flexion, inversion, and eversion. Assuming that fixation was solid and the wound is healed, begin deep knee bends five times a day for 20 minutes at 10 to 14 days with partial weight bearing (20 to 50 lb). When standing the patient is allowed to share the weight between both feet. Serial radiographs are taken and the patient begins progressively weight bearing starting at 6 weeks. The boot can be discontinued typically by 8 to 12 weeks depending on the bone quality, fixation, healing, and comorbidities.

COMPLICATIONS

Intraoperative complications are rare. In theory, the peroneal tendons or the sural nerve could be damaged. In a systematic review of eight case series (271 fractures) detailing the use of a minimally invasive approach to calcaneus fracture fixation, Schepers reported that there were no sural nerve transections and only one resolving sural nerve neuritis. We are unaware of any reports of peroneal tendon damage.[17]

OUTCOME

In general, the wound complication rate is much lower and the quality of fracture reduction is similar with a minimally invasive sinus tarsi approach compared to the extended lateral approach. Hospodar et al.[16] performed the sinus tarsi approach on 16 consecutive patients and compared the results to historical controls who received the extensile lateral approach by the same authors. There was no significant difference in the postoperative measurement of Böhler and Gissane angles. No major wound complications were seen in either group, but persistent pain and swelling were identified as problems with the extensile lateral approach.

Schepers compiled eight case series totaling 256 patients with 271 calcaneal fractures who underwent fixation through a limited lateral approach. Good to excellent outcomes were achieved in three-quarters of all patients. The mean minor wound complication rate was 4.1% and the major wound complication rate was 0.7%. The need for a secondary subtalar arthrodesis occurred at an average of 4.3%. Schepers concluded that both the functional outcome and complication rate of sinus tarsi approaches compare similarly or favorably to the extended lateral extensile approach.[17]

Gupta et al. performed calcaneal fracture fixation via the sinus tarsi approach on 32 consecutive fractures. There were two Sanders type I fractures, 20 type II fractures, and five type III fractures. Anatomic reduction of the posterior facet (<2 mm) was achieved in all but one fracture. Multiple radiographic measurements were performed. Postoperative Böhler angle, posterior facet angle, posterior facet depression, heel width, and calcaneal

height were significantly improved. There was only one wound complication related to the approach.[15]

Liu and Xu reported on a series of 31 patients with 32 intra-articular calcaneal fractures treated with open reduction and internal fixation through a small lateral incision. Of the 32 cases, 21 were Sanders type II fractures and 11 were type III fractures. After an average follow-up of 10.5 months, no soft tissue complications were found, and all had acceptable reduction. Both Böhler and Gissane angles were significantly improved. Postoperative outcome was assessed using the American Orthopaedic Foot and Ankle Society (AOFAS) Ankle-Hindfoot score. Two patients scored between 60 to 70 points, nine patients scored between 70 to 80 points, 16 patients scored between 80 to 90 points, and five patients scored between 90 to 100 points. The authors concluded that the small lateral incision approach is a good option for management of calcaneus fractures minimizing soft tissue damage without sacrificing outcomes.[18]

Ebraheim et al. reported favorable results on 106 intra-articular calcaneal fractures treated through a sinus tarsi approach with limited internal fixation (only pins). In this study, there were 71 Sanders Type II, 25 Type III, and 10 Type IV fractures. There was only a 3.8% superficial wound infection rate with no deep infections. At a mean follow-up of 29 months, the mean AOFAS score was 77.6. Outcomes roughly correlated with fracture severity. The authors concluded that a satisfactory reduction was achieved in type II and III fractures, but anatomic restoration was difficult to achieve in type IV fractures.[19]

In conclusion, the minimally invasive sinus tarsi approach is a safe and effective technique for calcaneal fracture fixation. Most reports demonstrate similar quality of fracture reduction with fewer wound complications when compared to the extended lateral approach. However, a randomized controlled trial comparing the two approaches is needed.

REFERENCES

1. Brauer CA, Manns BJ, Ko M, et al. An economic evaluation of operative compared with nonoperative management of displaced intra-articular calcaneal fractures. *J Bone Joint Surg Am.* 2005;87(12):2741–2749.
2. Buckley R, Tough S, McCormack R, et al. Operative compared with nonoperative treatment of displaced intra-articular calcaneal fracture: A prospective randomized, controlled multicenter trial. *J Bone Joint Surg Am.* 2002;84: 1733–1744.
3. Radnay CS, Clare MP, Sanders RW. Subtalar fusion after displaced intra-articular calcaneal fractures: Does initial operative treatment matter? *J Bone Joint Surg Am.* 2009; 91(3):541–546.
4. Benirschke Sk, Sangoerzan B. Extensive intraarticular fractures of the foot: Surgical management of calcaneus fractures. *Clin Orthop Relat Res.* 1993;(292):128–134.
5. Rammelt S, Zwipp H. Calcaneus fracture: Facts, controversies and recent developments. *Injury.* 2004;35:443461.
6. Sanders R. Intra-articular fractures of the calcaneus: Present state of the art. *J Orthop Trauma.* 1992;6:252–265.

7. Sanders RW, Clare MP. Fractures of the calcaneus. In: Bucholz RW, Heckman JD, Court-Brown CM, eds. *Rockwood and Green's fracture in adults.* 6th ed. Philadelphia, PA: Lippincott Williams & Wilkins: 2006: 2293–2336.

8. Sanders RW, Clare MP. Fractures of the Calcaneus. In: Coughlin MJ, Mann RA, Saltzman CL, eds. *Surgery of the foot and ankle.* 8th ed. Philadelphia, PA: Mosby Elsevier: 2007:2017-2073.

9. Zwipp H, Rammelt S, Barthel S. Calcaneal fractures–open reduction and internal fixation (ORIF). *Injury.* 2004;35 Suppl 2:SB46–SB54.

10. Zwipp H, Tscherne H, Thermann H, et al. Osteosynthesis for displaced intraarticular fractures of the calcaneus. *Clin Orthop Relat Res.* 1993;290:76–86.

11. Abidi NA, Dhawan S, Gruen GS, et al. Wound healing risk factors after open reduction and internal fixation of calcaneal fractures. *Foot Ankle Int.* 1998;19(12):856–861.

12. Lim EV, Leung JP. Complications of intraarticular calcaneal fracture. *Clin Orthop Relat Res.* 2001;391:7–16.

13. Palmer I. The mechanism and treatment of fractures of the calcaneus: Open reduction with the use of cancellous grafts. *J Bone Joint Surg Am.* 1948;30:2–8.

14. Essex-Lopresti P. The mechanism, reduction technique, and results in fractures of the os calcis. *Br J Surg.* 1952;39(157): 395–419.

15. Gupta A, Gahlambor N, Nihal A, et al. The modified Palmer lateral approach for calcaneal fractures: Wound healing and postoperative tomorographic evaluation of fracture reduction. *Foot Ankle Int.* 2003;24:744–753.

16. Hospodar P, Guzman C, Johnson P, et al. Treatment of displaced calcaneus fractures using a minimally invasive sinus tarsi approach. *Orthopedics.* 2008; 31(11):1112.

17. Schepers T. The sinus tarsi approach in displaced intra-articular calcaneal fractures: A systematic review. *Intl Orthop.* 2011;35(5):697–703.

18. Liu JH, Xu XY. Treatment of displaced intra-articular fractures of the calcaneus using a small lateral incision approach. *Chinese Journal of Orthopaedic Trauma.* 2006–2010.

19. Ebraheim N, Elgafy H, Sabry F, et al. Sinus tarsi approach with trans-articular fixation for displaced intra-articular fractures of the calcaneus. *Foot Ankle Int.* 2000;21(2):105–113.

CHAPTER 28

Minimally Invasive Operative Treatment of Proximal Fifth Metatarsal Fractures

Kathryn L. Williams   Robert B. Anderson

INDICATIONS

Proximal fractures of the fifth metatarsal are classified into three types based on anatomy and radiographic appearance. A zone I fracture occurs on the lateral aspect of the tuberosity, extending proximally into the metatarsocuboid joint, and represents an avulsion of the tuberosity. Zone II fractures, referred to as Jones fractures, include fractures that involve the metaphyseal–diaphyseal junction and begin laterally in the distal part of the tuberosity and extend obliquely and proximally into the medial cortex at the fourth and fifth metatarsal base articulation. Zone III fractures are distal to the fourth and fifth metatarsal base articulation and involve the proximal metatarsal shaft (Fig. 28–1).[1–3] Torg further classified the proximal diaphyseal fractures into three subtypes based on the age of the fracture and radiographic appearance. Type I fractures are acute with no intramedullary sclerosis, type II are delayed unions and have a widened fracture line with intramedullary sclerosis, and type III are nonunions, the medullary canal obliterated.[3]

The fracture type is important as the location of the fracture can have implications in ability to heal secondary to the blood supply of the fifth metatarsal. The watershed area present at the metaphyseal–diaphyseal junction creates an avascular zone, which can increase the risk of delayed union or nonunion (Fig. 28–2).[4–6]

In cases where surgical intervention is indicated, minimally invasive techniques for proximal fifth metatarsal fractures can be utilized. Typically this is best suited for athletes with acute type II Jones and Type III metaphyseal/diaphyseal fractures. Nonathletes with these fracture patterns can usually be managed with 6 to 8 weeks of non–weight-bearing cast immobilization. However, if there is little or no callous formation at the fracture site after this initial treatment, surgical treatment with minimally invasive techniques can still be pursued (Fig. 28–3A, B).

There is a subset of patients in whom initial surgical treatment should be considered. This includes not only athletes but also those patients with a refracture or postural abnormalities. Quill[7] reported high rates of delayed union, nonunion, and re-fracture in athletes treated nonoperatively, with up to a 50% nonunion or refracture rate and recommended intramedullary screw fixation in all Jones fractures. Josefsson[8] reported that

25% of patients with Jones fractures treated nonoperatively needed further surgical management for delayed union/refracture. Surgical treatment has been shown to decrease healing time. Clapper[9] reported a 100% union for seven Jones fractures treated operatively with a healing time of 12.1 weeks compared with 21.2 weeks for those treated with casting. Further studies also support early surgical treatment of acute Jones fractures in elite or high-performance athlete.[10–13]

The presence of prodromal pain prior to the presentation of an acute proximal diaphyseal fracture, the absence of prior treatment and radiographic evidence of a stress phenomenon indicates an etiology involving repetitive stress and a lower chance for successful healing with nonoperative treatment. Healing rates of 100% have been reported in proximal diaphyseal stress fractures using percutaneous screw fixation.[10–13]

Percutaneous or minimally invasive operative treatment of fifth metatarsal base fractures is not indicated for treatment of Zone I (avulsion fractures), as these types have a high union rate with nonoperative treatment.[9] It is also not indicated for those fractures that are localized to the distal half of the fifth metatarsal as these are best treated nonoperatively or with plate osteosynthesis.

In summary, minimally invasive operative treatment using percutaneous insertion of an intramedullary screw for fixation of proximal fifth metatarsal fractures is indicated for the treatment of acute Jones fractures in the elite or high-performance athlete, the patient with a diaphyseal stress fracture and radiographic evidence of nonunion or delayed union, and the informed nonathlete who prefers surgery rather than the risk development of a nonunion or refracture with nonsurgical treatment.

PATIENT POSITIONING

Surgery is performed as an outpatient and can be done with either a regional or general anesthetic. An Esmarch bandage placed at the midcalf level suffices as a tourniquet. General anesthesia is used if the surgeon desires a thigh tourniquet or bone marrow aspirate/graft from the iliac crest. The patient is positioned on a standard operating room table in the supine position. A radiolucent table may be used but is not necessary. The patient is positioned at the distal end of the table and a bump

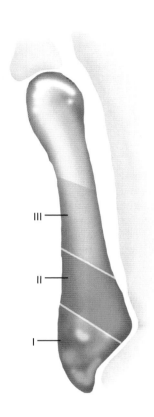

Figure 28–1. The three anatomic zones of the proximal fifth metatarsal.

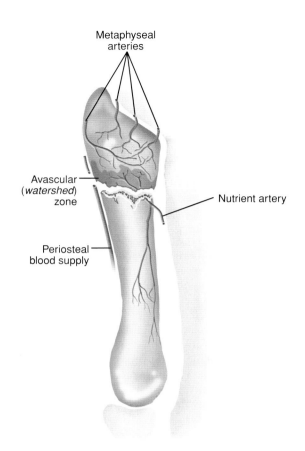

Figure 28–2. Illustration of the vascular supply to the proximal fifth metatarsal demonstrating the avascular (watershed) zone in the metaphyseal–diaphyseal region.

is placed under the ipsilateral hip in order to internally rotate the operative extremity. The patient's entire body is moved as far to the operative side of the table as safely possible so that the starting point can be accessed without obstruction. The ipsilateral knee must be able to be flexed in order to place the foot plantigrade on the edge of the fluoroscopy unit or the operating room table. A mini C-arm is essential and the physician should confirm that true oblique, AP, and lateral views of the fifth metatarsal can be obtained before prepping and draping the extremity.

If general anesthesia is used, a nonsterile tourniquet may be placed high on the thigh of the operative leg. As mentioned previously, a sterile Esmarch tourniquet may be applied either with general anesthesia or with an ankle/popliteal block and sedation. This latter method is our preference for most patients. The foot is prepped to the level of the midtibia or knee and draped using an extremity drape. The iliac crest is also prepped and draped if bone marrow aspirate or autologous bone graft is to be harvested. The surgeon stands on the injured side of the patient to access the lateral foot and the assistant or scrub tech stands at the foot of the bed. The mini C-arm is positioned on the injured side and brought in at an approximately 45-degree angle to allow for access to all three views of the foot (Fig. 28–4).

SURGICAL APPROACH

The base of the fifth metatarsal is palpated and drawn out with a surgical marker on the lateral foot for anatomic reference. In order to estimate the axial alignment, a Kirschner wire can be laid over the top of the fifth metatarsal and fluoroscopic images taken in the oblique plane. Using a surgical pen, a line can drawn on the skin along the wire proximal to the base. The axial alignment can also be visualized with fluoroscopy and the guidewire inserted in line with the fifth metatarsal shaft. A 1- to 2-cm longitudinal incision is made in line with the metatarsal approximately 2 cm from the base (Fig. 28–5A, B). Blunt dissection is done to protect terminal branches of the sural nerve, and should be protected during drilling and screw insertion to prevent injury and the potential for a painful neuroma. The peroneus brevis tendon may be encountered but usually lies superior to the insertion site of the screw. The soft tissues are carefully and bluntly spread in line with the incision down to the level of the bone to allow for insertion of the guidewire.

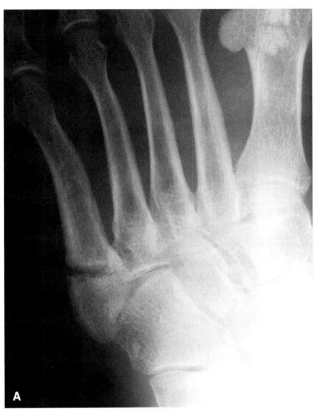
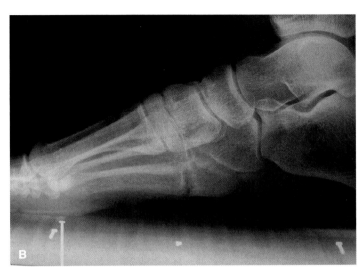

Figure 28–3. **A, B:** Oblique and lateral radiographs of a type II nonunion of the fifth metatarsal base.

REDUCTION TECHNIQUES AND FIXATION

A formal reduction is not usually needed as the correct placement of the Kirschner wire, tap and partially threaded screw allows for indirect reduction of the fracture. However, there is a definite order of steps that must be carried out to achieve appropriate placement of the screw and fracture alignment.

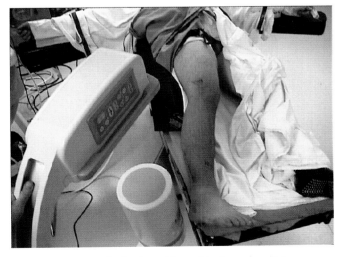

Figure 28–4. Patient positioned before draping.

A guide pin for the desired cannulated screw is chosen and inserted through the incision down to the level of the tuberosity of the fifth metatarsal. The appropriate insertion site is medial to the tip of the tuberosity, with the goal being to obtain a "high and inside" starting point, just lateral to the lateral border of the cuboid (Fig. 6A, B).

Under fluoroscopic guidance in the AP and lateral views, the guide pin is inserted down the center of the metatarsal shaft, past the fracture site and to the level of the isthmus, stopping before the metatarsal starts to curve. The proximal end of the pin should lie flush against the lateral skin of the heel while being advanced to prevent medial deviation (Fig. 28–7).

A tissue protector large enough to accommodate a 3.2- or 3.5-mm cannulated drill is inserted over the guidewire using a tissue protector (Fig. 28–8). The drill is advanced under fluoroscopic guidance to avoid penetration of the cortex, taking into account the intrinsic curvature of the metatarsal distally (Fig. 28–9A, B).

An alternative drilling technique is to use the cannulated drill to enter the proximal cortex only. The guidewire is removed and a solid drill of the same size (3.2 mm) is advanced under fluoroscopic control until the proper depth is obtained. This technique will help decrease the risk of perforating the cortex, while also helping to ensure that the entry site is in line with the diaphysis.

Once the intramedullary canal has been drilled past the fracture site, it must be tapped if a non–self-tapping

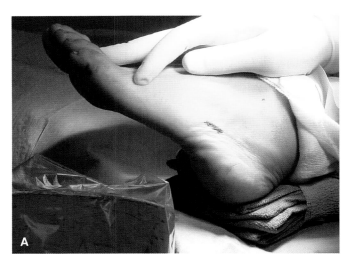 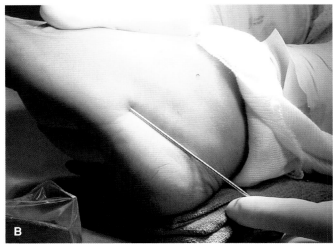

Figure 28–5. **A, B:** One to 2-cm longitudinal incision proximal to base of fifth metatarsal with the guidewire positioned along lateral border of foot.

screw is to be used. The guidewire is left in place or replaced into the bone and a solid or cannulated tap corresponding to the appropriate screw size chosen is used to tap to the intended screw length. A 4.5-mm tap with a tissue protector should be used initially but can be increased to the appropriate size based on the endosteal purchase of the threads. The tap should feel snug within the intramedullary canal and the distal fragment will begin to torque as the tap engages. This torque can be used as a measure of appropriate screw diameter (Fig. 28–10).

The screw length should be long enough so that all the screw threads pass the fracture site but not extend down the medullary canal past approximately 60% of the metatarsal length. Placement of an excessively long screw may cause the normal curvature of the fifth meta-

tarsal to straighten, thus displacing or creating a gap at the fracture.

The screw length can be measured with multiple methods. Some systems have grooves on the tap and with appropriate placement of the tissue protector against the bone, the screw length can be measured directly off the tap. Alternatively, and if available, the guide wire and depth gauge can be used.

Another alternative is to place a screw of the estimated length along the lateral border of the foot and use fluoroscopic imaging to check that the proper length was chosen. As mentioned previously, all threads should lie just distal to the fracture line and this is an easy and reliable way to ensure this happens. Our typical screw length is 40 to 50 mm (Fig. 28–11).

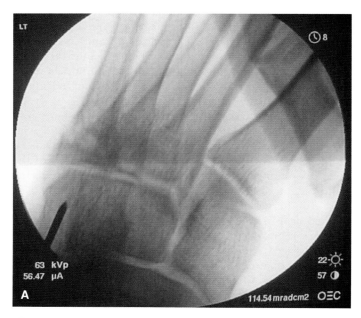 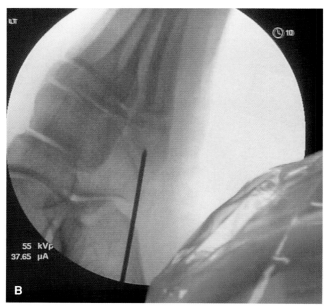

Figure 28–6. **A, B:** AP and lateral fluoroscopy showing "high and inside" starting point.

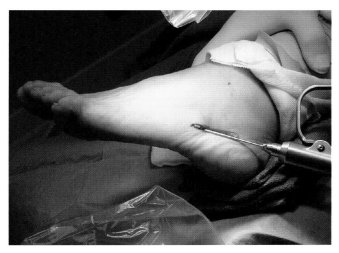

Figure 28–7. Insertion of guidewire with wire flush against the skin.

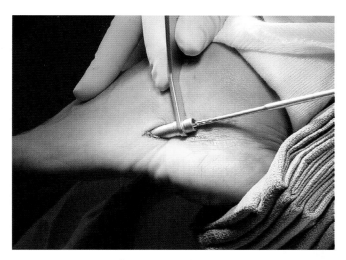

Figure 28–8. Drilling over guidewire with tissue protector.

A countersink can be used to prepare the insertion site. This may be desired if using a screw with a large head. Once the correct screw diameter and length is determined, the screw is placed under fluoroscopic guidance. Compression should occur as the screw threads are advanced past the fracture (Fig. 28–12). The distal portion of the fifth metatarsal and small toe may turn and torque, indicating that the endosteal bone is being captured distally. If gapping at the fracture occurs as the screw is advanced, the screw length and diameter should be re-evaluated. Final fluoroscopic images should be obtained in all three planes to ensure proper screw position and that diaphyseal perforation has not occurred (Fig. 28–13A, B). The wound is closed at skin level using interrupted nylon sutures, followed by application of a sterile dressing and short leg splint.

In general, the largest screw diameter that can be safely placed within the intramedullary canal should be used. The tap can be used to assess which size will have the best interference fit within the canal, obtaining endosteal bite with the threads. The screw diameter is frequently 4.5 mm or more, but there is no consensus on cannulated versus solid screws. DeLee et al's[11] original surgical technique described use of a 4.5-mm solid medial malleolar screw with 100% union rate. Subsequent studies have been unable to show superior results with fracture healing and refracture rate when directly comparing solid and cannulated screws, however Larson[12] reported refracture with cannulated screws in up to 40% of patients in one case series. Biomechanical studies have shown no difference in resistance to three-point bending when comparing 4.5-mm solid versus 4.5-mm cannulated

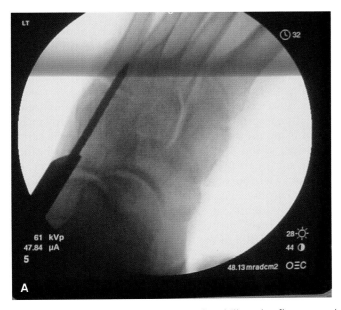

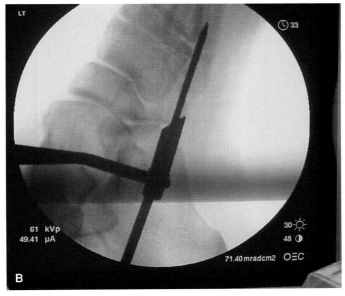

Figure 28–9.   A, B: Advancing the drill under fluoroscopic guidance to avoid penetration of the cortex.

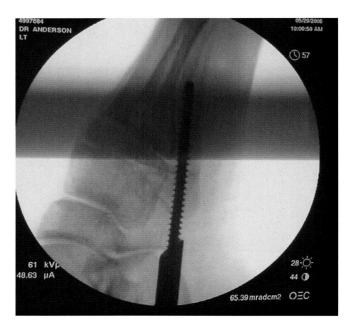

Figure 28–10. Advancing the tap under fluoroscopic guidance.

screws; and cannulated 4.5-mm versus cannulated 5.5-mm screws, but improved resistance to fatigue has been demonstrated in solid screws when using screws less than 4.0 mm.[14–16]

COMPLICATIONS

Intraoperative complications are usually due to an incorrect starting point and drilling angle when preparing the intramedullary canal and choosing a correct screw

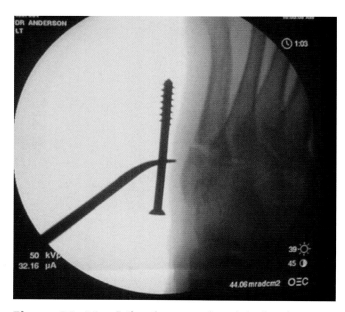

Figure 28–11. Estimating screw length indirectly.

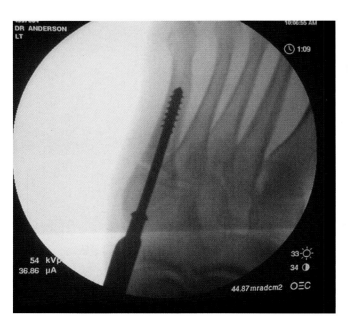

Figure 28–12. Placing the screw under fluoroscopic guidance.

length. It is important to avoid penetrating the medial cortex, as this will prevent true placement of an intramedullary screw, as well as create a stress riser. Keeping the starting point "high and inside," drilling under fluoroscopic imaging and advancing a solid drill bit on reverse will all help to position the screw appropriately within the medullary canal.

If the screw selected is too long, it may gap the lateral aspect of the fracture rather than compress across it. The screw threads need only to cross the fracture site. Fracture of the fifth metatarsal shaft or stress shielding can also occur if the screw length and diameter is too large.

Careful selection of the screw length is important and should be done with the techniques as outlined above. It is recommended that the screw be placed under fluoroscopic guidance so that length and size corrections can be made before a complication occurs.

During the approach, preparation of the canal and placement of the final screw the sural nerve is at risk of injury. In a cadaver study, Donley et al. demonstrated that after insertion of 4.5-mm screws in the fifth metatarsal using the approach as described above, the screw head was within 2 to 3 mm of the dorsolateral branch of the sural nerve. Injury to the nerve can occur at the time of insertion or removal of the screw and a sural nerve neuroma may explain persistent pain after screw removal. Patients with suspected sural nerve injury may have a positive Tinel sign and decreased sensation along the lateral border of the foot. Careful surgical technique, using drill guides, tissue protectors, and careful and gentle spreading of the tissues can decrease the risk of sural nerve injury. The use of loupe magnification has been suggested for the approach but is not routinely used by the authors.[17]

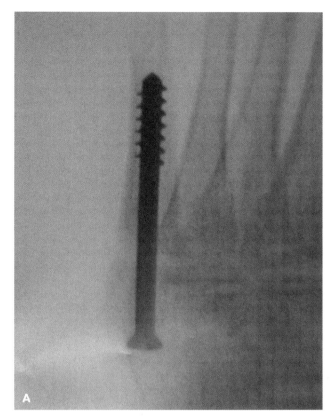
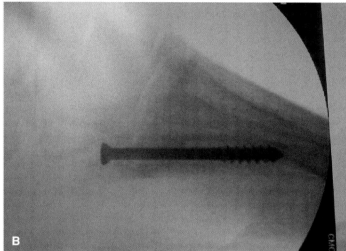

Figure 28–13.   A, B: AP and lateral views of final placement of screw.

Pain from a prominent screw head has been reported in up to 30% of patients. The use of a countersink can prevent the screw head prominence, but if the patient is symptomatic, shoe modifications such as moleskin padding or soft shoe liner can be used.[11] Screws with reduced head sizes are also available that decrease the risk of prominent hardware. Routine screw removal is not recommended because refracture after complete healing and screw removal has been reported.[8]

NONUNION AND REFRACTURES

Despite early intramedullary fixation of acute Jones fractures or after an appropriate period of nonweightbearing for those fractures treated nonoperatively, there are reports of nonunions and refractures in the literature. Wright et al. reported on six refractures after cannulated screw fixation with a screw size of 4.5 to 5.0 mm in athletes with Jones fractures. Because the refractures occurred on the day of return to full activity, they felt that a larger screw diameter was indicated in athletes with larger body mass and that functional bracing should be used initially.[18] Glasgow et al.[19] also reported six failures of intramedullary screw fixation with three delayed fractures and three refractures at 3.5 to 8 months postoperatively. Larson et al.[20] found that return to full

activity before complete radiographic union was predictive of failure. Altered biomechanics can play a role in nonunion and refracture. The foot posture should also be considered when nonunions and recurrent stress fractures occur as even mild cavovarus or metatarsus adductus can cause altered lateral column loading.[21–24]

Symptomatic nonunions and refractures after prior intramedullary screw fixation commonly require an open revision surgical procedure to attain bone healing. In this setting, the authors recommend removal of hardware if present, open debridement of the nonunion site, revision fixation with a larger diameter intramedullary screw, and autologous and/or allogenic bone grafting. The surgical set-up is identical to that for a primary intramedullary screw fixation, with the iliac crest prepped and draped for harvest of the autograft, if that site of bone graft harvest is chosen. The retained screw is removed through the previous incision. In the event of a broken screw, the proximal segment is removed through the previous entry site while the distal fragment can be removed through the nonunion or refracture site when it is opened as below (Fig. 28–14).

The fluoroscope is used to identify the fracture site. A 1- to 2-cm incision is made over the fracture site along the dorsolateral aspect of the fifth metatarsal. The soft tissues are bluntly dissected down to the bone and care is taken to protect the sural nerve. A small periosteal envelope

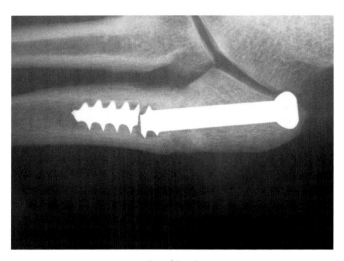

Figure 28–14. Example of broken screw.

is created along the dorsal and plantar bone around the fracture and the nonunion/refracture site is debrided with a curette. It is then drilled with the use of a drill guide, through the proximal incision with the drill on reverse so it acts like a reamer.

In the case of a nonunion that was treated nonoperatively, the starting point is established as described above. However, the canal may have significant sclerosis and this can be dealt with by advancing very slowly across the fracture site and alternating between forward and reverse. Successive taps are then used until sufficient torque is felt during tapping, which can be determined as described above by feeling the endosteal bite with successive taping. The appropriate screw length and diameter is chosen as above. In the setting of refracture after

intramedullary fixation, a larger screw diameter than was originally used is recommended.

As mentioned, autograft or allograft bone is recommended for nonunions and refractures. Autograft bone can be harvested from a number of sites including the iliac crest, lateral calcaneus, distal tibia, or proximal tibia and depends on surgeon and patient preference. It has been our preference to use the iliac crest with a minimally invasive technique, harvesting with a power trephine. We recommended avoiding harvesting from a weightbearing bone, particularly in the athlete, due to the risk of stress fracture. The fracture site will usually only accommodate 1 to 2 cc of graft. The graft is placed within the fracture and allowed to enter the medullary canal on both sides of the fracture. The selected solid screw can be advanced under fluoroscopic guidance either before or after the graft is placed. If the endosteal bite of the screw is not sufficient, consider going to the next tap to place a larger-diameter screw. For refractures and nonunions, a 5.5- or 6.5-mm diameter screw is typically utilized.[24,25]

In cases of delayed union with an intact screw, the authors may prefer to use bone marrow aspirate with demineralized bone matrix (BMA+DBM), which is available commercially. In these cases, the iliac crest is prepped and the bone marrow is harvested with the instruments supplied. The approach to the fracture site and development of a periosteal envelope is the same as described above. The BMA+DBM mixture is injected under fluoroscopic guidance. The space developed will only accommodate 1 to 2 cc of graft substitute, as one should be careful to not overstuff the area, as this can cause heterotopic bone formation and inflammatory response (Fig. 28–15A, B).

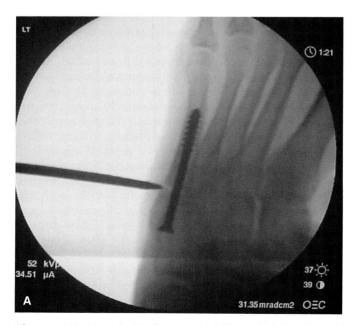

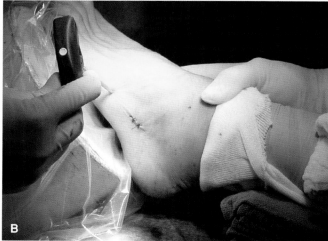

Figure 28–15. **A, B:** Placement of BMA+DBM (Ignite®, Wright Medical Technologies, Memphis TN).

REHABILITATION PROTOCOL

Immediately following placement of an intramedullary screw for an acute Jones fracture or diaphyseal stress fracture, a well-padded plaster splint is placed with the ankle in neutral dorsiflexion and the patient is instructed to be nonweightbearing. Our typical postoperative protocol is to keep the patient nonweightbearing for 2 weeks, followed by a walker for protected weightbearing for an additional 3 to 4 weeks. Radiographs are obtained at the initial postoperative visit and are repeated at 6 weeks postoperative. For athletes, return to play usually occurs with there is no remaining tenderness, typically between 8 and 12 weeks. As the radiographs will lag behind clinical healing, light jogging and increased activity will begin when the patient is asymptomatic with walking activity. The authors recommend leaving the screw in place indefinitely, as there is a high incidence of refractures after screw removal.[8] Custom orthotic devices are also utilized, especially in the athlete or those with underlying postural deformities, such a varus hindfoot malalignment. A varus unloading (lateral hindfoot and forefoot posting) orthotic insert is recommended to prevent refracture.[24] In large individuals, turf toe plates may also be added to shoewear to reduce the bending moment at the fracture site.

OUTCOME

A successful surgery can be defined as a radiographically healed fracture, and the patient returning to preinjury level of play with no limitations/symptoms or refractures.

REFERENCES

1. Dameron TB Jr. Fractures and anatomical variations of the proximal portion of the fifth metatarsal. *J Bone Joint Surg Am.* 1975;57(6):788–792.
2. Stewart IM. Jones's fracture: Fracture of base of fifth metatarsal. *Clin Orthop* 1960;16:190–198.
3. Torg JS, Balduini FC, Zelko RR, et al. Fractures of the base of the fifth metatarsal distal to the tuberosity: Classification and guidelines for non-surgical and surgical management. *J Bone Joint Surg Am.* 1984;66(2):209–214.
4. Carp L. Fracture of the fifth metatarsal bone: With special reference to delayed union. *Ann Surg* 1927;86:308–320.
5. Smith JW, Arnoczky SP, Hersh A. The intraosseous blood supply of the fifth metatarsal: Implications for proximal fracture healing. *Foot Ankle.* 1992;13:143–152.
6. Shereff MJ, Yang QM, Kummer FJ, et al. Vascular anatomy of the fifth metatarsal. *Foot Ankle.* 1991;11:350–353.
7. Quill GE Jr. Fractures of the proximal fifth metatarsal. *Orthop Clin North Am.* 1995;26(2):353–361.
8. Josefsson PO, Karlsson M, Redlund-Johnell I, et al. Jones fracture. Surgical versus nonsurgical treatment. *Clin Orthop Relat Res.* 1994;(299):252–255.
9. Clapper MF, O'Brien TJ, Lyons PM. Fractures of the fifth metatarsal. Analysis of a fracture registry. *Clin Orthop Relat Res.* 1995;(315):238–241.
10. Kavanaugh JH, Brower TD, Mann RV. The Jones fracture revisited. *J Bone Joint Surg Am.* 1978;60(6):776–782.
11. DeLee JC, Evans JP, Julian J. Stress fracture of the fifth metatarsal. *Am J Sports Med.* 1983;11(5):349–353.
12. Dameron TB Jr. Fractures of the proximal fifth metatarsal: Selecting the best treatment option. *J Am Acad Orthop Surg.* 1995;3(2):110–114.
13. Den Hartog BD. Fracture of the proximal fifth metatarsal. *J Am Acad Orthop Surg.* 2009;17(7):458–464.
14. Pietropaoli MP, Wnorowski DC, Werner FW, et al. Intramedullary screw fixation of Jones fractures: A biomechanical study. *Foot Ankle Int.* 1999;20(9):560–563.
15. Shah SN, Knoblich GO, Lindsey DP, et al. Intramedullary screw fixation of proximal fifth metatarsal fractures: A biomechanical study. *Foot Ankle Int.* 2001;22(7):581–584.
16. Reese K, Litsky A, Kaeding C, et al. Cannulated screw fixation of Jones fractures: A clinical and biomechanical study. *Am J Sports Med.* 2004;32(7):1736–1742.
17. Donley BG, McCollum MJ, Murphy GA, et al. Risk of sural nerve injury with intramedullary screw fixation of fifth metatarsal fractures: A cadaver study. *Foot Ankle Int.* 1999;20(3):182–184.
18. Wright RW, Fischer DA, Shively RA, et al. Refracture of proximal fifth metatarsal (Jones) fracture after intramedullary screw fixation in athletes. *Am J Sports Med.* 2000;28(5):732–736.
19. Glasgow MT, Naranja RJ Jr., Glasgow SG, et al. Analysis of failed surgical management of fractures of the base of the fifth metatarsal distal to the tuberosity: The Jones fracture. *Foot Ankle Int.* 1996;17(8):449–457.
20. Larson CM, Almekinders LC, Taft TN, et al. Intramedullary screw fixation of Jones fractures. Analysis of failure. *Am J Sp Med.* 2002;30(1);55–60.
21. Hetsroni I, Nyska M, Ben-Sira D, et al. Analysis of foot structure in athletes sustaining proximal fifth metatarsal stress fracture. *Foot Ankle Int.* 2010;31(3):203–211.
22. Lee KT, Kim KC, Park YU, et al. Radiographic evaluation of foot structure following fifth metatarsal stress fracture. *Foot Ankle Int.* 2011;32(8):796–801.
23. Theodorou DJ, Theodorou SJ, Boutin RD, et al. Stress fractures of the lateral metatarsal bones in metatarsus adductus foot deformity: A previously unrecognized association. *Skeletal Radiol.* 1999;28(12)679–684.
24. Raikin SM, Slenker N, Ratigan B. The association of a varus hindfoot and fracture of the fifth metatarsal metaphyseal-diaphyseal junction. *Am J Sp Med.* 2008;36(7)1367–1372.
25. Hunt KJ, Anderson, RB. Treatment of Jones fracture nonunions and refractures in the elite athlete: Outcomes of intramedullary screw fixation and bone grafting. *Am J Sports Med.* 2011;39(9):1948–1954.

Index